Second Edition

Communication Skills *for the* Health Care Professional

Concepts, Practice, and Evidence

Gwen van Servellen, PhD, RN, FAAN
Professor Emeritus
University of California, Los Angeles
School of Nursing

JONES AND BARTLETT PUBLISHERS
Sudbury, Massachusetts
BOSTON TORONTO LONDON SINGAPORE

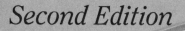

BP45

World Headquarters
Jones and Bartlett Publishers
40 Tall Pine Drive
Sudbury, MA 01776
978-443-5000
info@jbpub.com
www.jbpub.com

Jones and Bartlett Publishers
Canada
6339 Ormindale Way
Mississauga, Ontario L5V 1J2
Canada

Jones and Bartlett Publishers
International
Barb House, Barb Mews
London W6 7PA
United Kingdom

Jones and Bartlett's books and products are available through most bookstores and online booksellers. To contact Jones and Bartlett Publishers directly, call 800-832-0034, fax 978-443-8000, or visit our website www.jbpub.com.

Substantial discounts on bulk quantities of Jones and Bartlett's publications are available to corporations, professional associations, and other qualified organizations. For details and specific discount information, contact the special sales department at Jones and Bartlett via the above contact information or send an email to specialsales@jbpub.com.

Production Credits
Publisher: Michael Brown
Production Director: Amy Rose
Associate Editor: Katey Birtcher
Editorial Assistant: Catie Heverling
Production Editor: Tracey Chapman
Marketing Manager: Sophie Fleck
Manufacturing and Inventory Control Supervisor: Amy Bacus
Composition: Auburn Associates, Inc.
Illustrator: Accurate Art, Inc.
Cover Design: Brian Moore
Cover Image: © AlArt/ShutterStock, Inc.
Printing and Binding: Malloy, Inc.
Cover Printing: Malloy, Inc.

Library of Congress Cataloging-in-Publication Data
Van Servellen, Gwen Marram.
Communication skills for the health care professional : concepts, practice, and evidence / Gwen van Servellen. — 2nd ed.
p. ; cm.
Includes bibliographical references and index.
ISBN-13: 978-0-7637-5557-7 (pbk.)
ISBN-10: 0-7637-5557-5 (pbk.)
1. Allied health personnel and patient. 2. Interpersonal communication. 3. Communication in medicine. I. Title.
[DNLM: 1. Health Personnel. 2. Professional-Patient Relations. 3. Communication.
4. Patients—psychology. W 21 V2176ca 2009]
R727.3.V36 2009
610.69—dc22

2008015960

6048
Printed in the United States of America
12 11 10 9 8 7 6 5 4 3 2

6/13/11

Dedication

John Robert Dower

The first to suggest to me that communication comes and goes in many different forms but is always there to be expressed.

To our patients, families, and ourselves:

As miraculous as our ability to communicate is, not all patients and families can speak to be heard, listen to know, understand to respond appropriately and in a timely manner, or even remember what we write or say. In fact, the patient might tell us the same about the healthcare professional. The reasons are many, but it is always important to assume little and consistently assess the communication that has passed among patients, providers, and families. Let it be our goal to not miss one or more critical components that will result in compromised care.

What's New in the Second Edition?

This text is an excellent addition to a course on interviewing and therapeutic management of health provider and patient alliances. The revision of the text builds on previous strengths and adds considerable discussion to the evidence that healthcare communications are vital to quality care and patient well-being. The second edition maintains the same general structure but adds *four* new chapters to enhance the student's ability to understand the importance of communication skills and the link between healthcare communications and quality care outcomes. A *fifth* new chapter addresses the considerable needs and challenges of communication with patients with low health literacy in phases of prevention and treatment. As previously presented, each chapter provides a thought-provoking quote about the issues to be discussed in the chapter. Also, there are objectives for each chapter, key chapter terms in the updated glossary, and new references in the updated reference list.

- One new chapter is added to the new section on communications under challenging circumstances. This is Chapter 13, *Communicating with Patients with Low Literacy.*
- There are four additional new chapters making up a new section on expectations for healthcare communications, evidence for quality, and behavioral change:
  - *Health Communications and Quality Care* (Chapter 1)
  - *Health Communications to Enhance Behavioral Change* (Chapter 22)
  - *Internet Use and Communications of Patients and Providers* (Chapter 23)
  - *Altering Systems of Care to Enhance for Healthcare Communications* (Chapter 24)
- All other chapters have been revised and updated.
- Updated resources, including Web sites, provide additional references, background knowledge, statistics, and recommendations for evidence-based practice.
- New tables describe therapeutic communication approaches to managing such typical clinical challenges as nonadherence, low literacy, fears, and conflicts.
- Up-to-date evidence to support the impact of healthcare communications is detailed in a description of studies in the literature.

KEY FEATURES

In-depth discussion of the principles, practices, and evidence for effective communication approaches are provided and organized into logically presented sections: the importance and value of effective patient–provider communications and basic principles of communications (Part I); a discussion of therapeutic communication skills, one technique at a time (e.g., empathy, trust, questioning, use of silence, reflection, interpretation; Part II); skills needed to ensure therapeutic communications under challenging patient circumstances (e.g., patients in crisis, coping with chronic illness, and with limited literacy skills; Part III); communication patterns within and across providers and families (Part IV); ethics and healthcare communications (Part V); and finally, advanced issues (e.g., communications to enhance behavioral change, the use of the Internet in patient–provider communications, and systems of care that enhance or deter from effective communications; Part VI).

Key features of the text include learning objectives for each chapter, questions to address with respect to communication as a science, examples of dialogue from interactions between provider and patient, illustrations of the actual use of specific skills, explanations of the principles underlying the use of various skill sets, easy-to-read and -understand summaries in table format, notations about regulatory issues and standards of practice as appropriate, lists of resources pertinent to the subject of the chapter, and a complete glossary to assist students with definitions of terms.

Acknowledgments

As is the case for most extensive writing efforts, many people are to be thanked for their assistance along the way. Their names are not acknowledged on the cover, but their input was essential. Special thanks to faculty and students who offered their helpful advice and enthusiasm about what needs to be covered and how. Clearly, it was these individuals and the keen insight of Mike Brown, Publisher, who persistently asked about and saw the continued value of this material in educating health professionals. Those who granted permission to reprint excerpts of their work are appreciated. In some cases, the classic early work of those cited is invaluable to our in-depth understanding of communication processes. I would like to extend my appreciation to Katey Birtcher, Associate Editor of Public Health, Health Administration, and Clinical Nutrition, and those in the editing department of Jones and Bartlett for their extensive efforts in reviewing and recommending changes, including a tweaking here and a tweaking there.

Table of Contents

Preface

While healthcare communication skills and knowledge are the subject of many health professional educational programs, they might not receive the attention they deserve. These skills and knowledge are frequently taught—but only in the context of diagnostic interviewing. Until recently, there was little attention paid to ensuring that providers could not only conduct an assessment interview but could communicate well with a variety of patients. Even if providers have acquired the necessary skills, they might be concerned that within the current healthcare system, there is no time to use these skills, without recognizing that they cannot afford *not* to. Maguire and Pitceathy (2002) and others point out that providers (physicians in this case) do not communicate as well as they should. They summarize the case for better communication skill competency. Essentially, and this can be applied to all professional healthcare providers, good communication skills can help identify patients' problems more accurately, help patients adjust to the psychological stress of their illness, result in patient satisfaction with their care, and result in patients who are more likely to adhere to their advice and follow their treatment regimen; they conclude that even providers (doctors) have greater job satisfaction, and less work stress. Still, the majority of practitioners do not feel confident in their communication skills or perhaps had no formal training at all. If their skills were improved, the quality of care would improve, and the costs of this care could be reduced.

Effective communications are at the core of quality patient care. Patients require the help and support of other people. Every contact with a patient or potential patient requires courteous, considerate, respectful, and helpful communication. When patients get the responses they want, they feel good about their encounter with healthcare providers, and their need for positive interaction is satisfied. When patients feel good about their experience, they are more willing to cooperate and are more likely to repeat their contacts with us. If their experience is negative, however, they are likely to avoid and limit further contact. Depending on what is required to complete their care, patients' avoidance may have very serious consequences. It may cause them to avoid getting needed help, or it may cause them to ignore the healthcare instructions they have been given.

Negative communication experiences can cause anger and resentment toward providers and the healthcare system itself. If patients come to a healthcare facility, for example, and get routed to several providers without getting any real help, they will feel resentful about their encounter. One negative experience like this can require many additional positive interactions before its effects are completely erased.

The value of a positive provider–patient relationship, where good communication skills are practiced, cannot be underestimated. In addition to being the doorway to quality care, the patient–provider relationship built on sound communications is regarded as the most crucial component of the healthcare delivery system. Del Mar (1994), in an assessment of related literature over a 35-year period, showed that providers' good communication skills are associated with better care and even better health. This original study has been supported repeatedly in the literature.

Communications are best taught using a variety of teaching modalities. This text presents concepts, practice examples, and the evidence behind the importance of communication in patient–provider encounters. Practice experience, where students demonstrate and evaluate their skills, is enormously helpful in aiding learners to examine their expertise and where they need improvement. Student evaluations of courses aimed at teaching communication skills are usually positive, indicating that they do feel that their interviewing and communication skills are improved with course work. Undergraduate and graduate healthcare professional training programs that deny students formalized instruction in communication skills and principles produce an incompletely trained provider. A variety of skills are needed and should be in place if students are to effectively practice in today's complex healthcare environment.

The purpose of this textbook is to inform the reader about basic communication knowledge and skills, including concepts, practice, and evidence. Becoming proficient in communicating with a variety of patients and their families in varying healthcare settings and circumstances is a requirement of all healthcare professionals. Practicing effective communicative behavior with other health professionals is also mandated in this era of increased interprofessional collaboration. The literature—whether research reports, a review of the literature, consensus recommendations, affirmed experience, or any case studies and patient self-reports—is replete with examples of how communication can or did make a difference in the care that patients and their families received and the quality of care that was delivered.

Just reading about communication is not sufficient, however. Despite the abundant literature on communication and therapeutic response modes, communication knowledge and skills cannot be learned from textbooks alone. The critical test of providers' competency is how they put these principles and skills into practice with patients. Because of this, laboratory experiences in which students test out and practice therapeutic responsiveness is critical in their professional role development. Practice, patience, and feedback can significantly affect providers' attitudes about their abilities and feelings of self-efficacy.

Teaching staff who use this text will find the material detailed and informative. The text is intended to be applicable to upper-division undergraduate students as well as first-level graduate students and practicing health professionals. Most universities with health professional schools have an undergraduate core curriculum in which communication content and experiential learning is a requirement; therefore, the text is extremely useful to students who are entering the health professions but who have not yet encountered many patient–provider contacts. The text is designed to be useful cross-disciplinarily, and examples using these providers are used generously in the discussion. The importance of effective communication skills in all healthcare professions is undeniably important.

This text is dedicated to basic communication skills and concepts that are foundational to the healthcare professions. The chapter on human communications was enhanced by the analysis and synthesis of Gazda, Childers, and Walters (1982). I thank Dr. Rose Vasta for her contributions in elucidating the nature of selected therapeutic response modes.

Managing Care and the Implications for Healthcare Communication

The healthcare system's new tools will permit it to transfer both power and moral responsibility to families and individuals to manage their own health more effectively.
—Jeff C. Goldsmith

CHAPTER OBJECTIVES

- Identify factors affecting the current delivery of health care in the United States.
- Discuss health-promotion models that may establish and maintain health for the largest numbers of individuals in need.
- Identify how self-care, community-based programs, and interprofessional coordination are needed in today's healthcare climate.
- Discuss models of patient–provider communications and how these may reflect the current healthcare crisis.
- Identify typical stressors in patient–provider relationships.
- Identify potential patient responses to these stressors.

Powerful new tools emerging from the biotechnological revolution may soon render health care unrecognizable as we know it today. These changes will be felt in our methods of communicating with patients. The use of Internet sites, including provider–patient e-mail and the availability of health-related websites, is an example of how technology might affect the circumstances under which patient–provider encounters will take place. Healthcare communications are expected to be, on the one hand, more focused and, on the other hand, less direct as episodes of care are managed on the outskirts of the provider–patient relationship. Still, care may be more comprehensive than ever before. The compelling push in the opposite direction for managing patients' wellness over time and the need to actively engage patients in health-promoting behaviors emphasize a holistic approach. Providers' needs for skills in engaging, persuading, and facilitating change will remain critical.

Emerging in this biotechnological revolution are two primary issues: how will care be delivered, and what will be required of providers in these new delivery systems? How will communication between providers, clients, and families take shape? The first issue deals with healthcare delivery systems; the second, with the prevailing mode of interaction between provider and client.

Just what shapes health care and healthcare delivery systems and how these factors play a role in the evolution of health care in the United States is addressed in this text. A paradigm for viewing health care from a health-promotion model is presented. Implications for provider–patient and provider–provider relationships and communications are discussed. The role of communications in the provision of care is examined, and needs for commitment, caring, and partnership are highlighted. This text is addressed with multiple healthcare disciplines in mind.

The rigid boundaries that previously existed between professionals and professional training programs are no longer appropriate, and this text attempts to transcend assumptions of dissimilarity on such basic issues as patient–provider communications and therapeutic communications. In this section of the text, the history of the American system of health care is briefly summarized. The current crisis in healthcare delivery is discussed in detail, enumerating the basis for needed healthcare reform. It is important to understand potential threats to patient–provider communications as system barriers to adequate health care. The prerequisites for therapeutic alliances today include reassurances that problems at the system level will not govern the character of interaction between patient and provider. Encounter conflicts surrounding the availability and sensitivity of providers reflect generic problems with healthcare delivery.

HEALTHCARE DELIVERY IN THE UNITED STATES—1600s TO 2000s

If we were to trace the evolution of health care in the United States from its inception in the early 1600s to today's system of healthcare delivery, we might first conclude that because of so many differences—then and now—any comparison of these periods is impossible. Nonetheless, with closer examination, we can perceive certain common threads along with many differences. The evolution of healthcare delivery over the last 300 years is indeed significant. The healthcare system in the early colonial days (1620) was very different from the system we have today (2000s).

Factors Influencing Healthcare Delivery Systems

Those who study trends in healthcare delivery usually identify at least four elements that account for the character of delivery systems through time: (1) societal influences, (2) public health programs, (3) existing health problems, and (4) levels of technology. Forces affecting the evolution of systems of care in hospitals are depicted more specifically as (1) advances in medical science, (2) the development of specialized technology, (3) the development of professional training, (4) the growth of health insurance, and (5) the role of government.

For example, if we took a trip back in time to the colonial period (roughly 1620–1781), we would observe several factors that would account for the direction of health care. Society in the colonial period reflected small agricultural communities. Trade was important, and several port towns (Boston, New York, Charleston) were the chief points of entry for intercontinental trade. There were distinct health problems that reflected this social structure; epidemics were of concern and the port towns were seen as avenues for significant communicable diseases (e.g., yellow fever). Physicians and nurses were few but participated in initiating quarantine standards. The clergy played a significant role in caring for the ill, visiting patients and their families at home. Voluntary boards of concerned citizens were involved in public health concerns, but governmental involvement was negligible. Medical technology was insufficient to control health problems. However, ordinances were passed to control problems of sanitation, waste disposal, and public markets in the port towns.

In the 300 years that have ensued, vast changes in society and in health care make the problems and issues just articulated vastly outdated. Important social events such as the Civil War, and later, World War I and World War II influenced greatly what our healthcare delivery system became.

From the close of World War II through 1965, the delivery of care shifted dramatically to become the care of the infirm in hospitals. Urban areas became more prominent fixtures, and rural areas shifted to large farms. Housing improved and immunizations continued to improve our ability to fend off disease—this time, polio. With acute problems and infectious diseases more under control, chronic diseases came to the forefront. Diseases such as arthritis, heart failure, asthma, and diabetes drew our attention. In 1950 the government made its first significant contribution to health care, investing $73 million in medical research. While hospitals tended to dominate the delivery system, community programs were staffed to help patients and their families cope with chronic illness; these agencies included public health department programs and visiting nurses' associations.

The Vietnam War, extending from 1964 through 1973, influenced not only our social-political structure but also the structure of our healthcare system. Prevention of chronic diseases was still important, but the realization that these diseases would not be eradicated without significant changes in the health habits of the population prevailed. Health promotion programs to control smoking, diet, and substance abuse were stressed. By 1985 there were a total of 6,872 hospitals; the majority (5,784) of them were designated short-term acute-care hospitals. The federal government administered a mere 343 hospitals, while state and local governments administered only about 1,600 of the hospitals. While acute-care hospitals predominated, long-term care and nursing-home facilities also existed but in much smaller numbers. Home health agencies continued to deliver care to the chronically and terminally ill patient in the home.

Changes occurring from 1984 to date reflect tremendous shifts in health care. Public health problems continue to include environmental threats (e.g., pollution), but health problems once defined as disease and injury have shifted to include societal problems. What were once considered society's problems—teen pregnancy, drug abuse, domestic violence—are now being classified as significant threats to our nation. Along with the continual focus on the maintenance of the quality of life of those with chronic illnesses and disabilities, an environment for healthy living has become increasingly critical to the effective management of healthcare problems.

Current Healthcare Crisis

Traditionally, the American healthcare system has been organized around acute illnesses; the role of the healthcare system was to rescue us from these illnesses and take custody of us until we were well (Goldsmith, 1992a, p. 19). In the past two decades, this focus has been significantly shaken by our ability to manage health care on an ambulatory basis. The travesty is that we have built a vast and costly apparatus around this acute-care focus. Thus, the fit between healthcare needs and healthcare services has worsened significantly.

While Americans may disagree about issues related to the social problems that face our nation—including violence, homelessness, drug abuse, and teen pregnancy—there is general consensus that these social problems both affect and reflect the state of our nation's health and will have a significant impact on the future ability of Americans to stay healthy.

Most Americans agree that the healthcare system that exists in the United States today needs to be reformed. Public opinion polls have shown that only a quarter of the American public has faith in the current delivery system to meet our nation's healthcare needs. Healthcare reform was one of the major issues of the 1990 Conference of Governors (Kaplan, 1991). Healthcare reform was a major focal point in the 1992 presidential campaign and is retaining priority in recent presidential campaigns. Legislators continue to study and search for solutions to needed reform and acknowledge three basic deficiencies in our healthcare system: (1) affordability, (2) accessibility, and (3) accountability (IOM, 2004).

Affordability

To understand the problem we face in affordability of health care in the United States, it is important to examine how the costs of health care have escalated and how they are predicted to soar continually. In 1940 the nation spent $4 billion on health care. By 1950 these costs had tripled. The current situation is that healthcare costs keep rising and inequities in accessibility becomes clearer. In short, even with the advent of managed care, the nation's healthcare expenditures are high and headed higher.

What seems to be at the heart of the problem is the ability of insurance programs to deliver on the basis of need and recommended level of service. Those who pay for health care (frequently, employers) can no longer afford the same level of service formerly provided. The cost of care is exceedingly high in the United States. A recent report by the Institute of Medicine (IOM, 2004) called for the United States to implement universal health care by 2010. It is estimated that if some form of healthcare reform to reduce the costs of care does not occur in the United States, the economic viability of the United States will be significantly threatened some time in the 21st century. In this same report, it was stated that 43 million Americans are uninsured, and lack of health insurance causes 18,000 unnecessary deaths each year in the United States.

Accessibility

The enormous costs of health care are only part of the problem, albeit, a very serious part. A second significant challenge is healthcare accessibility. A 2001 report of the Institute of Medicine, *Crossing the Quality Chasm: A New Health Care System for the 21st Century*, called for a reform that centered on the needs of patients and assured they get the care they need in a timely manner. Despite the enormous costs of care, our current system of healthcare delivery does not equally provide for everyone.

Economists describing the problem of accessibility estimate that up to millions of people go uninsured despite the fact that the United States spends more of the gross domestic product (GDP) on health care than any other country in the world. The Institute of Medicine's report, *The Uninsured Are Sicker and Die Sooner*, explains that uninsured people are more likely to receive too little medical care and receive it too late, resulting in their getting sicker and dying sooner.

Essential guidelines that are continually considered include the following:

1. Healthcare coverage should be universal.
2. Healthcare coverage should be continuous.
3. Healthcare coverage should be affordable to individuals and families.
4. The health insurance strategy should be affordable and sustainable to society.
5. Healthcare coverage should enhance health and well-being by promoting access to high-quality care that is effective, efficient, safe, timely, patient-centered, and equitable.

How can this be? Despite the fact that the American healthcare system is one of the most technically advanced in the world and that so much is spent on health care, a substantial proportion of the population is locked out of the system. This problem is described as one of both the uninsured and underinsured. This, however, is not the only basis for the problem of access. Surely the lack of healthcare services in rural areas, and even in some urban areas, contributes to the problem of accessibility and therefore healthcare disparities.

The first and extremely invalid assumption that the public makes is that these people are largely the unemployed. This assumption is incorrect. Those people who are locked out of health care are employed, often at very low wages, but the employers cannot afford the high costs of health insurance.

The problem is also not distributed evenly over all groups. The elderly, for example, do not fall into this group. Since 1965, they have been covered under Medicare. The indigent are not part of the group either. Medicaid provides for them if they are poor, blind, and disabled. Although Medicaid helps the indigent, the services provided under Medicaid are being curtailed, and fewer poor people are assisted.

The criticism around Medicaid has included arguments that some groups are favored over others, and the favoritism that exists may further enhance the nation's social problems. Consider, for example, teenage pregnancy. In 1980 the only way to obtain health insurance (through Medicaid) if you were poor was to become pregnant. Most states allow low-income families eligibility if those families support small children. The issue of inequities in the provision of services has become a political football more than once.

What appears to be the case, at least people fear it is the case, is that health care is a luxury. This luxury is provided only to certain groups. And the luxury that does exist makes the absence of care appear even more unfair.

The recent IOM report on healthcare disparities indicates that research has extensively documented the pervasiveness of racial and ethnic disparities in health care. In 1999, as part of a national effort to eliminate healthcare disparities, Congress required the Agency for Healthcare Research and

Quality (AHRQ) to produce an annual report to be called the National Healthcare Disparities Report (NHDR). The report includes tracking disparities in access to quality care. The American Medical Association (AMA) summarized the problem: although there have been improvements in the health of U.S. residents, racial and ethnic minorities remain disadvantaged and experience a lower quality of health services and are less likely to receive routine care and have higher rates of morbidity and mortality than nonminorities. These disparities in health care were said to be present even when controlling for gender, condition, age, and socioeconomic status.

Accountability

The third and less frequently discussed issue surrounding healthcare delivery today is the problem of accountability. It is shocking to realize that despite the extremely large amounts of money expended for health care, we know relatively little about its outcomes. Is it effective? Is it even safe? Is it efficient? (We already know that it is too costly!) Well, this is changing; there is an emerging effort to identify outcomes and to examine where problems exist. An example of this is the emphasis on assessing medication errors in health care, their source, their costs, and how they may have been prevented.

Can you imagine the Chrysler Corporation not knowing the quality of its product or IBM not improving on its products and services? Not very likely, you would say. Well, why does the healthcare industry not know what a successful product is or how much it should cost to deliver the best product to the greatest number of people?

The most difficult piece of evidence to explain is the great variability in healthcare provisions with the resultant outcomes being the same, or at least much the same. We observe variation in practices. For example, some patients are provided more tests, but they do not necessarily survive any longer than less-tested individuals with the same healthcare problem. For example, at a Veterans' Administration hospital in California, 40% of the patients received an angiogram following myocardial infarction (MI). Those MI patients in the same geographical region, but privately insured, were reported to receive angiograms 80% of the time. It was reported that there was no evidence to suggest that those who were treated more aggressively (with angiograms) were any better off, given the survival rates of these patients (Kaplan, 1991). Other examples have shown that more frequent hospitalizations, or hospitalizations that cost more, are not more effective in prolonging life. We have even been shown the contrary—that certain medical intervention was not only unnecessary but could have put the patient at significant risk for other problems. As surprising as it seems, especially in light of the high costs of care and the advancement in technology that has occurred, we cannot establish with more exactness what treatment yields what outcome.

Those who predict or try to influence the shape of healthcare reform usually recognize that any change that does occur will have to address all three elements—affordability, accessibility, and accountability—simultaneously. Most important, we are now not only faced with healthcare problems as we have known them for years, we are faced with a "sick" system as well. Altering the sick system will be as important as treating illness and promoting health.

A PARADIGM FOR ENSURING BETTER HEALTH TO LARGER NUMBERS AND EMERGENT DELIVERY SYSTEMS

The challenge of ensuring better health to larger numbers of people and delivering that care equitably raises several complex issues: What is health? How is it established and maintained? How is this objective met with the largest numbers of Americans?

Needs for Reform and Health-Promotion Models

Older notions of public health and individual entitlement tend to deemphasize the dynamics of several factors that affect the health status of most persons. A social ecological orientation to health considers the interaction of numerous social, political, and environmental as well as physical and emotional conditions that affect individuals' quality of life. At the risk of being too abstract, a paradigm that ensures better health to larger numbers includes all of these factors and affects and is affected by public policy.

A basic assumption behind such a paradigm is that health is a multifaceted phenomena encompassing emotional well-being, physical health, and social integration. It is a model that recognizes the interplay among individuals, families, and groups that are set within particular socio-culturally defined fields. It is a model that views health and illness on a continuum and estimates years of health based on projections of life span. When years of health are the aim, the effect of medical treatment on everyday functioning and a person's quality of life must be evaluated. We should then be able to assess the particular impact of a drug or surgical procedure on the quality of life of the patients we see.

A critical departure in the adaptation of a health-promotion model is the adherence to concepts that are foreign to more traditional medical approaches. For example, the traditional medical model stresses patho-physiology. Specific disease processes, characteristic of both illness and injury, are judged in relation to body systems and specific clinical evidence, such as lab tests and blood pressure. Opinions about intervention based on these clinical measures may produce different, even contradictory, conclusions. Medical interventions (e.g., medications to lower blood cholesterol) aim to reduce death due to coronary heart disease. Biological models are used to justify this choice of treatment, and the model argues that there is a benefit to this treatment because it reduces deaths from coronary heart disease. Interestingly enough, in controlled experimental studies, the overall outcome—morbidity—for this group of patients (from all causes) is not affected. A clearer example of the problem of the traditional medical model becomes apparent when the issue is surgical intervention. The benefits of surgery are usually stressed without equal attention being given to the complications that can occur. In contrast, a quality-of-life health-promotion model will give significantly more weight to a variety of factors, including treatment benefits, estimates of the relative value of treatment versus no treatment, and side-effects that occur in relation to the treatment chosen. Decisions about treatment become quite specific with clarification of what intervention is essential, very important, or only valuable to certain groups of individuals.

The Promotion of Self-Care and Community-Based Programs

The demand for inpatient care is predicted to decrease, not disappear. Acute care will not remain the model for the American health system; the ultimate focus will be outside the hospital. Goldsmith (1992b) points out that planners and public health policy makers have come to realize that community-based systems, whether founded on a public health model or medical group practice (or some combination of the two), are the foundation for an effective new system of care. This model will stress health promotion and active participation on the part of patients who are no longer the passive recipients of health care.

An outcome associated with newer health-promotion models is the achievement of high levels of self-care potential. Self-care refers to the actions performed by patients (or their significant others) directed at alleviating the effects of illness and its treatment. These actions, taken with the interest of protecting and promoting health and well-being, reflect many sociocultural interpretations that the patient places on his or her current illness and future goals. One of the variables repeatedly cited in providing quality of care through health promotion is the character of the patient–provider relationship, particularly that between physician and patient. Features of this relationship that were associated with positive patient behaviors were (1) the friendly and accepting attitude of the provider, (2) patients' perceptions that the physician had spent time with them, (3) patients' feelings that they had control in the interaction and input in their treatment programs, (4) patients' satisfaction with the care they received, (5) a treatment program that was actually tailored to them as individuals, (6) situations in which patients felt that information was willingly shared with them, (7) absence of formal disagreement with patients, and (8) continuity of the specific provider–patient relationship. Although the largest proportion of these data focused specifically on patient–physician encounters, the conclusions have validity for encounters between other health providers and patients.

It is clear from current projections of trends in healthcare source delivery that not only the patient will be instrumental in deciding the impact of healthcare reform, whole communities will shape the manner in which this care will be rendered. Less care will occur in acute-care hospitals; more care will occur in brief urgent-care centers. An increasingly significant proportion of the care of the very ill will occur in the home. Providers will be asked to assist in this transition.

In truth, the American system has few alternatives; inpatient hospitalization is too costly and the advent of diagnostic-related groups (DRGs) no longer permits the extended hospital stays enjoyed a little more than a decade ago. The de-institutionalization of healthcare delivery will characterize the major shifts in delivery systems. Rather than just inpatient or outpatient service, there is likely to be a flexible flow in the use of a variety of services extending through the course of disease and illness to include end-of-life care.

Managed Care and Interprofessional Collaboration

Adapting a health-promotion model of care has direct implications for the collaborative relationships of health providers.

If we endorse a broad concept of health and recognize the value of the quality of our patients' lives, we depart from tendencies to view patients through the narrow channel of disease or illness. Once open to health in the broader context, not just the absence of disease, we automatically recognize the importance of multiple health and human service providers. The overall goal—maintaining the patient's optimal level of health and increasing the patient's years of freedom from disease and absence from disability—frees us to think out of the box, not only of formal approaches to cure and care administered by physicians, nurses, dentists, pharmacists, and many other providers, but we are also encouraged to consider the multitude of alternative health care approaches and strategies that lie outside scientific medicine.

This health-promotion perspective emphasizes both the advantages and the appropriateness of multilevel interventions. Many of these interventions are complementary. Reducing stress, for example, can occur through meditation; it can also be attained through relaxation and massage programs. Others are synergistic, building on one another to produce the desired results.

What concept of interprofessional teamwork is appropriate? Under the old disease-oriented approach, providers were relegated to positions of importance with respect to their role in ridding individuals of disease. Physicians, under this model, are at the top of the hierarchy for several reasons. They had the authority to cure disease. Under this model, because disease is paramount in directing healthcare providers, physicians automatically assumed the primary leadership role.

Managed care has been considered as a potential solution to containing healthcare costs, and at the same time, ensuring equitable care to all Americans. The managed care model is expected to be the prevailing form of healthcare delivery now and in the future. According to many providers, managed care of the ill will require, at the very minimum, multidisciplinary teams consisting of physicians, nurses, home-care providers, and ambulatory-care practitioners. Under managed care, the aim is to provide a range of services in such a way that these services and their costs will be scrutinized and controlled. Three basic managed care programs exist at present: health maintenance organizations (HMOs), preferred provider organizations (PPOs), and fee-for-service plans.

HMOs and PPOs have been criticized for their drawbacks. Despite the fact that they were designed to provide preventive healthcare services and to improve the continuity of quality of care, the results reveal problems. Healthier individuals are favored by managed care systems over those who are at high risk, those who require high-cost procedures, and those who are chronically ill and need long-term care. Managed care has also been criticized for overlooking quality of care in order to meet the basic aim of cost containment. Also, low-income populations are often not served by these plans.

Managed care systems and case management are being hailed as the primary solution to needed healthcare reform. Skills and knowledge that are necessary to function in these systems of care are being defined. The real and potential importance of effective communication skills is clear, particularly as they relate to healthcare assessments, disease management, and multidisciplinary collaboration. The outcomes of health care are clearly a reflection of the provider's command of effective communication skills and knowledge as they are executed in new roles.

Managed Care versus Case Management

Managed care is a system of managing and financing healthcare delivery to ensure that services are needed, are efficiently provided, and are appropriately priced. Through a variety of means, including preadmission certification, concurrent review of necessity of services, and financial incentives, managed care attempts to contain costs, ensure optimal patient outcomes, and maximize the efficient use of service utilization.

As previously indicated, managed care is one system of delivery that is proposed to correct the problems in healthcare delivery that were, and continue to be, out of control. Managed care is rapidly changing traditional approaches to health care. The managed care industry can be understood by segmenting the industry into three distinct options. Current and future developments in managed care suggest that it has fulfilled its promise in supporting quality care and cost containment concerns remain. Still, problems remain and have led to erosion of the system with cost increasing significantly after the turn of the century (Lagoe, Aspling, and Westert, 2005).

Frequently associated with the concept of managed care is the term **case management**. Although managed care and case management are sometimes used interchangeably, they refer to distinctly different phenomena (see Figure I–1). Managed care generally denotes the way care is structured for reimbursement. Case management, however, is a technique used to monitor and coordinate treatment, usually for specific diagnoses. Traditionally a utilization review process, case management means that care is closely monitored and coordinated, particularly with regard to high-cost service-intense diagnoses. Case management includes activities of assessment, treatment planning, referral, and follow-up to ensure that comprehensive and continuous services are provided. Case management oversees reimbursement for care in that it ensures that the coordinated payment and reimbursement of services is properly executed.

The emergence of managed care is congruent with case management because both aim to ensure quality and control costs. Managed care systems have been widely endorsed as necessary options in health care reform. The goals of these organizations—to ensure maximum value from resources—is congruent with the

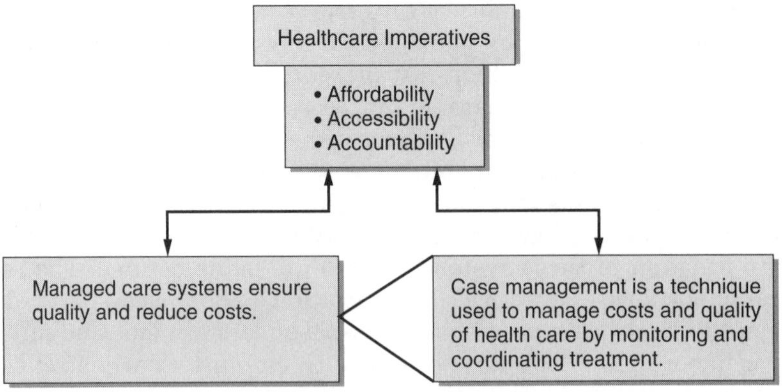

Figure I-1 Needs for Healthcare Reform and Managed Care Systems.

basic philosophy of health care professionals (Hicks, Stallmeyer, and Coleman, 1992). This philosophy holds in high esteem a focus on the total needs of an individual, not just on the disease process and on maintaining health to minimize the need of future expensive healthcare intervention.

Underlying Problems and Issues with Managed Care and Case Management

Healthcare reform is not new and different; reform can be traced back in time to the health initiatives of President John F. Kennedy's New Frontier and President Lyndon B. Johnson's Great Society. Because healthcare reform spans several decades, we can safely conclude that reform in the United States is a continuous process.

Managed care, though, has come under severe criticism. Primarily, this criticism is leveled at the premise that accessibility, affordability, and accountability in health care are realistic. Some providers claim that addressing any one of those three elements will inevitably compromise another (Kissick, 1994). Choices need to be made, and these choices may preclude the possibility of simultaneous significant improvement in all areas.

Managed care is not altogether new, but neither is case management. Case management is not new to our concept of professional practice because disease management has been a familiar approach of providers in their caregiver roles. Controlling costs is also not a unique idea, because providers have been historically motivated toward this aim. Case management, though, has undergone widespread criticism. The case manager is sometimes viewed as an extension of an already extensive bureaucratic system, adding yet another layer to the healthcare delivery system. It is felt that quality of health should be provided and managed by healthcare professionals. The reliance on those other than healthcare professionals—particularly clerks in insurance offices who, in some cases, decide treatment options—defies our ability to ensure quality.

These issues have generated a great deal of debate: (1) What professional is best suited to be a case manager? (2) What added expertise is needed to function in this role? (3) What approach is best suited to execute the role with arguments for and against direct contact versus telephone triaging of patients?

In part, concerns about case management have surfaced because of the rapid proliferation of case management systems. The current managed care industry is criticized because it is felt that case managers were needed before adequate planning for their preparation could occur. Essentially, the professionals managing care may not have the expertise to execute their roles. No real data, however, are available to judge the quality of care under case management. While data about patients' responses to case management are limited, patients are said to value the system because it eases their burden in managing their own care.

Shifts in Care Delivery

In keeping with the need for healthcare reform and the methods used to secure accessibility, affordability, and accountability, certain predictable trends are shaping health care. These trends have particular implications for provider encounters with patients and their families.

Community Ambulatory Care

Diminishing hospital use and vast expansion of ambulatory care are occurring. Health promotion and disease prevention—high-priority aims in healthcare reform—are achieved largely in community ambulatory care settings.

Disease Management

These predicted shifts in the focus of care clearly indicate that the majority of services will occur in the community ambulatory care setting. This does not, however, mean that disease is no longer a concern. A new term, *disease management*, describes a community approach to treating chronic conditions. Diseases such as HIV and other chronic, severely debilitating conditions are examples. The care processes of disease management include prevention and health promotion. Early identification of disease; assessment of problems secondary to disease; and development, implementation, and evaluation of a plan of care are encompassed in this approach to disease management.

Disease management consists of taking a single problem such as AIDS, cancer, diabetes, or cardiac and psychiatric conditions (conditions known to be chronic) and applying regular interventions for consistent outcomes. Early identification is critical to patients who can benefit from early detection. The individual's unique needs are understood to be the essential part of assessing the problem as well as developing care plans. Care is to be individualized and patient-centered. In plan development, the protocol for care is based on defined medical practices that promote health rather than those that simply treat disease. The plan is put into action using health-promotion strategies prior to such anticipated periods and routine illness treatment. Plan evaluation occurs regularly but is not confined to measures of treatment. Rather, evaluation also includes measures of the level of health maintained over time.

Interprofessional Collaboration and Consultation

Interprofessional collaboration and consultation are necessities of both managed care and case management. To develop and implement successful managed care approaches, support from key participants—administrators, physicians, nurses, and other healthcare providers—is required. The ability to work with other individuals on a continuous basis is essential to the success of case management. Case management within and outside hospitals requires consultation with finance personnel, administrators, and various providers (e.g., dietitians, physicians, social workers, physical therapists, and nurses) to obtain relevant information about potential problems.

The idea is to collaborate with many in order to design strategies for solving problems. Ideally, case managers are professionals—nurses or physicians. These professionals communicate with provider groups to identify problems, plan strategies, and evaluate progress within patient care critical pathways as well as to evaluate the overall impact of these actions. Within case management, therapeutic relationships with patients and families are important. Case managers rely on those relationships to derive mutually acceptable outcomes. Consultation with patients and families and the development of a collaborative relationship with these individuals are said to be as important as the collaboration and consultation that occur within colleague relationships.

THE SKILLS AND KNOWLEDGE OF PROVIDERS IN A MANAGED CARE ENVIRONMENT

Generic to All Providers

The skills and knowledge that are necessary for providers who work in managed care environments are defined, in part, by the expected outcomes of managed care and case management approaches.

Managed care includes a commitment to reduce cost, make services accessible, and control and monitor quality. Managed care should (1) positively affect the cost of service, (2) improve provider consultation and communication, (3) engage other key providers in participating in care planning, and (4) improve continuous quality improvement through the design of critical-care pathways. Additionally, patients should be positively affected in that their care is coordinated for them and that there is a reduction in unpredictable outcomes. Thus, they should be more knowledgeable and better prepared to understand and participate collaboratively in the planning and evaluation of their care.

Although there are a variety of case management models, common to all are the following service components:

- Client identification and outreach.
- Individual client assessment and diagnosis.
- Service planning and resource identification.
- Linking clients to needed services.
- Actual service implementation and coordination.
- Monitoring service delivery activities.
- Patient advocacy to reduce problems of access to care.
- Evaluation of these activities and their expected outcomes (Allred, Arford, Michel, Dring, and Carter, 1995).

To accomplish these goals, providers need to function as both multidisciplinary and multi-service integrators. Integrators operate at the hub of the wheel as they bring together and coordinate broad-based services.

Roles Specific to Case Manager

Case managers in managed care organizations steer, guide, and track patients through a variety of care activities, thus enhancing continuity of care. A major instrument in this tracking process is the critical-pathway analysis imbedded in the patient's plan of care. Critical pathways and critical-path tools were so coded based on the Critical Path Method (CPM), a part of the Program Evaluation Review Technique (PERT) developed by the U.S. Navy and Lockheed Aircraft Corporation.

The patient-care plans that are developed identify a "critical pathway" of key events (activities and interventions) that must occur as projected if the desired patient outcomes are to be achieved within a specified time period. The case manager oversees these pathways and facilitates interventions to ensure that patients progress appropriately and satisfactorily. The coordination and collaborative consultation that occurs requires skillful assessment and negotiation.

The specific facets of the case manager role have been detailed in the literature. A thorough account of this role for nurses is presented by Hicks, Stallmeyer, and Coleman (1992). Patient advocacy, patient education, resource and risk management, benefits interpretation, and provider liaison are all aspects of this role.

The Role of Communication in Delivery of Health Care

Exploring the issue of the importance of communication skills and knowledge to providers is somewhat like discussing the need for eyes in order to see. Most providers would not argue either the relevance or importance of these skills and knowledge. The issue is rather what communication skills and knowledge are needed and how will they be acquired. Additionally, in this era of evidence-based practice, providers can no longer be satisfied with knowing how to do it, they must understand why and what evidence there is to support benefits of these approaches.

In this text, dimensions of the phenomena of human communication and, more specifically, healthcare communication are explored in depth. Essentially, every provider needs a foundation in the basic anatomy and physiology of communication. Providers need to know the variables that affect reception, processing, and expression. They need to understand the relationship of communication to quality care outcomes. They also need to understand the multicultural context in which communication occurs. Providers deliver healthcare services, all of which—disease prevention, health promotion, health screening, and health education—require foundations in therapeutic communications. Therapeutic response modes are needed not just to successfully assess individuals and families, they are needed to manage care and to increase patient awareness and capacity for personal health management and self-care. Specialized knowledge and skill are needed to relate effectively in these capacities when crisis or prolonged chronic illness are the subjects of healthcare management.

To participate fully in interprofessional managed healthcare teams that are collaborating with other providers and patients and their families, knowledge of the dynamics of group and family communication patterns is required. Communicating effectively with all relevant constituencies—patients, providers, and regulatory agencies—calls for effective negotiation skills. The ethical precepts of communicating in managed care, particularly with regard to patients' rights to informed choice and informed consent, must serve to critically guide our practice in these emerging models that now dominate healthcare delivery. Finally, advanced issues (e.g., communication and models of behavior change, communication and the use of the Internet, and communications as a function of systems of care) further extend the coverage of the topic of how the provider will use and alter factors that enhance communications.

CONCLUSION

In summary, vast changes have occurred in the American healthcare system over the past 300 years. These changes have reflected many factors, including the advancement of medical technology, the American social structure, and threats to health and equitable healthcare delivery that have plagued us over time. With a seemingly unwavering belief in the American system of health care, the American dream became one that included absence of disease and, if that was not possible, remarkable chances of recovery from extraordinary debilitating conditions. This American dream is quickly becoming a significant nightmare as we attempt to assure all Americans of the privilege of health and absence of disease. Recognizing our goals and concomitantly restructuring our delivery systems while containing costs is the challenge for healthcare reform.

Affordability, accessibility, and accountability are major recurrent system barriers to the delivery of effective healthcare services. They are not isolated problems; they affect providers' one-to-one encounters with patients. Patients' reactions to providers reflect their fears and concerns that basic health care is costly, may not always prove adequate, and is frequently administered by a nonresponsive system. These fears and concerns are translated into communication difficulties where patients mistrust providers' intentions and the system as a whole.

Attitudes of mistrust and fear of neglect, if they do exist among patients, are not without basis in reality. Previously, they may have been described as an anticipated set of concerns felt by most patients but without much substance. Still, there is a new context for patient anxiety, and it can hardly be ignored. Thus, it becomes even more imperative that providers be guided by sound principles of interpersonal communication.

Healthcare reform will include new goals for health promotion where patients fulfill certain self-care behaviors never before expected of them. Reform will occur outside the hospital, in neighborhoods, and in community settings. It will require new concepts of interprofessional collaboration. Finally, it will require a growing sensitivity and awareness of patient–provider encounters that work and do not work. Certainly the trust, confidence, and security that providers evoke in their encounters—an element of professional practice always held in high esteem—will play a critical role in the reform that takes place at the system level. To this end, the parameters of good interpersonal communications are the "handbook" for all health professionals. Provider–client communications are both a determinant and a by-product of successful healthcare delivery. Exhibit I–1 describes some patient perceived difficulties critical to correcting communication deficits.

Exhibit I–1 Patients' Descriptions of Difficulties in Communicating with Providers in Inpatient Settings: Verbatim and Implied Reactions

"Having to tell my story over again."
Please save me the energy and humiliation.

"Not having doctors get together on their opinions—each one telling me something different."
If my doctors are not together, how can I trust what they do?

continues

Exhibit I–1 Continued

"The RNs, doctors, and physical therapists communicate poorly (to one another) . . . and they do not follow-up on the information they give."
Do they think I don't notice this and worry?

[What is difficult is] "wanting to speak to someone who really cares (and not having anyone)."
I'm lonely and isolated, somebody recognize me.

"I get frustrated, irritated when nurses are not able to respond because they are 'overwhelmed.' "
What is their work if it isn't to care for me?

"When nurses say, 'I'll be back in 5 minutes' and don't come back at all or it takes a long time."
How can I trust what they say to me?

"Having nurses lie to me (e.g., about not having blankets)."
What can I really believe?

"The nurses didn't involve my family (in discharge planning)."
My family needs support and counseling—I'm afraid they won't get it.

"I rarely ask for a nurse unless I really need one—nurses don't come when you call them—I ask the nurse for minor things and don't get them."
Will I always know when I need a nurse?

"I don't know what is expected of me—I don't want to be a bother."
If I ask them what is expected, will I bother them?

"Night nurses don't answer call lights."
Sometimes I wonder if there really is someone out there behind the door.

"I'm beginning to feel like an inmate—not a patient . . . staff are more concerned about hospital procedures than patient needs."
I feel locked up, punished by the way they treat me.

"People are nonentities—I feel like a prisoner, alone in my room."
Nonentities are not entitled to anything.

"People come into your room without permission."
"People come in and don't identify themselves. I feel like a guinea pig."
How can I tell if they should be here or not? What are they going to do to me?

"Some nurses are more professional than others—some bring their problems to work. Their attitudes are reflected in their work . . . causes you to wonder if they really care about you. You feel dependent and worry if they really care. You feel helpless."

If they can be both professional and unprofessional, how can I make sure I get the professional one?

"When I ask one member of the medical team a question, he always answers, 'You'll have to ask Dr. D.'—don't get information when I want it."
Does he know the answer—why is he withholding it?

"(Staff) were not present to support my wife with the stress she is experiencing due to my illness."
I don't think they realize how she must feel.

"Medical students who don't know what they are doing—come in at 2:00 a.m. to take my blood, drop equipment, say 'my resident/teacher will probably tell me to go back and try it again.' "
Are medical students given experiences they can do right?

"(I worry about) morale and high turnover. I don't want to worry about my care—but some nurses work two or three shifts in a row."
How can they be up to speed? Will I suffer because of this?

"Lack of communication between doctors, hospital, and volunteers. More competition than cooperation."
"Too many different doctors and nurses are involved in my care . . . I worry that they might not be communicating . . . that orders from one doctor might conflict with orders from another."
"It is very bothersome when I have to fill a doctor in on the aspects of my care."
What would happen if I wasn't able to monitor my own care?

"Not always understanding doctor's answers to my questions, I ask a question and get a nonanswer for an answer. I am supposed to be satisfied with that!"
Do they think they are really helping by treating me that way?

"When you push the call light and the nurse doesn't come—a volunteer comes instead. This happened with my roommate: My roommate yelled all night for the nurse."
What does it take to get a nurse?

"I've tried to get a vegetarian diet. I'm still getting a regular diet despite five days of asking for a change, talking to the dietitian, etc."
I can't get through to them no matter what.

"The nurses don't think about how it must feel to be a patient."
They are insensitive to my needs.

"I'm afraid my doctor is not telling me the truth (cancer diagnosis)."
I can't trust what he says.

continues

Exhibit I–1 Continued

"The nurse got mad when I told her I couldn't take my pill with water."
Why is she mad at me? Doesn't this ever happen with other patients?

"There is really only one nurse who takes the time to talk to me."
I must make sure I get that nurse.

"Not having answers about why I'm sick."
Do they know and are just not telling me?

"Too many different nurses; hard to form a relationship with a nurse—causes you to hesitate to open up and confide (in them)."
"Doctors not knowing what's wrong with me—not taking my symptoms (diarrhea) seriously."
My communications don't count. I don't count.

Healthcare Communications: Foundations for Understanding Communications in Healthcare Settings

Part I of this text introduces the foundations for understanding communications in healthcare settings. This introduction is critical to grasping the importance of addressing communications in a textbook on healthcare relationships and why it is essential that communication skills are not only taught but retained. There is much to know about the phenomena of communication. Interpersonal communication is one of the most important of the basic life skills (Gazda, Childers, & Walters, 1982). Effective interpersonal communication skills are said to be the gateway to the development of other important life skills. Successful professional role development depends on our knowledge and understanding of communication concepts, practice, and evidence. In no other professions are interpersonal communication skills more important than in the health professions. As such, they have been studied extensively. Knowing which communications promote health behaviors is basic to provider role development. But, there are principles and concepts of communication that are even more generic and critical to patient–provider relationships.

Chapter 1, Health Communications and Quality Care, examines the relationship of communication to desired patient care outcomes. This chapter illustrates what is known about the importance of provider communication and selected outcomes: adherence to treatment, healthcare utilization, trust and satisfaction with healthcare providers, and improvements in health status. The years have passed that we teach and train providers to practice communications solely for the sake of adhering to professional values. While these values are foundational to our professional practice, there is an equally important role for this training and education—to ensure that our patients get safe high-quality patient care. There is a growing body of knowledge that addresses the importance of patient–provider communications in achieving better health outcomes. This knowledge creates not only a professional imperative but a scientific necessity. Chapter 1 presents evidence of the importance of the nature of provider–patient communications and illustrates how these communications have implications for healthcare outcomes.

Chapter 2, Principles of Human Communication, addresses the "anatomy" and "physiology" of human communications. The sensory modalities, information processing functions of the brain, and the role of memory and concentration are reviewed. The verbal and nonverbal dimensions of communications; the meta-communicative value of messages; and the basis for deficits in perception, processing, and transmittal of messages are discussed.

Chapter 3, The Nature of Therapeutic Communications, addresses the inevitable consequence that provider communications can either be therapeutic or nontherapeutic. How to distinguish between these phenomena, enlisting therapeutic response modes, and resisting nontherapeutic responses are addressed. Therapeutic and nontherapeutic response modes have either helpful or deleterious outcomes; the rationale behind certain therapeutic response modes is presented.

Chapter 4, Cultural Similarities and Differences and Communication, discusses the process of avoiding cultural blurring and effectively communicating in cross-cultural contexts. In this chapter the importance of cultural competence is stressed. Examples of specific responses are discussed because they carry different interpretations across groups. Communication fluency across groups is presented as a continuum; with cultural incompetent behaviors at the negative end of the spectrum and cultural competence at the valued opposite end of the spectrum.

It is not necessary to deliberate very long about the importance of communication to our roles as providers. What providers generally do not comprehend is that communication is a science as well as an art. It is inconceivable that any text on applied communications would ignore the basic principles and concepts that have been culled from years of study of human communication.

CHAPTER 1

Health Communications and Quality Care

Quality is never an accident; it is always the result of high intenions, sincere effort, intelligent direction and skillful execution; it represents the wise choice of many alternatives.
—William A. Foster

CHAPTER OBJECTIVES

- Discuss the relationship of communications between patient and provider and the goal to achieve quality patient care.
- Discuss the Institute of Medicine's definition of quality care.
- Identify the aims identified in the *Crossing the Quality Chasm* report.
- Demonstrate the "teach-back" approach.
- Using a specific chronic condition and particular standard medication to treat this condition, describe the consequences of treatment nonadherence.
- Discuss what is meant by "white-coat adherence."
- Identify selected communication approaches to improve treatment adherence.
- Identify selected principles of communication that would facilitate the development of trust in the patient–provider relationship.
- Discuss communication approaches to assess and monitor symptom severity.
- Discuss how you would determine factors that influence patient utilization of healthcare services.

Communication across all sectors of the health arena is critical to quality care. Further, improving the quality of communication is tantamount to improving patient outcomes. Communication between provider and consumers affects every facet on the health continuum—from health promotion and disease prevention to assessment, diagnosis, and treatment. An overriding interest in the area of communicating with patients and their families is the degree to which these communications result in quality care outcomes. Beyond the idea that communication reduces malpractice risk is the notion that it actually does have something to do with quality care. There is evidence that communication between patients and providers, directly or indirectly, determine the extent to which patients:

Experience fewer adverse medical events.
Exhibit higher levels of adherence to their treatment regimens.
Trust their care and their providers.
Are satisfied with their care and their providers.
Practice effective self-management behaviors.

Experience less symptom severity.
Suffer less morbidity and mortality.
Access and utilize available health resources.

This chapter will focus on communication and its relationship to desired healthcare outcomes. This chapter will describe what is known about the importance of provider communication and selected patient and healthcare outcomes: adherence to treatment, healthcare utilization (including retention in care), trust and satisfaction with healthcare providers, and improvements in health (selected documented findings in chronic illness). In each of these sections, what has been found to deter effective communication as well as contribute to effective communication strategies will be highlighted and described. Important linkages will be proposed that document how communication affects quality care. For example, when the provider's communications include listening and involvement in decision making, trust may be higher. If trust is high, patients are more likely to return for treatment and adhere to their treatment regimen.

QUALITY CARE

A landmark report of the issue of quality care in the United States was issued by the Institute of Medicine (IOM) in *The Chasm in Quality: Select Indicators from Recent Reports*. This report identifies clear areas in need of attention if healthcare quality is to be improved. In this report, statistics about health care in the United States are provided, including the number of persons who die from medical errors annually, whether patients receive the recommended care, the prevalence of worse outcomes in the uninsured, the number of patients who die each year from illnesses such as heart attack because preventive care was not adequate, the incidence of death due to medical errors, and the prevalence of mismanagement of patients with select chronic disease. The question raised here is to what extent, and how, problems in patient–provider communication are directly or indirectly related to quality care indicators.

The topic of quality care has been addressed in length. In a recent IOM report, quality care was defined as:

> The degree to which health services for individuals and populations increase the likelihood of desired health outcomes and are consistent with current professional knowledge.
>
> (*The Chasm in Quality*)

Since the development of this work, a series of IOM quality reports have been published and include: *To Err Is Human* (2000), and *Keeping Patients Safe* (2004a). The intention was to identify the scope of the problem of quality of care in selected arenas and propose plans to alleviate these problems over time. In 2001, the Institute of Medicine released the landmark report, *Crossing the Quality Chasm: A New Health System for the 21st Century.* This report concluded that the U.S. healthcare system is in need of fundamental change, and it recommended strategies for achieving substantial improvements in the quality of health care.

The Quality Chasm's framework consisted of six aims:

1. Making health care more safe.
2. Making health care more effective.
3. Implementing a patient-centered approach to health care.
4. Delivering care in a timely manner.
5. Increasing efficiency.
6. Insuring equitable health care for everyone.

In addition to these aims, 10 rules were set forth to guide the redesign of health care:

1. Care based on continuous healing relationships.
2. Customization based on patient needs and values.
3. The patient as the source of control.
4. Shared knowledge and the free flow of information.
5. Evidence-based decision making.
6. Safety as a system property.
7. The need for transparency.
8. Anticipation of needs.
9. Continuous decrease in waste.
10. Cooperation among clinicians.

These recommendations were made in the context of an extensive review of the evidence available that suggested quality needed to be enhanced. Data were categorized as indicators of deficits in quality of care.

For example, *The Chasm in Quality: Select Indicators from Recent Reports* (IOM) indicated that medical errors account for more deaths per year than breast cancer, AIDS, or motor vehicle accidents (citing data from the Institute of Medicine, 2004b; Centers for Disease Control and Prevention, National Center for Health Statistics: Preliminary Data for 1998, 1999). The question that must be raised is to what extent do patient–provider communications contribute to these statistics and others. Otherwise, to what degree, and how, communications are related to quality care outcomes.

OPERATIONAL DEFINITIONS OF QUALITY CARE

Within the IOM framework, which calls for safety, effectiveness, efficiency, patient-centered, timely, and equitable care, are a number of operational definitions of quality care. These definitions have been used as outcome measures to determine the extent to which care is higher in quality. Additionally, these indicators have often been used in clinical trials to provide evidence of quality outcomes. The following discussion highlights studies using these quality indicators.

Adverse Outpatient Drug Events

While much attention has been placed on the problem of inpatient adverse drug events (ADEs), less attention has been given to arenas in which the patient is self-managing his or her care and communication difficulties result in adverse outpatient drug events. Adverse drug events are serious instances in which errors can lead to morbidity, mortality, or hospitalization. The potential for these errors are great. According to Cherry, Woodell, and Rechtsteiner (2007), reporting on an analysis of data from the 2005 National Ambulatory Medical Care Survey, an estimated 963.6 million outpatient visits to physician offices occurred, with an overall average of 331.0 visits per 100 persons. Medications were provided, prescribed, or continued in 679.2 million visits, accounting for 70.5% of all office visits. At 40.2% of all visits, two to seven drugs were recorded, and at 5.6% of visits, eight or more. With medication therapy being the primary reason for physician visits and at the tune of high numbers, it is not surprising that drug errors and communications surrounding medication taking would be of considerable concern.

Medication errors are harder to assess in the outpatient setting for a variety of reasons. Documenting the incidence of outpatient medication errors is difficult because the problem is somewhat "invisible." Still there have been attempts to document the prevalence of outpatient medication errors. In the IOM 2006 report *Identifying and Preventing Medication Errors*, it was estimated that about 530,000 medication-related injuries occur annually among Medicare recipients seeking care in outpatient clinics. This does not include outpatients who are not Medicare patients and who are from different age groups. It does not include errors that do not result in an identifiable injury. Altogether, because outpatient errors are more difficult to detect and document, this figure may be more than double that reported.

Once the incidence of outpatient errors is revealed and described, the task is to identify those categories of patients at higher risk for medication errors. At this point, more needs to be known about the factors that place individuals at risk for medication errors. Where and how these problems arise can be summarized to some extent but require a multifaceted perspective. The independent and interactive effects of several variables affect whether certain groups will be at higher risk. Age, disease severity, cognitive deficits, presence of a support system, complexity of the medication regimen, and communications between provider and patient all play a role. Take, for example, the elderly patient who is living alone, has poor nutrition and hydration, has certain comorbid conditions such as impending renal failure. She is taking multiple medications for a variety of conditions received from a number of different specialists who did not communicate well with each other or the patient. These medications were filled at different pharmacies. This scenario is a "prescription" for danger. Now suppose the patient decides to take more medication after becoming aware of increasing but nonspecific symptoms. There are many opportunities for effective communication to improve the situation and protect the patient from drug errors. Table 1–1 depicts several communication strategies to minimize drug errors. Additionally, given that the delivery system had something to do with the resulting problem, the patient needs to be prepared to deal with potential confusions while navigating the system.

What did the patient need to know? Who needed to communicate what and when? How should potential problems be addressed? These are all important questions. The patient is in a position to have an adverse drug event, something that is occurring more often because people are living longer with the

Table 1–1 Communications to Minimize Drug Errors

Principle	*Example*
Assessing what the patient population will need to know and what might be difficult for them to understand is the first step in organizing an approach to the patient.	"What do you know about this medication/treatment? What is most difficult for you to understand?"
Identifying practical and psychological barriers (poor memory, distraction, cognitive impairment, lack of education, language facility). Instruction will be more effective if cognitive and motivational problems are taken into account.	Assess and plan to address these problems with visual aids, reminders, simple instructions, and use of community caregivers where appropriate.
Using medication lists[a] may help in anticipating difficulties.	Patient medication lists can provide accounts of all medications, schedules, over-the-counter remedies, potential drug interactions, side-effects, prescriber, purpose, what monitoring is required, and date plan should be reviewed.
Encouraging patients to ask questions and give information (using a shame and guiltfree line of inquiry) will more likely provide critical information with which to individualize your approach.	"Many of our patients don't understand why they are taking this medicine and what will happen if they forget to take it; how about you?"
Anticipating that patients may expect information without specifically asking; check out what they understood you to say and where the confusion lies.	Use "teach-back" approach. "Let's see how clear I was; can you tell me what you would do if you missed a pill?"
Fears are a basis for not entering into dialogue. Encouraging the expression of fears and concerns will allow for better assessment.	*"It is common to have questions now or later . . . we are together in making the treatment work . . . I can help you better if you tell me what you are afraid of or what bothers you about taking your medication."*
Encouraging full disclosure will reveal potential safety issues.	"There are many things that patients do when they can't make a decision about their medicine . . . they don't fill their prescription, they don't refill it, they don't take the right amount, at the right time, they might stop taking the medicine without telling us, they might take someone else's medication because they ran out or can't afford it . . . these decisions can cause problems . . . let's talk about whether they might happen in your case."
Communicating clearly and simply about medications will lessen the chance of error.	*Avoid the use of jargon: "use as directed."* *Don't use abbreviations: use "daily" instead of "QD."* *Avoid use of decimals: instead of 0.5 gm, use 500 mg.* *Use pre-typed prescriptions and instructions.*

[a]*See Massachusetts Coalition for the Prevention of Medical Errors; MEDLIST.*

chance of having more than one chronic illness. Living longer means more medications. There are more likely to be several different providers and/or specialists involved who may or may not be communicating effectively.

In a paper identifying problems associated with outpatient adverse drug events, Brown, Frost, Ko, and Woosley (2007) identified several psychological and practical barriers patients face in their everyday lives that may result in ADEs. In this study, prescriber–patient miscommunication factors were considered among the most important. They represented 30% of all factors identified by patients. These factors related to how the provider expressed information, elicited information, and the level of exchange. It was noted that 85% of the reported miscommunication factors related to patients' failure to give information or ask questions of the provider.

Lack of motivation to disclose or ask for information and expecting the provider to tell the patients what they needed to know were also important factors that, together with the factors of fear of negative consequences, fear of being rude or inappropriate, and a poor relationship with the physician, made up about 45% of the miscommunication factors. Additionally, 17% of factors related to patients' inabilities to give pertinent information, including poor memory, being distracted, cognitive impairment, and lack of education or language facility to communicate. Brown and colleagues (2007) proposed a model to account for the many factors patients reported. The model, based on patient self-reports, included psychological and barriers of everyday life, as well as those shown in the literature in the domains of patient, provider, and system of care: literacy of the patient, lack of health information, beliefs and attitudes, multiple drug use, communication skill deficits, limited capacity of provider to track medications, time and technology constraints, provider–patient communication, access to health care, and lack of funds.

Treatment Adherence

As has been commonly posited, communication is more likely to be at the root of the problem than any technical aspects of medical care. Communication is directly associated with treatment adherence. As Travaline, Ruchinskas, and D'Alonzo (2005) state, patients who understand their providers are more likely to fully disclose their problems, understand their treatment and its options, modify their behavior, and follow their medication regimens. While these outcomes are not solely due to the character of the provider–patient communications, the content and manner in which providers communicate is very important.

It is well known and documented that adherence leads to better health outcomes and nonadherence places the patient at risk for poor recovery and disease progression. Nonadherence has been identified as a contributing factor in cases of adverse events. Such is the case for women who do not follow up on abnormal Papanicolaou (Pap) smears who lacked follow-up for two or more years (Khanna & Phillips, 2001). Avoiding follow-up in this case leads to more advanced cancer presentation when presenting for care.

Nonadherence does not always lead to adverse events, but the likelihood that treatment will be compromised is high. Treatment adherence refers not only to medication adherence but compliance with appointment schedules, diet and exercise regimens, or lifestyle modifications. Irrespective of adverse events, maximal benefits from any treatment plan will not be achieved if individuals discontinue interventions before completion of the treatment. Even if the patient sees the plan through to its completion, less than full adherence to one or more aspects can limit the benefits of the treatment plan, and in some cases, make the patient more susceptible to complications, mortality, and morbidity. Disengaging from treatment or drop out rates are serious and can limit overall effectiveness of the intervention.

Medication adherence refers to the extent that the patient complies with the dosage, schedule, and instructions provided by the provider. Within this context there is room for a great deal of error that may not be immediately recognized by patient, family, or provider.

Drugs don't work in patients that don't take them.
— C. Everett Koop, MD

The exact number of medication errors made by patients receiving outpatient treatment is not fully known, but it can be estimated with figures from studies of outpatient visits in which medications are prescribed. The public's reliance on medications has risen dramatically. The Kaiser Family Foundation (2007) reported an increase in the number of medications purchased from 2.1 billion in 1994 to 3.6 billion in 2006, an increase of 71%. The percentage of the population with a prescription drug expense in 2004 was 59% (for those under age 65) and 92% (for those 65 and older). It was estimated that the average number of retail prescriptions per capita increased from 7.9 in 1994 to 12.4 in 2006 (Kaiser Family Foundation, http://www.imshealth.com). Previous studies of patients experiencing a wide range of chronic conditions have reported that medication adherence is problematic and that even in clinical trials adherence might be as low as 43% (Osterberg & Blaschke, 2005).

In the treatment of all major chronic illnesses (arthritis, asthma, hypertension, major psychiatric illness, diabetes, pulmonary disease) adherence to medication regimens is concerning. While the standard of 80% dose adherence (usually taken as the number of pills taken relative to the number prescribed) is sufficient in some cases, this standard is not acceptable in other cases (e.g., HIV/AIDS), where less than 95% adherence may result in health status decline and disease progression. All patients are at risk for poor adherence patterns. Taken as a whole there is a phenomena that has been observed in patients with many types of chronic disease. It has been documented that patients do better just before an office visit *(white-coat adherence)* and worse when they tire of the demands of the regimen. Also, patients pick and choose which medications out of several they might follow more exactly. They do not adhere equally across all medications. These observable phenomena suggests that it is important to find ways to talk about nonadherence patterns and the likelihood medication adherence will wax and wane over time.

Another instance requiring special attention is when patients are prescribed new medications for the first time. Although the provider may describe the medication, the need for it, and how to take it, there may be pitfalls in this encounter. First, the patient may not know the questions to ask the provider about the new medication nor understand the answers given. Second, when provider and patient enter into a discussion, communications may be ambiguous. Things may be left unclear because neither understands where the other is coming from. Despite the fact that information can be communicated clearly and briefly to increase the patient's understanding and adherence to the medication regimen, this does not always occur. Expecting to eventually understand, the patient and the provider could wait in anticipation for the next cue but nothing tangible surfaces, and both are thus resigned to the situation. The patient might be left with uncertainty and the provider with not knowing what the patient has gathered from the conversation.

To alleviate uncertainty and as time passes, patients are faced with a decision about the uncertainty they experience. Do they decide to take the medication how they remembered the provider telling them? Take the medicine how they *think* the provider would want them to take it? Call the provider's office and wait for a call back? Take a portion of it—some is better than none and probably wouldn't be harmful? Call someone and ask them how they take it? Look the medication up on the computer and take the recommended dose? Ask the pharmacist? Do nothing until seeing the provider at the next visit two weeks from now? Go see another provider and see what they say? Consult a family or folk healer? Maybe do a combination of things?

Identifying the patient's personal circumstances about what they need to know and how they will best receive this information is the patient-centered approach that is advocated within medical circles (Khanna & Phillips, 2001). Recognizing and responding to patients who may be displaying problems with adherence is critical to providers' roles.

Providers are not necessarily proficient in identifying when someone is having a problem with adherence (Osterberg & Blaschke, 2005). In fact, adherence is very difficult to measure. Patients who are more adherent are probably more likely to remember their conversations with providers about adherence. However, providers often overestimate the degree to which patients are following the plan. There are several reasons for this. First, the provider may not know how to ask about adherence. If the provider asks: "Are you taking your medications?" The response is likely to be a short "yes" without further clarifying what problems the patient is having. Posing a close-ended question with the underlying message: "of course you are," yields a simple answer—and one that matches what the patient thinks the provider wants to hear. Additionally, the provider may not know how to explore the possibility of nonadherence without creating shame or guilt. "Remember what I told you last time, you have to take your medications all the time, not just when you can remember to" creates the feeling that if one forgets it is not OK and they are not doing their part in getting better despite the concern and attention of the provider. Osterberg and Blaschke recommend, instead, the approach of presuming nonadherence issues and asking, "How often do you miss taking them?" Table 1–2 summarizes key principles and examples of interventions to improve adherence behaviors.

Trust and Patient Satisfaction

The relationship of trust between patient and provider is built on the effectiveness of their communications. Mutual trust is essential to quality care out-

Table 1–2 Communications to Improve Adherence Behaviors

Principle	*Example*
Providers are not proficient in identifying patients' problems with adherence.	Make the assumption that there is some problem or some pattern that results in some level of nonadherence and that your assessment of adherence might underestimate the problems the patient is having.
Open-ended questions will elicit clarification and expansion.	"What problems are you having with taking your medication?" or "Since your last visit, what problems have you had taking your medications?" not "Are you having any problems taking your medication?"
Statements and questions that minimize shame and guilt will encourage self-disclosure.	"Many of my patients have trouble taking their medications, how about you?" not "You have to tell me if you are not taking all your medications."
Patients may not know what is incorrect about what they are doing.	Use "teach-back" and return demonstration to pinpoint problems the patient might not recognize by using the medications in their prescription bottle to assess how they are interpreting the directions.
When patients receive a new medication, some degree of passive reluctance may inhibit clear exchange.	"What does taking this medicine mean to you?" "What more could I tell you that would help you to know more about the medication/treatment?"
Everyday life and competing priorities may interfere with following the treatment or medication regimen.	Problem-solve with the patient about what the barriers might be and how each barrier could be minimized in their case. For example, "Knowing that it is difficult to remember to take your medication when you are so busy all the time, what could you do? There are typical things we can do: provide a pill box reminder, refrigerator magnets, help you remember by picking a specific time each day to take your medicine . . . would any of these help?"

comes, particularly to adherence and adaptation of changes required when one is ill or at risk for developing disease or illness. Trust and patient satisfaction are intimately related, but what comes first and what follows is not as clear. One might question how the patient can be satisfied with his or her care if there is not a basis of trust in medical care and the provider(s) that are rendering this care. Likewise, how can the patient trust the healthcare system and provider without a basis of satisfaction with the care received?

Trust in the context of patient care and the relationship between patient and provider refers to the extent that the relationship and partners in this relationship can be relied upon and take the interests of the other in mind. Trust can contribute to the healing forces in the interaction between provider and patient by contributing to an increased sense of safety and security if not overall well-being (Lee & Lin, 2008; Hall et al., 2002). Providers want patients to trust them and the system. They know that this will get the patient to seek health care earlier rather than later and that positive outcomes are more likely. Most providers agree that trust must be mutual to build a successful working relationship.

Some discussions of the quality of trust in the patient–provider relationship has been likened to religious belief rather than a strong level of confidence that the provider is to be trusted. The idea of "blind trust" translates at the societal level where health providers are trusted in general in their role of "healers." Trust in a provider leads to a sense of comfort, security, and safety. On the contrary, the reverse, "I can't trust the healthcare system," may lead to a sense of anguish and despair—turning individuals away, setting them on a course of finding their different solutions. Rather than a sense of blind trust, which historically has been the case, it can be argued that the public has grown to have a realistic perspective on trusting health providers. The media and wider experiences with health care have increased the public's awareness that errors do occur and providers are sometimes at fault. Until recently, the vehicle for trust building has been the ongoing relationship of one provider to one patient (Saultz & Albedaiwi, 2004). It has been suggested that by the nature of advances in technology, today it is not so easy to build and sustain a trusting relationship.

Patient satisfaction, a term formerly used to describe satisfaction with inpatient care, is now commonly used to describe the quality and perceptions of outpatient services as well. There is no real consensus about what patient satisfaction is, and the multitude of surveys to measure this phenomena suggest a lack of agreement (Saultz & Albedaiwi, 2004). Although it is thought to be ill-defined, patient satisfaction has frequently been used to mean patients' perceptions of the affective and technical aspects of the provider's performance (Meredith, Orlando, Humphrey, Camp, & Shelbourne, 2001). Otherwise, patient satisfaction encompasses perceptions of both the manner in which the patient is addressed (how the provider treats the patient) and the technical competence the patient believes the provider to have (how much the provider really knows what they are doing). Regardless of its measurement, the patient's level of satisfaction reveals something about the patient's preferences and expectations of care received within the realities of the care environment. Patient satisfaction stems from the expectations of the patient relative to the experience of care and how well the two match (McKinley, Stevenson, Adams, & Manku-Scott, 2002).

There are key indicators that seem to be associated with patient satisfaction, and these are addressed in multiple patient survey instruments. The following questions/statements are examples of frequently asked questions and give some idea of how communication plays a role in the patient's valuation of the care received. These survey items are usually presented with the option to reply yes or no, strongly agree to strongly disagree, all the time to not at all, or some variation of these choices.

"How satisfied are you with the information the provider (physician) provided?" (very to not at all)

"Did the provider use language that you could understand?" (yes or no)

"Was your doctor good at explaining the reason for medical tests?" (yes or no)
"Doctors act too unfriendly and disinterested." (strongly agree to strongly disagree)
"Doctors' explanations are easy to understand." (strongly agree to strongly disagree)
"Doctors and the medical staff listen carefully to what I tell them." (all the time to none of the time)
"Doctors and the medical staff spend enough time listening to me." (strongly agree to strongly disagree)
"The nurses and doctors sometimes ignore (don't listen) to what I tell them." (strongly agree to strongly disagree)
"The doctor / medical staff don't give me a chance to ask questions." (agree or disagree)
"The staff treat me with respect and courteously." (all the time to none of the time)
"The medical staff / physician doesn't really care about what I think." (strongly agree to strongly disagree)

One can see that the way the question is worded and the reply options offered can influence the results considerably.

Participatory roles in health care are critical in encounters with health providers to build trust and satisfaction. Essential to advancing participatory provider–patient roles is the underlying importance of mutual trust and patient satisfaction. Basic to this proposition is the acceptance of the principle that patient–provider communications mediate the positive relationship between health orientation and relationship satisfaction (Dutta-Bergman, 2005).

These participatory roles are not easy to come by, depending on the previous experience and fears of some patients. For example, populations that have experienced health disparities may encounter any number of concerns: lack of access to care, inadequate insurance coverage, fears of hospitalization, death, and experimentation by health providers. They may not relate to the system as one that will serve their needs; thus, to enlist them in participatory roles will require discovering and acknowledging these concerns.

In discussions of patient satisfaction and patient–provider communications, several aspects of the communication have been reported as essential: does the provider actively listen, explain the treatment in a manner to address fears and misconceptions, and demonstrate empathy through an understanding of the patient's experience and concerns? In traditional views, these dimensions of the interactions between provider and patient are best achieved in the ongoing continuity of the patient–provider (or providers) relationship.

There is currently debate as to whether continuity is necessary or, if necessary, if it is practical. Theoretically, with continuity of relationship, there is an increased opportunity for meaningful explanations and teaching. This teaching is likely to be more patient-centered in that the provider hypothetically knows more about the patient, not only about the presenting problem, but about the patient's fears, beliefs, social resources, and psychological well-being. These are the pieces of data that help tailor the patient's treatment and take into account factors in the patient's everyday life that affect responses to treatment and acceptance of the treatment regimen.

Table 1–3 provides a list of principles and practices that help build trust and satisfaction in the provider–patient relationship.

Effective Self-Management

Effective self-management is the extent to which the patient manages disease and illness effectively to elicit healing and promote health. It is estimated that 50% of those with chronic illness are getting appropriate medical intervention. It has also been estimated that 50% are managing their illness and treatment successfully. The Centers for Disease Control and Prevention (CDC)

Table 1–3 Communications to Improve Adherence Behaviors

Principle	*Example*
Listening to the patient will increase the patient's perception that the provider cares and hears the patient's concerns. Restatement of what the patient says further reinforces that the patient has been listened to and has been heard building trust and satisfaction.	Demonstrating active listening: "I have been listening to you tell me about your fears about taking this medication. Let's talk about them."
Building on the continuity of the relationship will increase the perception that the patient is truly heard and the provider is willing to include the patient as a partner.	Building on continuity and restating: "The last time I saw you you were afraid that the medication would make you feel too drowsy and you would feel 'spacey' . . . tell me how you have been feeling since you started this new medication . . ."
Recognizing the barriers, both everyday stressors, and major constraints that affect the patient's response to utilizing healthcare advice will build an empathetic relationship, which in turn will engender trust and satisfaction.	Examining stressors: "People we take care of have many demands on their time. What demands on your time might prevent you from remembering to get your prescription refilled?"
Trust and satisfaction are related to expectancy; determining what the patient expects from care will help build a working relationship.	Discover and address the patient's expectations: "When you came in, you asked me about if you still needed to take so many medications. I talked about your Lipitor. But let's get back to what you wanted to talk about . . . the many medications you are taking and if you still need to take so many."
In caring for disadvantaged populations, lack of insurance, inadequate access, fears of the medical system, fears of being experimented upon, and fears of hospitalization may influence their trust of health providers and the healthcare system in general.	Acknowledge and address fears and disparities that bring the patient to treatment late: "It must have taken a lot to get you to come for a checkup . . . not easy at all . . . were you afraid that something bad would happen?"

estimates that of all health conditions, chronic diseases are particularly prevalent, costly, and preventable (CDC, http://www/cdc.gov/nccdphp/overview.htm). These diseases (primarily heart disease, stroke, cancer, and diabetes) require considerable self-management by those who have them. The CDC estimated that 7 out of 10 Americans who die each year in the United States (more than 1.7 million people) die of a chronic disease.

> Self-management is defined as the tasks that individuals must undertake to live well with one or more chronic conditions. These tasks include having the confidence to deal with medical management, role management, and emotional management of their conditions. Self-management support is defined as the systematic provision of education and supportive interventions by healthcare staff to increase patients' skills and confidence in managing their health problems, including regular assessment of progress and problems, goal setting, and problem-solving support. (IOM/NAS. 2004, ch 5, p 57)

The prolonged course of illness and disability from such chronic diseases as diabetes and arthritis results in extended pain and suffering and decreased quality of life for millions of Americans. Chronic, disabling conditions cause major limitations in activity for more than 1 of every 10 Americans, or 25 million people. More than 90 million Americans live with chronic disease, and 7 of every 10 Americans who die each year, or more than 1.7 million people, die of a chronic disease (CDC, http://www/cdc.gov/nccdphp/overview.htm).

The importance of effective self-management as a component of quality health care is quite clear. While the issues of disease self-management have been addressed, the focus has been disease-specific and focused on one condition (e.g., diabetes, arthritis, or asthma). There is reason to believe that self-management strategies can be viewed across chronic diseases. Chronic diseases then would be those illnesses that have in common a prolonged course requiring self-management behaviors by patients and their caregivers. While self-management is not new to chronic disease, the role of the patient and caregiver is becoming a more active participatory one and this requires substantially improved communication between providers and those affected. The role is one of partnership, and the expectation is that a power differential is less important than the patient accepting leadership on behalf of living successfully with a prolonged condition. For example, with increasing potential for home monitoring, there is a greater role for patients to play in adjusting their medications, problem solving and making treatment decisions. New communication strategies that link providers and patients in different ways may be the direction of the future. See Chapter 23 for a more in-depth discussion of electronic and telephonic interventions linking providers and patients.

The realm of supportive self-management in chronic illness is a growing area of research and practice. The chief questions stem from understanding the appropriate mix of supportive relationships and information that will maximize the patient's ability to live as comfortably as possible with a chronic disease. Table 1–4 presents a series of steps that promote communications which enhance effective patient self-management. Provider–patient interactions have been associated with positive self-management and health outcomes.

Table 1–4 Communication and Effective Self-Management: Guides to Supportive Self-Management

- Assess the patient's own views of barriers, beliefs, and fears surrounding the chronic condition.
- Ensure that the patient and family know what is needed and why.
- Assess the patient's motivation for lifestyle changes to support disease management.
- Assess the social support and social network of the patient to determine adequate supportive relationships to achieve management goals.
- Identify the patient-specific strengths and limitations that may affect the patient's self-management practices.
- Identify with the patient and caregivers strategies they have used that worked.
- Focus on setting goals and solving problems, using action plans or personal contracts when appropriate.
- Mobilize and link patient and caregivers to community resources to assist the patient and family to manage the disease and its social, spiritual, psychological, physiological, and quality-of-life issues.
- Provide for seamless, continuous care delivery that promotes effective self-management.
- Provide systematic follow-up with provider phone calls and visits to monitor progress toward the goals.

Caregiving communications and information exchange is also critical to effective self-management. However, it is not clear that strategies that work well with certain groups work equally as well across ages, ethnicities, genders, and persons coming from diverse social/economical communities.

> Coleman and Newton (2005) stress the importance of supporting self-management in patients with chronic illness. They add that this kind of support exceeds traditional knowledge-based patient education to include patient problem-solving, self-efficacy, and application of knowledge to real situations that matter to the patient. The important distinction is that information is not enough; what is increasingly clear is that the patient's perceived self-efficacy is important and that this aspect is to be evaluated on an ongoing basis as often as level of knowledge.

Symptom Severity

Symptoms will be identified, monitored, and treated effectively provided the provider and patient address symptoms in depth and the patient can partially, if not fully, describe his or her experiences. The problem here is that the provider and patient use different languages to describe what is happening. It follows that if the patient or caregiver does not discuss symptoms regularly with the provider, the symptoms may persist or go unchecked. Attention must be placed on the quality of dialogue between provider and patient that will elicit this information. The connection between management of symptom severity and patient–provider communication has been made. Donovan, Hartenbach, and Method (2005) reported on a study of 279 women experiencing multiple symptoms associated with active ovarian cancer. They reported an average of 12 concurrent symptoms; however, only 61% of these women had discussed their most noticed symptom with their healthcare provider in the past month. Only half reported that they had received symptom management recommendations. While it would be nice to believe that symptoms and symptom management is fully addressed in patient visits, this might not be the case.

Why would patients not discuss their symptoms with providers? There may be several potential reasons for this, including patient-specific, patient–provider relationship, and healthcare system factors. It is possible that patients might not know how to describe their experience, and in the absence of bleeding, swelling, or pain, these signs and symptoms are vague phenomena for which the patient has no words. They might talk about symptoms using metaphors:

> *"Sharp like a needle-stick."*
> *"Hard like a baseball . . ."*
> *"Itchy."*
> *"Scratchy."*
> *"Tickles . . . like a feather."*

Patients' use of metaphors can be useful. Patients are pleased when the provider matches this language because it is an expression that the provider is engaged in the attempt to find out what is going on, regardless of the difficulty the patient is having providing adequate detail. Otherwise the provider might want to use the same terms as the patient rather than revert to medical jargon (Skelton, 2002). It has also been suggested that it might be best when patients cannot think of words to describe their symptoms that they be encouraged to use metaphors. "When you get that feeling . . . what is it like?" "It's like bugs are running all over my body." The provider then has the advantage of using the metaphor to ask further questions: "When you get that feeling that bugs are running all over your body . . . is it hard for you to breathe?" Part of the relief that patients experience in the moment of tension of not knowing how to talk about their experience is that there is someone who cares and is patient enough to help them figure it out. While using patient metaphors initially, it is important to eventually use the medical language with which patients need to become familiar.

Another dimension of the problem of assessing and treating symptoms is the quality of the provider–patient discussion. This involves the provider's training and expertise, basic assessment and interviewing skills, and interpersonal style. In a National Institutes of Health (NIH) news release in 2002, it was stated that cancer-related pain, fatigue, and depression are undertreated in cancer patients (http://www.nih.gov/news/pr/jul2002/od-17.htm). Sometimes providers confine their attention to symptoms most frequently associated with the disease, ignoring important sequelae or co-morbid conditions that interact with symptoms of the presenting condition. It has been reported, for example, that few physicians ask patients about suicidality associated with chronic life-threatening disease when they are significantly prevalent and should be assessed. The National Cancer Institute (http://www.concer.gov/cancertopics/pdq/supportivecare/depression/HealthProfessional/) brings attention to the need to carefully assess for suicide in cancer patients, particularly when contributing symptoms (e.g., pain needs to be controlled). An example would be:

"Many patients with cancer at some point think about suicide . . . like doing something if it gets too bad. Have you had any thoughts like these?" Providers' training needs to include comfort with discussing a wide array of symptoms from those that are easy to discuss, those that might be embarrassing and those that are "taboo."

Education for an open discussion of symptoms should begin with the health and disease identification process. Symptom discussions should be integrated in all visits and conversations. The repetitive nature of these discussions will improve on patients' abilities to express themselves and will make the provider more familiar with how the patient experiences symptoms. Emphasis should be placed on the patient's perception of the symptoms, not just an objective measure of presence/absence or severity of symptoms. Table 1–5 summarizes specific communication strategies to assess and monitor symptom severity.

Morbidity and Mortality

While the data are limited in this area, providers are likely to admit there is some relationship between effective communication and morbidity and mortality. Rather than "Is provider–patient communication associated with morbidity and mortality?", the question may be, "To what extent and through what pathways are communication and morbidity and mortality related?" *The Chasm in Quality* report emphasized that indicators such as deaths due to medication errors, lack of preventive care, and poor management of patients with major medical illness care are of concern and that progress must be seen on these indicators. Earlier in this chapter, the question was raised about how the connection between such indicators and patient–provider or provider–provider communication provide such alarming results.

More and more, the emphasis on patient self-management skills and patient empowerment to engage in active partnership with providers have been presented as necessary to combat such outcomes of increased morbidity

Table 1–5 Communications to Assess and Monitor Symptom Severity

- Assess and monitor character and severity of the symptoms (intermittent or persistent; mild, moderate, or severe).
- Assess and monitor over time.
  - "Has your coughing been better or worse since your last visit?"
- Assess how symptoms have affected functional status.
  - "In the last two weeks, how often have you had problems with awakening at night because of coughing, problems with symptoms after exercising, etc.?"
  - "How many days from work or your normal activities have you lost since your last visit?"
- Monitor communications with patient:

  "What questions have you had that you wanted to ask about?"

  "Has anything interfered with getting your questions answered or with talking to me or the staff?"

  "How can we help you to improve your management of your care?"

  "What things have we worked on that have helped you?"

and mortality. If effective delivery of health care depends on efficiency and effectiveness of communication, then it follows that patient–provider communication is associated with outcomes (Teutsch, 2003).

Let's examine one possible connection. Effective communication is associated with adherence to medical regimens, satisfaction, and trust in the provider. Adherence is necessary to prevent the progression of disease and morbidity associated with the disease, such as in diabetes. In certain cases, as with HIV/AIDS, adherence to medication regimens is closely associated with the success of disease progression and even death because of the link between medications and viral suppression. If the communication between patient and provider is effective and efficient, these outcomes are more likely—thus the connection between mortality and morbidity.

In almost every care encounter, providers are pressed for time to address patient needs and relay complex information in an emotionally charged context. Under everyday circumstances, the likelihood that this communication will be adequate and result in patient trust and satisfaction is threatened, and the consequences may result in lack of operational knowledge and/or uncertainty about the "what-fors." Any or all of the following interact to increase the risk of poor management: errors in carrying out the regimen, misconceptions about the disease or treatment, feeling tired or overburdened with the regimen without telling the provider, inadequate self-management support, lack of awareness of the need to monitor and why, and turning to substitute sources of information that may misguide the patient.

Healthcare Utilization and Retention

Quality health care depends on healthcare utilization patterns and retention in treatment. *Patterns of utilization* refers to both the frequency of utilization and the services that are utilized, suggesting that patients might use services but under- or overuse certain services in inappropriate ways. An example of this is patients' overuse of emergency care when the problem could be addressed in outpatient visits. Healthcare utilization patterns do not provide data on the adequacy of care received. Healthcare utilization refers to a person's behavior in reaching out to and complying with existing available healthcare services.

Race / Ethnicity

It has been estimated that by 2050 one in every two Americans will be African American, Hispanic, Asian American, Pacific Islander, or Native American (Modlin, 2003). There are clear and significant disparities in health and treatment of ethnic and minority populations, suggesting that more attention must be given to providing culturally competent care. The disparities that do exist are due in part to the level of cultural competence of the clinician. Some of the suboptimal care received is due to these deficits in competence. Care and care providers that are neither trustworthy nor satisfying to patients are likely to turn potential recipients away and or cause them to discontinue care prematurely. Cultural beliefs and health practices play a significant role in utilizing health services and remaining in the healthcare system. One needs to consider how treatment and approach are consistent or inconsistent with previously held beliefs or conceptions of disease and treatment. Without sufficient appreciation or attention to the beliefs of the patient one cannot expect adherence or retention in care.

In an important piece of research focused on Latino satisfaction with communications with health providers, it was reported that Latino Spanish-speaking respondents were significantly more dissatisfied with provider communication than either Latino English-speaking or white respondents (Morales, Cunningham, Liu, Brown, & Hays, 1999). The investigators conclude that these individuals may be at increased risk of lower quality of care and poor treatment outcomes, and even dis-enrollment.

Gender

Gender, communication, and what keeps people coming back has been addressed in the literature in a number of ways. First, studies have examined the difference in character of communication when the provider is female. Weisman (1986) studied patients' responses to female physicians. Both the behavior of female physicians and responses to them differ from the case of male physicians, pointing out that female physicians might be better communicators and more empathetic. A number of studies have focused on the concordance in the dyad; that is, female patients and female physicians versus female patients and male providers. The effect of the provider's gender on the satisfaction of services received is inherently important in the utilization of healthcare services and recidivism. Further, Weisman concludes that physician–patient dyads, where both parties are of the same sex, might be important in cases where sex-specific conditions are the focus, the condition is highly sensitive; or in the treatment of chronic conditions over protracted periods of time, when a long-term relationship is required.

Age

The warning: "Don't go back. . . . you'll just get sicker (it will be worse)" might be a function of several patient characteristics. But it has relevance to the age of the patient for many reasons. Adolescents and young adults might feel and express such sentiments. For example, youth who are prescribed an antidepressant may not like coping with the side-effects of their medication: "I feel different." Young people may also be concerned about peer perceptions. Who wants to carry an inhaler in football practice? In studies of youth, the following disease frustration issues were observed: not wanting to take the medication at school, feeling that it gets in the way of their activities, not wanting other people to know they are taking medication, not liking what the medication does to their appearance, feeling tired and forgetting to take it, and feeling tired of living with the medical condition (Simmons & Blount, 2007). If youth and providers do not discuss these issues, they may passively dis-enroll.

In the elderly, health literacy, cognitive decline, and worsening illness affect patients' abilities and willingness to seek treatment and continue care over time. Problems with transportation can affect attendance at follow-up appointments and, if these problems are not discussed with providers, might lead to disengaging when in fact they should be seen frequently. The lack of accessible and affordable transportation is a major barrier to health care. It is an issue of availability as well as affordability. Of particular vulnerability are the elderly who may not be able to drive. (Compared with all other age groups, people 75 and older have the most medical visits. It is unknown whether this group has a significant dis-enrollment issue that is a function not only of age but of many other sociodemographic factors.)

Illness

Illness affects utilization of care in complex ways. Communication abilities affect how well an individual can describe his or her need for care. Persons with communicative disabilities primary or secondary to their condition require special attention. Most obviously, medical conditions affecting speech, vision, reception, and interpretation of data are extremely important to communication effectiveness. Disorders of this kind would include speech impairment, visual impairment, deafness, and cognitive disabilities and/or mental disorders. These conditions are often referred to as *disabilities*. The problem of communication and keeping patients with disabilities in the loop for basic health promotion and health care has been acknowledged, and attention to altering services has received ongoing attention.

People with disabilities include a large and growing population that needs access to services. It has been noted that while more than 54 million Americans may have been identified as "disabled," the actual number of people living with a disability in the United States today is unknown. However, many people with disabilities do not seek out or receive the quality of care they need. Consequently, they may only access care for emergencies, thereby reducing important contributions of health promotion and disease prevention. There are many reasons people with disabilities do not seek healthcare services early on: provider ineptness and lack of resources, patient embarrassment and fear of losing more independence, and staff and patient experience of frustration in communicating.

In the important document entitled "People First: Communicating with and about People with Disabilities" (http://www.health.state.ny.us/nysdoh/promo/people.htm), principles and practices for communicating with people with disabilities were identified. They include (1) treating all with respect; (2) making sure an offer of assistance is accepted before continuing; (3) speaking directly to the person without using an interpreter, until the patient requests that you use one; (4) always identifying yourself before speaking; (5) listening attentively when talking to someone who has difficulty speaking; (6) getting the attention of someone who is deaf using touch; and (7) relaxing about responding inappropriately (there is the chance that you will be understood and accepted for what you say). Further, there are words or expressions that are preferred (e.g., using *person who is blind,* not *blind man*). Other terms (e.g., spastic, retard, gimp, and cripple) are hurtful and should be avoided when talking to or about patients.

In a brief report by Berren, Santiago, Zent, and Carbone (1999) focusing on healthcare utilization by persons with severe and persistent mental illness, mental patients were more likely to use urgent care settings than counterparts without mental disorders. Additionally, among typically frequent urgent care users, patients with severe and persistent mental illness used urgent care to higher degrees. The investigators point to the necessity of mainstreaming these patients in routine outpatient services. There are many reasons these patients use urgent care, including system, patient, and provider factors. When providers are not skilled to work with this population, do not like working with this population, and where the psychiatric patient's symptoms interfere with clear and unambiguous communications about symptoms and history, urgent care might be perceived to be the only answer. Indeed, as Berren and colleagues point out, the use of urgent care under the existing circumstances may be adaptive, especially when the patient's support system is weak or nonexistent. This pattern of utilization would be categorized as inappropriate, but the inappropriate use of care services is perhaps more the result of the system and provider deficits.

CONCLUSION

Clear healthcare communication is the foundation of healthcare delivery. It affects every aspect of the health–illness continuum from prevention and health promotion, to assessment and diagnosis of disease and illness, to the adequacy of treatment and the continued self-management of chronic or life-threatening diseases. The question raised here is to what extent and how problems in patient–provider communication are directly or indirectly related to quality care indicators.

The purpose of effective communication is to bring both the patient and health providers to a level of understanding that will aid the provider in delivering patient-centered care and the patient to management of health and illness over time. Quality of care is seen through the patient's eyes and measured professionally through the lens of best practice procedures. Quality has been defined in many ways and recent IOM documents released the landmark report, *Crossing the Quality Chasm: A New Health System for the 21st Century.* This report concluded that the U.S. healthcare system is in need of fundamental change and proceeded to identify key indicators that serve to guide the assessment of our current and future healthcare systems: making health care more safe, making health care more effective, implementing a patient-centered approach to health care, delivering care in a timely manner, increasing efficiency, and ensuring equitable health care for everyone. In the context of these goals several indicators measure the likelihood that we will reach these aims. The degree to which change must be made to ensure a meaningful level of success is unknown, but what is clear is that providers' communications are directly or indirectly important in addressing any deficits that are present.

In this chapter, the link between quality and communications was described using available literature that, while mixed, supports the premise that with better patient–provider communication comes quality care.

CHAPTER 2

Principles of Human Communication

It is obvious that communication is a conditio sine quo non of human life and social order. It is equally obvious that from the beginning of his (her) existence a human being is involved in the complex process of acquiring the rules of communication, with only minimal awareness of what this body of rules, this calculus of communication, consists of.
—Paul Watzlawick, Janet H. Beavin, and Don D. Jackson

CHAPTER OBJECTIVES

- Identify and describe the sensory modalities.
- Describe the process of sensory awareness and sensory receptivity.
- Describe how the sensory modalities transmit messages to the brain.
- Describe ways in which perceptions affect the emotional experience of individuals.
- Describe how learning is a stimulus-processing activity.
- Discuss the function or utility value of interpersonal communication.
- Discuss ways in which communication is an outcome of interpersonal processes.
- Discuss the principle of the multidimensionality of communication (i.e., the levels of communication).
- Describe how human communication is inevitable.
- Identify how punctuation functions in the delivery of interpersonal messages.
- Discuss how interpersonal communication may be either symmetrical or complementary.

Human communication is the product of a combination of numerous physiological, psychological, and environmental influences. Patterns of communication are indeed difficult to understand without knowing the origins and intricacies of communication in their relationship to neurological functioning—particularly the workings of the central nervous system but also the dynamics of communication in the interpersonal context.

Several principles and concepts of human communication increase our knowledge of this high-level capability. From the standpoint of biophysiology, these include how sensory reception of information occurs, the basis for distortions of sensory experience, the processing function of the brain, and sensory and feedback mechanisms and learning. Axioms of human communication that address the origins of communication in interpersonal interactions are also discussed.

SENSORY AWARENESS AND SENSORY RECEPTIVITY

The Sensory Modalities

Recognition that sensory awareness and sensory processing is critical to understanding human communication leads us to consider basic concepts and principles about sensory modalities. While all senses play a role, the most salient sensory modalities to complete our understanding of human communication are the visual, auditory, and kinesthetic. Some individuals are particularly adept with the use of one modality (i.e., are better at picking up visual rather than auditory clues); others are multimodal, exhibiting strength in more than one modality. We are not exactly the same, and our capacities are capable of changing over time and in the context of our experience.

Studies of the relative strength of one modality over another suggest that age and maturation influence whether individuals are strong in only one modality or have mixed modality strength (Gazda, Childers, & Walters, 1982). The debate continues, with some researchers declaring adults to be primarily visually oriented versus their being multimodal. So while age might make a difference in our sensory strengths, it might be the same for all people.

Early on, Goldman (1967) conducted a well-designed experimental study comparing individual preferences for a sensory modality: visual, auditory, or haptic (defined as a combination of kinesthesis, pressure, and tactile sensation). He concluded that adults, as well as first- and third-grade children, preferred an auditory modality; the adults chose the visual over the haptic; the children were equally divided between the visual and the haptic.

Along these lines, another theory is that there is a sequence to the development of modality strength. Children have shown a developmental sequence of modality strengths (Barbe & Milone, 1980). In the early grades, children have more well-defined strengths and tend to be auditory rather than visual or kinesthetic. As they progress through elementary school, their modalities become mixed and interdependent, shifting toward the visual and kinesthetic. By adulthood, many people have mixed-modality strength. Other researchers, however, contend that vision is the dominant modality of the species (MacLean, 1973).

Of course, in the process of communication, all modalities work together to influence self-expression and understanding of the environment. A clear delineation of the strength or weaknesses within a given person may be difficult to establish. Still, researchers, particularly educators, are interested in the issue of modality variability and dominant modality in hopes of being able to predict and engage patterns of communication and patterns of problem solving when teaching different age groups.

Perhaps one of the most misunderstood aspects of sensory awareness is the assumption that the purpose of our sensory apparatus is to give us complete information about all the stimuli in our environment. In truth, our sensory capabilities are not designed to give us information in this way; the major purpose is to give us a very select range of feedback that is most useful to us. From studies of nonhumans (e.g., bees and other insects as well as bats), we know that some sights and sounds that are perceived by other species are not available to us. And, like many animal species, humans tend to be sensitive to only a certain range of stimuli—the stimuli most useful to their way of life. What distinguishes humans from other species is that humans can generally access a wider range of stimuli and this stimuli is unique to our way of life.

Even humans, however, have been shown to have selective perceptual abilities despite the fact they may have a broader range. For example, we can taste the sweetness in certain foods and the bitter taste of some poisons (at low concentrations), but we fail to be able to discern other tastes that are neither harmful nor helpful. Our sense of smell is highly attuned to many gases but insensitive to others such as nitrogen. In short, our capacity to perceive through our senses is biologically regulated, and these capacities are largely determined by the information that would be most helpful to us.

This principle of utility also applies to how and why we become selective throughout our lives. Utility for certain information changes as we grow. Consider for a minute the infant's capacity to perceive separation from a nurturing figure. While other stimuli are not meaningful, distance or nearness of the nurturing figure is critical to the infant. Our training and occupations can also influence our perceptual range. Law-enforcement professionals are keenly aware of and even exceedingly perceptive about certain environmental threats. These capacities are not inherent in others; however, repeated exposures to life-threatening conditions reinforce the need to accurately and quickly perceive environmental clues that may suggest danger. Our keen awareness of a patient about to experience a life-threatening change is a function of our exposure to these situations and why we become more acutely aware of the cues with experience.

Another important example of selective perception among groups of humans is that of pain. We know that the sensation of pain has strong motivational properties. In general, pain is to be avoided. Still, the perceived intensity and quality of pain varies a great deal. We know that pain stimuli can be the same, yet they affect people differently. We also know from observations of athletes that serious injuries may be experienced with little pain. There are still other people who report extreme levels of pain when the injury or illness does not seem to justify it. Does this also mean that some patients will require more medication than others with the same pain stimulus? This question is answered by the fact people experience pain differently but also that the same pain stimuli will be perceived differently by the same person, depending on time and context, even when the stimulus for pain has not changed at all. We also know that healthcare professionals can manipulate patients' experiences of pain by changing patients' perceptions of the stimuli. When dentists say to a patient, "You're doing fine—just a little more (drilling)," they are manipulating the patient's perception of the character of the stimuli. If a provider suggests that a pain experience is "a tug," "a needle prick," or a dull sensation, the character of the sensation of pain might change. Additionally, the suggestion that pain will subside and the patient will experience relief affects the patient's perception of whether the pain stimulus is overwhelming or within his or her control. Understanding that the pain is not out of control enables the patient to relax. Relaxation reduces the negative experience of the pain. Fear is a mediating condition that, when eased through relaxation or reassurance, will influence the experience of the sensation of pain. Most providers understand their role in helping patients manage discomfort and pain and will use the power of suggestion in helping their patients cope with pain stimuli.

Patients are thought to be able to alter, at least in part, their experience by altering their perceptions. In the arena of cognitive psychotherapy, examples of reframing one's interpretations of situations has relevance here. One can perceive his or her life or relationships as "hopeless." Feelings of hopelessness generally increase anxiety and depression related to the observation and interpretation of his or her situation. However, if the perception of one's life situation is changed (e.g., a challenge is not hopeless), negative feelings of depression and anxiety seem to lessen, and the patient is able to adopt a more positive approach to problem solving. The idea is that if we can modify cognitions, assumptions, and beliefs, we can change our emotions and behaviors accordingly. Critical to a full analysis of the role of perception is knowledge of how stimulus awareness is processed in the brain.

PROCESSING STIMULI AND THE BRAIN

Through the Sensory Modalities to the Brain

When physical energy such as light, sound, heat, or cold reaches the sense organs, it must be converted to a form that can be processed in the brain. The information processing that goes on within the brain has three distinct steps.

The first step is simply *reception*: the absorption of physical energy. *Transduction* is the second step and refers to the conversion of physical energy to an electrochemical pattern in the neurons. Finally, *coding* takes place (Figure 2–1).

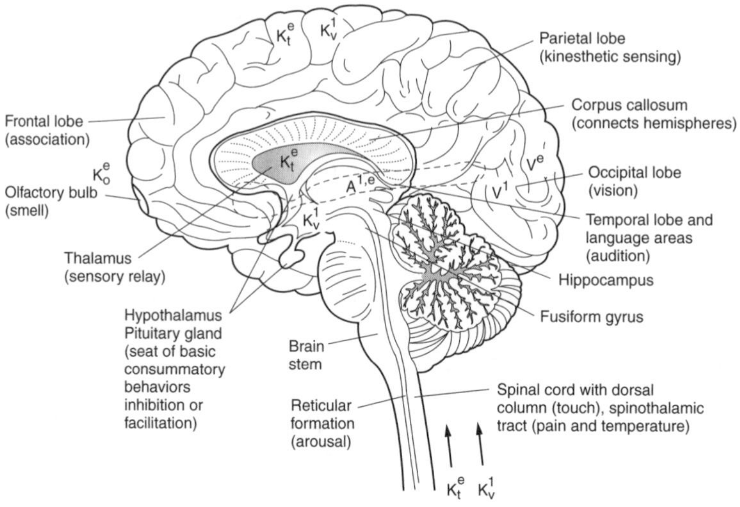

This medial aspect of the brain and spinal cord of the central nervous system includes a surface view of the temporal lobe, with language areas illustrated in dotted lines. Projection sites for receiving information through the sensory modalities are plotted with the following abbreviations:

$A^{1,e}$ = auditory input, both internal and external.

V^e = visual input in the occipital lobe, external.

V^1 = visualization in the deeper striate layers of the occipital lobe or temporal lobe.

K_o^e = kinesthetic input from sense of smell, external.

K_t^e = kinesthetic input from touch, external. The nerve signals move up the spinal cord in the dorsal column, are relayed through the thalamus, and are projected to the sensory cortex of the parietal lobe.

K_v^1 = kinesthetic input from pain and temperature, internal, visceral. The nerve signals move up the spinal cord in the spinothalamic tract, are processed in the hypothalamus, and are projected to the sensory cortex of the parietal lobe.

Figure 2–1 Medial View of Brain and Spinal Cord. *Source:* Reprinted from G. M. Gazda, W. C. Childers, and R. P. Walters, *Interpersonal Communication—A Handbook for Health Professionals*, p. 30, © 1982, Aspen Publishers, Inc.

Coding is the one-to-one correspondence between some part of the physical stimulus and some aspect of the nervous system. For example, light rays that strike retinal receptors (reception) are converted due to a change in the receptors' membrane polarization (transduction). The resulting train of impulses in the optic nerve has a frequency that increases as the intensity of light increases. This is evidence of coding. It should be remembered that sensory information is coded so that the brain can process it, and, interestingly enough, it may have little resemblance to the original stimuli. The idea that what is perceived is not exactly what actually is, is an extremely important principle of human communication. The proverb: "Believe half of what you see and nothing of what you hear" has some basis when we consider the fact that we always perceive selectively.

It is possible, for example, to create optical illusions. Optical illusions exist because what is perceived is actually different from what is actually there. One very common example of an optical illusion is provided in Figure 2–2. If we look at one line with one eye and the other line with the other eye, the illusion is apparent. This optical illusion, the Müller-Lyer illusion, suggests that one line may be longer than the other; usually line B is reported to be longer than line A. In fact, these lines are of the same length. Various theories used to explain optical illusions generally agree that what causes optical illusions is within the brain, not within the sensory organ (eye). To experiment with your own response to optical illusions, online examples are available through the Web (search for keywords Illusions and Paradoxes: Seeing Is Believing).

The important principle to understand is that our perceptions are not the same thing as the stimuli that are picked up by our sensory receptors. An important line of study is the appearance of hallucinations in individuals experiencing mental illness (e.g., schizophrenia). Hallucinations are involuntary and can occur in the absence of any external stimuli. Thus, a person sees or hears something that is not there. How is this possible? Silbersweig and Stern (1998) explored these questions in human auditory neuroimaging studies. They were able to gather information about normal and abnormal conscious and unconscious brain states. Their work was important in understanding how the brain can literally create its own reality . . . it can be conscious of something that is not even there. This raises the issue of whether and how the brain responds to internal stimuli versus external stimulus.

When sensory information reaches the brain, higher and more complex processing takes place. The human brain is complex, consisting of as many as

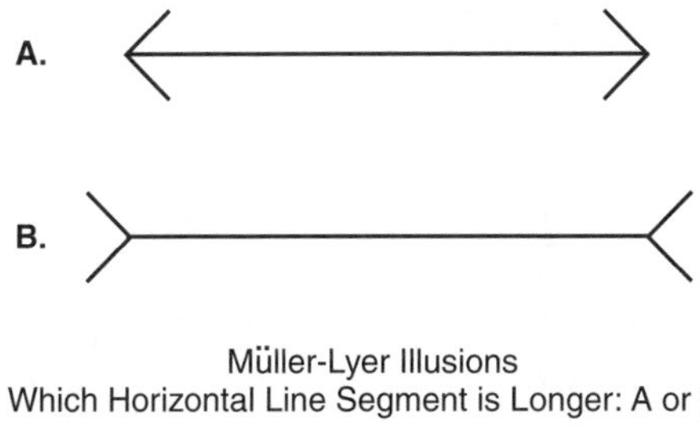
A.
B.
Müller-Lyer Illusions
Which Horizontal Line Segment is Longer: A or B?

Figure 2–2 Optical Illusions Perceptions Are Not Direct Reflections of Stimuli.

100 billion neurons varying in size from 4 microns (0.004 mm) to 100 microns (0.1 mm) in diameter. Neurons are cells that send and receive electrochemical signals to and from the brain and nervous system.

These neurons are not haphazardly arranged; they are assembled in discrete areas of the brain, and these areas have their own specialized function. Still, we have the experience of unity. Thus, although our brains are divided into many parts, each containing many neurons, our consciousness is as one. The unity of consciousness comes from the many connections between various brain parts.

The brain performs its information processing primarily in two domains. It is concerned with (1) language-related elements or the theoretical symbols and (2) thought-related elements or the qualitative symbols (Mullally, 1977). Processing different types of symbols is dependent on functions that occur within the left and right hemispheres of the brain.

The theoretical symbols—such as visual-linguistic elements, or the written word; auditory-linguistic elements, or the spoken word; visual-quantitative elements, or written numbers; and auditory-quantitative elements, or spoken numbers—are processed primarily in the left hemisphere of the brain. Qualitative symbols of a sensory nature, such as sounds, taste, or visual pictures, are associated with cultural codes or the meanings that are received from observing nonverbal expressions. These symbols are processed primarily in the right side of the brain.

The bilateral symmetry of the brain provides that sights and sounds, which bring information in from the external environment, are processed by using both hemispheres together. The two hemispheres are connected by the corpus callosum for the transfer of information of different sensory modalities (Brodal, 1981). In the normal brain, it appears that any information reaching one hemisphere is communicated regularly to the other, largely to corresponding regions.

Until the early 1950s, the function of the corpus callosum was not known. In the past it was, on occasion, cut by a neurosurgeon (e.g., to treat epilepsy or to reach a deep tumor in the pituitary gland). Scientists and researchers have reported anatomical, physiological, and behavioral discoveries about the specialization of the cerebral hemispheres. Bakan (1971) discusses the directions of conjugate lateral eye movement (CLEM) and the inherent duality of human behavior and experience. The neurological pathways that come from the left side of both eyes (the left visual field) are represented in the right cerebral hemisphere and vice versa. Thus, when parts of the left cerebral hemisphere are stimulated, the eyes move to the right; when parts of the right hemisphere are stimulated, the eyes shift to the left.

Day (1964) identified right-movers and left-movers—persons who tend to look to the right or left while reflecting. Right movement presumably activates the left cerebral hemisphere and its specialized functions that are verbal, analytic, digital, and objective. Left movement is presumed to activate the right cerebral hemisphere with its special functions that are preverbal, synthetic, analogic, and subjective. Individuals tend to look up and away when a question has been posed and the answer must be retrieved (Gur, 1975).

Singer (1976) reported experimental research findings to support the conclusion that if an individual is involved primarily in attending to visual images and fantasies, the person is less likely to be accurate in detecting external visual cues. Similarly, if internal processing is primarily oriented around auditory fantasies (i.e., imagined conversations or music), then the person is less likely to be accurate in detecting external auditory signals.

In both cases, the individual is better at detecting external cues in the modality other than the one in which the person is attending to internal images and fantasies. Such experiments suggest that a private internal image or fantasy in a given modality uses the same brain structures or pathways as does the processing of an external stimulus in that same modality.

Individuals look to the side or down to eliminate visual stimuli, especially the meaningful and reinforcing face of another person that might interfere with a train of thought. Dilts and colleagues (1979), in their book *Neurolinguistic Programming*, illustrate the eye positions for visual, auditory, and kinesthetic accessing of information. They also identify each eye position with its particular body posture, breathing pattern, and hemispheric specialization (see Figure 2–3).

The right movements of the eyes access the left hemisphere for constructed images (V_c), for visualization of novel and abstract patterns, or for constructed auditory (A_c), putting an idea into words. The eyes looking down and to the right access an awareness of body sensations (K_{vto}) and kinesthetic information, including the visceral, tactile, and olfactory. The left movements of the eyes access the right hemisphere for remembered images (V_r), for visualization of eidetic patterns from past experiences, or for remembered auditory experiences (A_r) and sounds and tape loops of messages from past activities. The eyes looking down and to the left are representative of an internal auditory dialogue (A_{id}), talking to oneself, probably in short cryptic commands and suggestions and simple sentence messages (see Figure 2–3).

The left cerebral hemisphere is associated with the development of speech and language. The temporal lobe is larger on the left side than on the right in about two-thirds of the brains examined (Geschwind & Levitsky, 1968; Witelson & Pallie, 1973). The left side is best developed in the brain of the fetus and newborn infants, suggesting that asymmetry does not result from environmental or developmental factors after birth.

Electrophysiological experiments using auditory (click) and visual (flash) stimuli were designed to measure the evoked responses in the brains of both

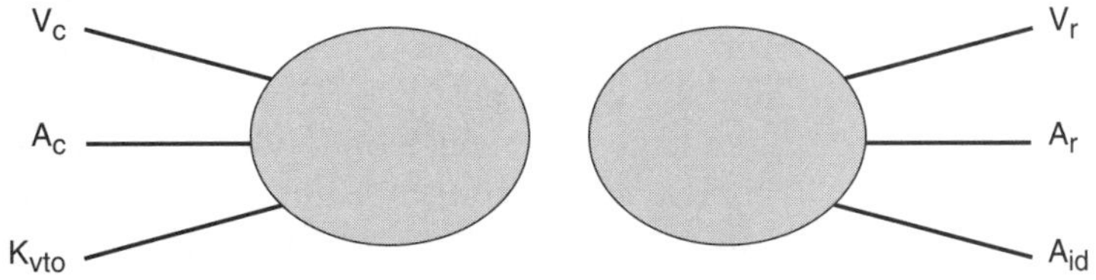

Figure 2–3 Eye Positions for Accessing Information. Visual accessing cues for a normally organized right-handed person: V_c = visual constructed; A_c = auditory constructed; K_{vto} = kinesthetic visceral, tactile, or olfactory; V_r = visual remembered; A_r = auditory remembered; A_{id} = auditory internal dialogue. *Source:* Adapted with permission from R. B. Dilts, J. Grinder, R. Bandler, J. DeLozier, and L. Cameron-Bandler, *Neurolinguistic Programming I,* © 1979, Meta Publications.

adults and five-week-old infants (Wada, 1977). The results show that auditory responses are significantly greater in the left hemisphere and visual in the right. It appeared that the fundamental auditory neurocircuitry needed for the growth of speech and language is biologically and asymmetrically designed for both initial acquisition and for further development.

Early research indicated that the right ear outperforms the left ear in hearing and identifying competing digits, a reflection of left-brain dominance for language (Kimura, 1961). The right ear has better access to the left hemisphere because of the crossed auditory pathways. While the right ear connects directly to the left hemisphere (language area), the left ear's route to the same area first must go to the right hemisphere and then cross over to the left side and the language area. However, a clear left-ear advantage was found for all melodies and environmental sounds (Krashen, 1977). It appeared that the left ear has direct access to the right hemisphere, and the right brain is dominant for music, chords, and nonverbal sounds.

It was evident from studies with patients who suffered brain damage to the right hemisphere that the right brain makes an important contribution to human performance, having functions complementary to those of the left hemisphere. The right side of the brain probably processes information differently from the left, relying more on visual imagery than on language. The right hemisphere of the brain specializes in perceiving and remembering faces, unfamiliar and complex shapes for which there are no ready names, and drawings of incomplete gestalts in which parts are missing. Its importance is to spatial orientation and visuospatial relationships. It is thought to provide the neurological basis for the ability to take fragmentary sensory information and convert it to a coherent organization of the outside world. Nebes (1977) referred to this as a sort of cognitive-spatial map by which individuals plan their actions.

Ordinarily, the left and right hemispheres exchange information when each hemisphere has access to the information that passed initially to the opposite hemisphere. All this occurs through the large bundle of fibers, corpus callosum, as well as several smaller bundles of fibers. What happens if the corpus callosum is injured? Clearly, any damage to the corpus callosum will result in impaired exchange of information. We know, for example, from those who have had surgery to interrupt severe epilepsy, that epileptic seizures can be limited to only one side of the body. This is a positive outcome of the disruption in information flow. When seizures are so severe that they cannot be controlled by customary antiepileptic drug treatment, surgery has been performed to cut the corpus callosum. This results in preventing seizures from crossing from one hemisphere to another. Thus, when seizures occur, they are less severe because they affect only one side of the body. Interestingly enough, these surgeries have brought unexpected positive results because the seizures not only occur with less severity, they also occur less frequently.

The marvels of coordination between right and left hemispheres are also seen in other cases where split-brain phenomena has been observed. Observations of the roles of right and left hemispheres have led to many speculations: for example, is one sphere more important or more dominant? When it was first determined that the left hemisphere controls speech, the right sphere was viewed as subordinate. Its role was seen as one of support to the left sphere. Through further research, however, particularly with studies of patients whose corpus callosum was damaged (commonly referred to as split-brain patients), it became clear that the right hemisphere is capable of many more functions than was first thought. For example, the right hemisphere does understand simple speech, although it cannot control speech. It can also perform certain functions better than the left hemisphere, such as the control of emotional expression. It has been shown that after damage to the right hemisphere, people not only have trouble forming facial expressions that depict emotions, they also have trouble understanding others' emotions. Also, people who have suffered damage to the right hemisphere speak with less-than-normal amounts of inflection, suggesting impairment in emotion. Also, the right hemisphere seems to be specialized for complex visual and spatial tasks. For example, people who have damaged their right hemisphere have difficulty finding their way from one place to another.

Perceiving to Emoting

Does everyone have emotions, even if they appear to have none? Let's say you have been asked to care for young children, 7 to 12 years of age, who, you have been told, possess "inhuman destructive capabilities." They seem to have superhuman powers and state that they are on an important mission. They have been placed on Earth for the specific purpose of destroying the existing social structure so that a new system can be established. Their eyes are opaque; they have platinum hair, and they look alike. Although they have faces, they have no recognizable facial expressions. Do they have emotions? Are they aware of feelings?

The question is not whether they have emotional experiences similar to other humans, such as anger, happiness, or sadness. You cannot know what it feels like to be like them. Indeed, they may not have any conscious experience of feelings. You are looking for familiar behaviors that suggest that they have emotions. Emotion, for you, is defined as temporary changes in inflection or in the intensity of behavior. Thus, from your point of view, if they attack another person and increase the intensity of their behavior to do this, they are showing emotion. Movement, which shows no change in intensity, is, for you, lacking emotion. You observe that they attack people, but the intensity of their movements stays the same. This scenario may sound like a script from a science fiction movie; still, the question is relevant: how do we know whether this group of children (or any human beings, for that matter) has feelings and emotions and experience them in ways like ourselves?

Emotion has been studied as a function of autonomic arousal. The intensity of behavior is largely governed by the functions of the autonomic nervous system (ANS). The ANS has two systems: the sympathetic and parasympathetic processes. Both regulate the involuntary processes of the body. The ANS is named as such because it is thought to operate autonomously. There are many feedback loops in the body, and these continually send and receive information about individuals' experience. Wilhelm Reich perceived the reciprocal action of sympathetic and parasympathetic systems (Buhl, 2001). Essentially, these two parts of the ANS function reciprocally. The sympathetic system controls arousal and the fight–flight mechanism, and the parasympathetic involves relaxation. The parasympathetic system comes into action after stimuli have been acted upon. It allows us to wind down while the sympathetic system governs arousal that occurred initially. Otherwise, the sympathetic nervous system prepares the body for intense vigorous response while the parasympathetic system increases digestion and other responses associated with relaxation. The most compelling reason for the arousal of the parasympathetic system is frequently the removal of a stimulus that excited the sympathetic system in the first place. The example of people fainting after intense arousal illustrates this point. When something life-threatening happens (e.g., almost getting run over by a car), the sympathetic nervous system is excited. When the threatening stimulus is removed, a rebound effect—overactivity of the parasympathetic system—occurs. Thus, some people might collapse or faint after this initial intense sympathetic nervous system response.

Reaction from the sympathetic nervous system occurs not only because of initial stimulus to the sympathetic system but also as a result of the individual's interpretation of the stimulus. Individuals' interpretations of the stimulus are critical. This is why it is difficult to predict reactions when people perceive a threat or challenge. For example, predicting stress levels by simply counting stressful life events may be highly unreliable. More accurate measures are those that factor in a valence or the perception of the stimulus. For example, changing jobs is generally regarded as stressful. Just how stressful can vary a great deal from one person to another, based on their perception of the change. They may not even regard it as a significant event. Because of this, we need individuals to tell us how they perceive the change—for example, on a continuum from +7 (being extremely positive) to −7 (being extremely negative). To have a total hysterectomy may be perceived as very traumatic and threatening to some women but not to others. Would it be an error then to approach all women having this surgery with expressions of deep sympathy for their condition? The surgery itself may not be the stressor; rather than the surgery, the confinement and separation from her children might be most worrisome. By discovering the unique distressing elements, we can respond more appropriately.

In the previous section, we alluded to the importance of being able to alter perceptions of events. The power of individual interpretations of stimuli has been described in certain cognitive approaches to counseling (e.g., Cognitive Behavioral Therapy [CBT]). Questions about the neurocognitive effects of psychological counseling have been explored. Some researchers have suggested that CBT has the potential of modifying certain dysfunctional circuitry associated with, for example, anxiety disorders. The implications are that this form of counseling can functionally "rewire" the brain. This has been illustrated in the work by Paquette and colleagues (2003) in experiments to regulate fear associated with spider phobia.

It is believed that the mammalian brain continually rewires itself, suggesting that the brain is undergoing change many times within a single day. Do we have the capacity to rewire our own brains? In the field of psychology, attribution theory suggests that when stimuli or events are perceived to be negative but also judged to be global (affect many parts of one's life), the experience can be more emotionally painful. Recurring or enduring stimuli produce feelings of hopelessness. Conversely, when these same events or stimuli are perceived as manageable, they elicit feelings of hopefulness. We know that the way in which stimuli or events are interpreted has a great deal to do with the way in which people respond. People who engage in actions of "mind over matter" are using their abilities to master challenges by reinterpreting the meanings of the stimuli. Making the stimuli (perceptions of the stimuli) less threatening is their way of modulating stress-related reactions. Thus, any given event or stimuli may produce a great deal of sympathetic nervous system arousal, a moderate amount, or very little. It depends on the individual's interpretation of the event and the way he or she processes the perception of the stimuli.

For a long time, it was thought that it was impossible to exert direct control over stress, including heart rate and other biologic processes affected by the ANS. With the advent of science and practice of various versions of biofeedback, it has been found that people can control their responses to stress by progressively relaxing their skeletal muscles—as their muscles relax, their emotions become calmer. Voluntary control over responses like heart rate does not seem to be possible; however, indirect effects through the process of the progressive relaxation of skeletal muscles—possibly with biofeedback—do seem to reduce stress and promote calmness.

Emotions and the expression of emotions depend largely on an area of the brain called the limbic system. MacLean (1970) used this concept to refer to this area of the brain; "limbic" comes from the Latin word *limbus*, which means border. Parts or structures of the limbic system form a border around certain midline structures of the brain. The brain area most important for emotions and emotional expression, *the limbic system*, is a circuit that includes the amygdala, the hypothalamus, parts of the cerebral cortex, and several other structures.

MacLean (1973) identified this enlarged lobe as the connecting structure between the visual system and the limbic system of emotional behaviors. He suggested that the fusiform gyrus gives rise to the weepy feelings that people may experience upon witnessing an altruistic act:

> Primates, above all other animals, have developed a social sense which in man becomes conspicuous for its altruistic manifestations. As evidence that a charitable social sense is still in evolution we need only recall that the word altruism was coined as lately as 1853 by the philosopher Comte . . . and that the word empathy was introduced into our language by Lipps . . . about 1900. Altruism depends not only on feeling one's way into another person in the sense of empathy. It also involves the capacity to see with feeling into another person's situation. (p. 42)

Emotional behavior may be understood in part by studying the behaviors that are necessary for self-preservation and procreation. One list of such behaviors (modified from Denny & Ratner, 1970) is resting, eliminating, water balance, thermoregulation, feeding, aggressive-defensive behaviors, sexual behaviors, and care of the young. Animals, including humans, fulfill their basic needs in cycles that include an appetitive phase, a consuming phase, and a post-consuming phase (Denny & Ratner, 1970).

Even under the most normal circumstances there is a rise and fall in body activities (brain, digestive system, senses of taste and smell, etc.). This cyclical rise and fall is referred to as facilitation or inhibition, respectively; emotional behavior may be represented as exceptional states of facilitation or inhibition. Each of the several basic consuming behaviors has its own normal range of arousal and may also show a range of overreaction (extreme facilitation) and underreaction (extreme inhibition). The language used to describe feelings and emotions usually refers to these extremes. Examples of inhibitory words for underreaction are *depressed*, *helpless*, *lonely*, and *discouraged*; facilitory words for overreaction are *excited*, *angry*, *panicked*, and *passionate*.

The limbic system is said to consist of the structures in the brain that are essential to emotion. It has been described as a response-modulation system on a continuum of inhibition to facilitation for consuming behaviors that meet physiological needs (McCleary, 1966). The visual structures of the brain have connections to the limbic system in the prefrontal cortex and in the occipitotemporal lobe and the fusiform gyrus. There is evidence that these connections function to help individuals gain insight into the feelings of others—to see with feeling. MacLean (1962, p. 300) writes that in the complex organization of these evolving structures "we presumably have a neural ladder, a visionary ladder, for ascending from the most primitive sexual feeling to the highest level of altruistic sentiments."

MacLean (1973) also suggested that these large capacities of the brain may be incapable of being brought into full operation until the hormonal changes of adolescence occur. If this is so, it would weigh heavily against the claims of those who contend that the personality is fully developed and rigid by adolescence, if indeed not by the age of five or six.

Another condition previously believed to be related in part to damage in the limbic system is autism. Because the limbic system is in charge of emotions, lack of emotional response characteristic of these children was thought to be limbic system related. However, the exact explanations for the cause of autism are not yet known. According to the National Institute of Mental Health (NIMH) and National Institute of Neurological Disorders (NIND), autism is a developmental brain disorder characterized by three distinctive behaviors. Autistic children have difficulties with social interaction; have problems with verbal and nonverbal communication; and exhibit repetitive behaviors or narrow, obsessive interests. Scientists are not certain what causes autism, but it is likely that both genetics and environment play a role. Variations in many genes, influenced by one's environment, seem to interact during brain development to cause vulnerability.

Individuality in response processes is well studied. Each individual learns to depend on one sensory system or another as a means of perceiving and understanding the world. This dependence on particular sensory modalities is characteristic of human beings and generates patterns of experience that differ between and within individuals.

All normal humans have essentially equivalent sensory organs and structures, both anatomically and physiologically. The neurological pathways that serve the senses are presumed to be similar in all human brains. So what makes for the individuality? Despite the similar "equipment," no two individuals understand a particular occurrence in exactly the same way because of the differences that are learned through selective attention to sensory input channels and with variations of experience with the senses (Bandler & Grinder, 1982; Bateson, 1972).

"Selective attention to sensory input" means that at any one time individuals usually attend to (are conscious of) one, or possibly two, of their sensory channels, and their attention is limited to only seven "bits" of information. Miller (1956) reported that the span of absolute judgment and the span of immediate memory impose severe limitations on the amount of information people are able to receive, process, and remember. *Relearning* is recognizing something similar to what we knew previously. Thus relearning a subject, say, a foreign language (French), that we have previously studied is easier and more rapid than learning a completely new subject. Although there are similarities between present experiences and memories, there are always differences.

Interference can occur if the mind gets confused about the similarities and differences between memories of previous experience and these new experiences. Using the example of learning unfamiliar languages, attempting to learn two new languages at the same time, alternating back and forth, will tend to confuse you in areas in which the two languages are similar. Imagine that you are trying to learn Spanish and French at the same time. You previously understood French after two years of college-level French. You would be relearning the French you knew before and learning Spanish for the first time. Would this be more confusing than only relearning French or only learning Spanish for the first time?

The study of how much information can be processed and retained is interesting. "Bits" and "chunks" of information have been measured and quantified by several researchers to ascertain how much individuals can know at any one time. Much discussion has centered around the idea that the amount, while varied, is fairly constant. The number 7 [e.g., the number of bits of information (7 ± 2)] is constant for the absolute judgment of inputs into one sensory channel. We know, however, that there may be quite a bit of variance in what is processed and retained. The ability to focus attention is thought to be important in protecting the brain from the bombardment of too much information, which results in confusion.

Learning from internal sensory representations includes how to pay attention to the feeling states of emotion, the visceral and proprioceptive cues for breathing and digestion, and the visual imageries of day and night dreams. Individuals "listening," so to speak, to their own bodies are knowing themselves through internal kinesthetic sensory information (K_i). Along these lines, people in states of meditation can pay selective attention to the responses occurring in the deeper recesses of the brain. They can monitor the rise and fall of emotional responses, particularly aggressive-defensive or sexual behaviors. They can identify "gut reactions" and catching the breath as kinesthetic-sensory responses to stimuli.

So, one reason individuals have different experiences despite similar genetic endowments of the brain and body and despite similar environments is that, characteristically, each one attends to different aspects of the self and of the environment. "It is something like a cooking class. Since each of us selects some similar and some different ingredients in similar and varying proportions, we each end up with something different to put into the oven" (Gordon, 1978, p. 215).

Several factors affect any one individual's attention and processing of stimuli. Some of these factors have been mentioned previously, including damage, injury, or even irritation such as that caused by epileptic seizures. However, both drugs and diet can have an effect as well, and because they can decrease the synthesis or release of serotonin, they are potentially mood-altering substances. This is one reason drugs and diet are seriously considered when explanations of violent outbursts, anxiety, and the inability to experience pleasure are studied.

Learning: A Stimulus-Processing Activity

Sensory information taken into and processed by the brain may have both short- and long-term effects on our behavior. Still, are all aspects of sensory information retained? Our memories have a lot to do with our knowledge of the world and what we need to do. Memory, however, is fragile and does not always serve us in the way that we need it to. We are subject to forgetting, and our recall of information is not always as accurate as it needs to be to function properly. What we generally mean by memory is what scientists call *explicit memory*. This is our conscious, intentional awareness of previous experiences that come to our conscious awareness in our everyday living. It is possible for us to construct memory out of the interaction of previous experience and incoming current information (Schacter, 1990).

How do patients, for example, remember to follow our advice exactly as we instructed? Their memories may be faulty; thus, we provide a number of recurring stimuli to help activate more accurately what we told them. In the case of medication adherence, we provide pill boxes, refrigerator magnets, timers, pictures, and medication logs. Hopefully, these aids enhance conscious recollection of their previous experience with us during the time we gave them instructions.

Over the course of the study of the mechanism of memory and response, many theories of learning have been put forth. Perhaps one of the most well-known is found in Pavlov's theory of higher nervous activity (Chilingaryan, 2001). His classic conditioning theory emphasizes the role of reward. Underlying this theory is the notion that the learning process is successful because it increases the probability of a desired outcome. Pavlov proposed that learning consists of transferring a reflex from one stimulus to another; in this way, a stimulus that would normally elicit a response could be replaced with a new stimulus that would, in turn, elicit the same response. This theory, merely an inference, suggested that pairing a conditioned stimulus with the unconditioned stimulus caused the growth of a new or strengthened connection between a conditioned stimulus center in the brain and an unconditioned stimulus center in the brain. However, neither Pavlov nor his colleagues could actually observe this hypothesized growth of connections in the brain.

Pavlov's theory, like those of many other theorists of the time, was overly simplistic in many ways. First, it presumed that learning about stimuli was not related to those stimuli (i.e., learning about tastes is the same as learning about temperatures). Second, the immediacy of the learning experience was viewed as important but was not examined in the context of the situation. It is known that certain learning (e.g., eating certain foods and getting sick), happens with a single instance. It does not take several trials to realize you should avoid this food. Also, learning to avoid the food that caused you to become sick can happen even if the taste of the food and illness are separated by short or long durations. In sum, learning can occur differently, depending on what is to be learned.

It is generally believed that during learning, some change must take place in the neurons in the brain. But, this change could take many forms, from the growth of a new axon, to new connections among neurons, to increased or decreased release of synaptic transmitters, and so on. And, it is generally believed that the mechanisms differ, depending on the particular learning task. That is, the mechanisms are not the same for all instances of learning.

In summary, learning is often attributed to changes made over large areas of the nervous system. No matter how much of our brains participate in the process of learning, what is always required is change at the cellular level. For learning to occur, cells (neurons) must change their properties. Studies that address single-cell changes attribute changes to biochemical changes. Impaired learning is often associated, then, with chemical deficiencies in the brain. Theories of this kind have demonstrated that certain drugs might impair or improve learning through different biochemical processes. Studies of memory, for example, suggest that certain proteins must be synthesized. Some drugs and hormones have been shown to facilitate memory, and while the specific action is not known or well understood, the biochemical transmission at synapses is the focus of attention.

As has been shown in this discussion of the neurophysiological basis for communication, several processes and structures are involved, ranging from small, molecular changes to larger regions of the brain and the entire central nervous system. These dynamics, in and of themselves, are exceedingly complex and are addressed in a great deal of depth in other discussions of brain topography and brain chemistry. The reader is encouraged to explore the fascinating world of neurophysiology and the progress that has occurred in understanding perception and learning. Neurolinguistics is a specialized science that studies how people receive information through the senses, process the information in neurons and neural pathways in the brain, and express the information in language and behaviors. Still to be described are the interpersonal and relationship principles of communications that come to us largely from the behavioral science fields.

INTERPERSONAL FOUNDATIONS FOR HUMAN COMMUNICATION

Communication has been said to be a conditio sine quo non of human life and social order (Watzlawick, Beavin, & Jackson, 1967). Communication (see Figure 2–4) occurs on three levels—intrapersonal (or that which goes on within an individual), interpersonal (referring to that between individuals or within groups), and mass communication (that which is transmitted publicly).

It is also clear that from the beginning of our existence, we are not only refining our neurophysiological capacities to communicate, we are equally

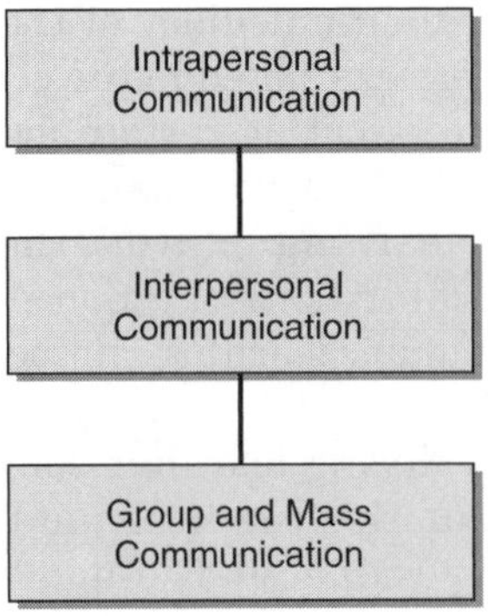

Figure 2–4 Human Communication Contexts—Within, Between, and Across People.

engaged in the process of acquiring the social rules of communication. Historically, much of what we know from science comes from the study of communication as a one-way phenomena. Knowledge of communication was largely gleaned from studies of speaker-to-listener communication; communication as a function of the process of interaction was virtually ignored. Now we operate with a much higher level of understanding about communication. We no longer think of communication singularly, as a single communicational unit or message. We think of communication as a series of messages (interaction) and as patterns of interaction (transactions). The principles and concepts presented in this discussion will address aspects of communication that are interpersonal and interactive.

Human communication is of two types: digital and analogic (Gazda et al., 1982). When we refer to something by name, we are employing *digital communication*. The same object can also be described as a representation or likeness; this represents *analogic communication*. The following example may help us differentiate these two types. When we are visiting a foreign country and we listen to people speak, we may not understand any of the language. However, if we watch the people while they are speaking—for example, their intentional movements—we may understand at least some of what the communication is about. This latter form of communication, which often includes the nonverbal content and the context of the interaction, is analogic communication. Humans are the only species known to use both digital and analogic communication. Although we rely heavily on digital communication, there are times in which we rely almost exclusively on analogic communication. With messages that we perceive and send to define relationships, we predominantly use analogic communication. Some say that emotionally disturbed children and animals are keenly aware of analogic communication. The special intuition that these groups are believed to possess makes it very difficult to deceive them. Because we use and receive both types of communication, we are constantly translating from one to another. It is like having two languages—Spanish and French—and, as sender or receiver, having to flow between them. Our abilities to translate from one mode to another is vital. To talk about our relationships, we must translate largely analogic data to the digital form (e.g., by choosing words to describe our feelings for another person). And when we translate from the digital to the analogic, we risk the loss of information that cannot be communicated symbolically.

The Principle of Function or Utility of Communication

As in the biological sciences, the study of communication in the social sciences has led to understanding communication by the identification of its *function*. This is to say, what people perceive and express is influenced by their need to perceive and express.

Everything we learn, for example, is relative unless it has a point of reference. The point of reference may be described as human needs. We know, for example, that survival and, from an interpersonal standpoint, security are basic needs. What is generally agreed is that this principle of function holds true for virtually all perceptions and expressions. Sensory and brain chemistry suggest that only relationships and patterns of relationships can be perceived and that these form the basis of human reality. So, in one way or another, functionality is predominant in our communications; we do not just perceive an event, we scan an event looking for meaning related to our needs. In this way, objects or people are not the target of our perceptions, rather they are functions. This is an important principle because it depicts the fact that our perceptions are not random events but are organized around our perception of meaning. Thus, it is possible to say that our initial awareness, and any subsequent rectification of this awareness, is highly influenced by our awareness of ourselves and the needs we experience.

The Principle of Process

The second major concept of human communication in an interpersonal context is that of *process*. When we think about how communication occurs in relationships, we observe that no statements can accurately reflect a communicative exchange if not first analyzed from the standpoint of function and then analyzed from the standpoint of an ongoing and ever-changing process. Messages sent and received are products of a continuous process; they are not independent of other stimuli in the interpersonal environment. Communication, then, is a mutually interdependent activity among two or more individuals in a changing environmental context.

The interpersonal communication process consists of a dynamic exchange of energy among two or more individuals within a specific sociocultural context. Literally, communication is a process in which individuals share something of themselves, whether it is feelings, thoughts, opinions, ideas, values, or goals. This process, when it happens in effective interchange, helps make individuals feel more human, more in touch with reality, and more capable of social intimacy. Also, the ability of individuals to influence one another and thereby exercise power, and even control, should be considered an important impetus for interpersonal communication. The communication process has frequently been depicted in a linear fashion but has now been replaced by more complex conceptual models. Figure 2–5 illustrates this phenomena.

A concept critical to understanding communication as a process, then, is that of feedback. *Feedback* is a series of responses that depicts change. It is not a

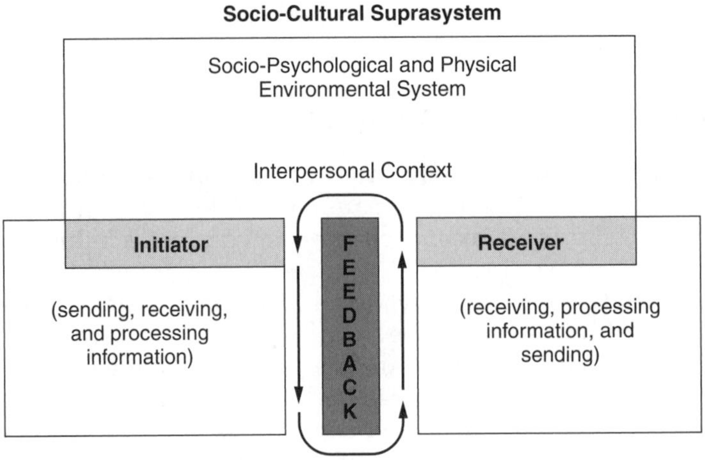

Figure 2–5 Functional Components of the Communication Process.

linear chain of events, e.g., event A affects event B, and B affects C, C, in turn, affects D, and so on. Rather, D leads back to A. Therefore, the process is circular. Feedback plays an important role in establishing, modifying, and stabilizing relationships. The concept of feedback is frequently addressed as a loop; that is, in relationships, the behavior of each person affects and is affected by the behavior of each other person. Systems that engage in feedback are distinctively different from those that do not; they generally display higher degrees of complexity. In open systems theory, open systems are generally differentiated from closed systems by the process of fluidity and permeability achieved to a great extent through the process of feedback (see Figure 2–6).

We know that some very closed systems, (e.g., cults) restrict feedback, both within the system and between the system and the larger suprasystem—society-at-large. It can be postulated that the reason that feedback is not allowed is that feedback and the exchange of information across the boundaries of the system would result in the disruption of the system. Thus, to maintain homeostasis, the cult (system) disallows open exchange with the external environment. There is no feedback. This scenario can be contrasted with the open system. Functional families, for example, display intricate levels of feedback and information processing. Family decisions may require members to voice their preferences to one another in ongoing, continuous ways. These decisions are a direct result of multiple views—not the opinions of one or two members. Decisions occur as a result not only of people voicing their views but also because these views are reactions to the views of others. Fluidity is one characteristic of these systems, and information can flow easily from member to member and between the family and its external environment. This process is transactional because individuals in an interaction affect others and are affected themselves.

When looking at theories of causality, it is appropriate to speak about the beginning statement and the results (at the end of the chain). When applying the principle of the feedback loop, this explanation is faulty: A may not cause B; the beginning is arbitrary and depends on where one enters the loop.

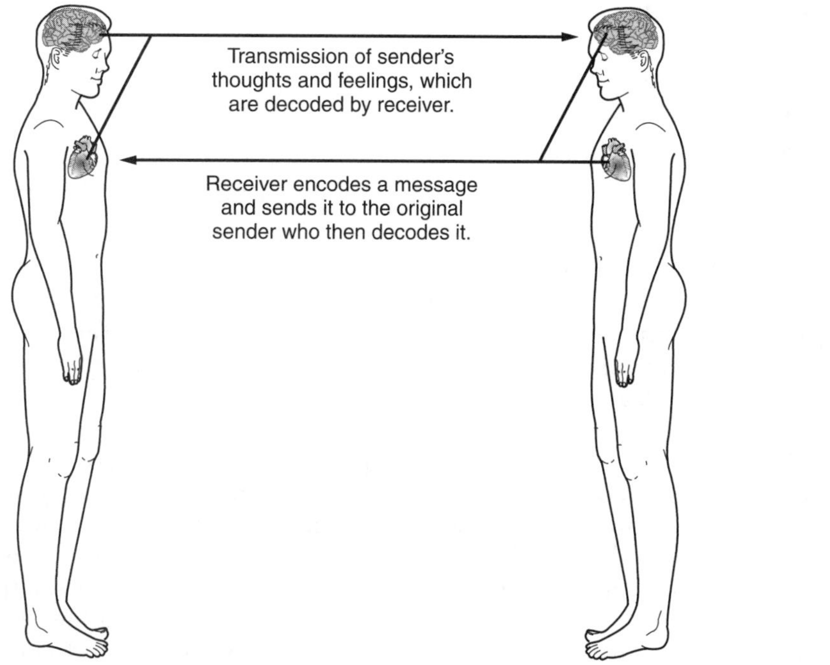

Transmission of sender's thoughts and feelings, which are decoded by receiver.
Receiver encodes a message and sends it to the original sender who then decodes it.
Sender-receiver
The sender encodes his thoughts and feelings into words and gestures and transmits them to the receiver via sound, touch, sight, and smell. At the same time, the sender is receiving messages from the person with whom he is communicating.
Receiver-sender
The receiver deciphers the sender's transmission. He determines what request the sender is making of him after he decodes the sender's cognitive and affective messages. Simultaneously the receiver is sending messages to the other person.
Feedback
Feedback refers to the circular process by which Sender and Receiver influence one another.

Figure 2–6 The Reciprocal and Circular Nature of Interpersonal Communication. *Source:* Adapted with permission from S. Smith, *Communications in Nursing,* 2nd edition, p. 5, © 1992. Mosby Yearbook.

The Principle of Multidimensionality

A third important principle of interpersonal communication is that it is *multidimensional* (see Exhibit 2–1). What does this mean and what are the dimensions? Usually when speaking of the multidimensionality of communication, we perceive two distinct levels: (1) the content dimension and (2) the relationship dimension. Watzlawick and colleagues (1967), recognizing that communication has at least two dimensions (content and relationship aspects), suggested that we cannot fully understand communication until we know something about both aspects. The relationship aspect may be more hidden, while the content aspect more transparent (Crowther, 1991). Some clinicians describe three levels: (1) the content level, (2) the feeling or emotional level, and (3) a level that describes the perceived relationship of one communicant to

Exhibit 2–1 Multidimensionality of Human Communication

- The content dimension
- The feeling or emotional dimension
- The relationship dimension

---

another. This model incorporates the idea that every message has a separate emotional quality that further clarifies both the content and the relational levels of the communication. Regardless of whether we differentiate two or three levels, it is clear that communication is used not only to exchange information (e.g., facts or ideas), it is also used to address the interpersonal relationship dimension.

Consider the command: "Take this pill now with this water." The explicit message or content aspect of this expression is the obvious: you need to take the pill. However, suggested here, through both verbal and nonverbal clues, is evidence about the relationship and even what feelings one holds about the other. The command communicates authority: one person (provider) perceives herself in an authority relationship with the other (patient or client). One has power over the other, and this is enacted in the exchanges that occur. Somewhat subtle is the underlying attitude: I have expectations of you, and if you do not do as I say, you will let me down. Further, my expectations are legitimate.

Said in a somewhat different way, one aspect of a message conveys information; this is synonymous to the content of the message. It may be about anything regardless of whether it is true or false, valid or invalid, or even indecipherable. The command quality of the message, however, describes how the message should be received and, therefore, describes the relationship of the communicants. Putting these relationship aspects in words, they would say: "This is how I see myself in relationship to you, you in relationship to me or how, at least, it should be." Consider these two expressions that seemingly communicate the same directive: "Take this pill with water—it'll be easier," and "If you refuse the water, you won't be able to take this pill." While these statements communicate approximately the same content (i.e., you need to take this pill with water), they define somewhat different relationships with the patient. The first example suggests a supportive, facilitative relationship, while the latter suggests a supervisorial, somewhat skeptical relationship.

Sometimes the distinction between levels of communication are depicted in descriptions of meta-communication and meta-information. *Meta-communication* is a term frequently used to identify communication about the communication. It is communication about how a message is supposed to be received. The report aspect of the communication conveys the data; the command (meta-communication or meta-information) describes how this communication should be taken. "You better take me seriously" is one verbal translation of the meta-communication in this message: "If you think I'm going to take out the garbage, you're crazy!" The relational or meta-communicative aspects can also be expressed nonverbally; by frowning or piercing looks; or through the context of the encounter, as when people criticize each other in front of strangers.

Communication about the relational aspects, or feeling dimension, sometimes occurs at the nonverbal level.

This brings us to still another important axiom of human communication: Communication is both verbal and nonverbal (see Figure 2–7). Sometimes verbal communication is the term used to describe the content level of a message. Otherwise, what did the sender say? This is the information or direct message intended. Nonverbal aspects of communication—facial expressions, gestures, positioning—are perceived by those who receive our messages and are considered part of the communication or interaction. Nonverbal aspects frequently disclose the feeling or relational dimension of the communication as evidenced in photographs of individuals' facial expressions (see Figure 2–8).

Can you imagine being in a relationship where you cannot have access to the nonverbal content of the interaction? Facial expressions, posture, and movement would not be available data. How would you draw conclusions about the emotional and relational aspects of the interaction? You would need to rely almost exclusively on the spoken word, together with evidence of inflection, pace of speech, and tone of voice, to establish the other person's feelings about you. Would you be secure in your judgments or satisfied with your data? Most likely the answer is, not really. What is characteristic of human communication is that meta-communication (communication that classifies the relationship) is extremely important. A great deal of what is communicated through nonverbal channels is symbolic. Facial expressions or body movements are symbolic representations of the nature of the relationship between communicants. Not only do humans rely heavily on nonverbal aspects, they are trained to use these aspects to communicate more effectively and efficiently.

Discrepancies between verbal and nonverbal communication (messages) are generally picked up in human dialogue. Discrepancies can occur in many ways, for example, in different verbal reports or in differences between verbal and nonverbal messages. Consistency in communication is important because it provides a foundation for trust. Should communication be inconsistent or two opposing messages be delivered, there is reason to mistrust the other person and the relationship. In most relationships we do not look for or search for inconsistencies across verbal messages or between verbal and nonverbal messages. However, if given a reason to mistrust someone, we have the capacity to

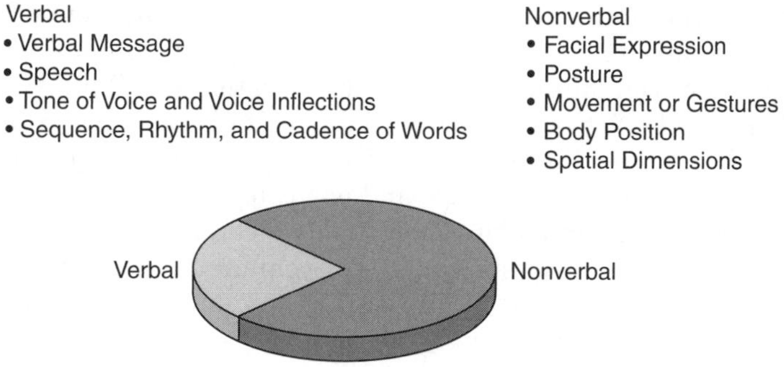

Figure 2–7 Categories of Verbal and Nonverbal Communication.

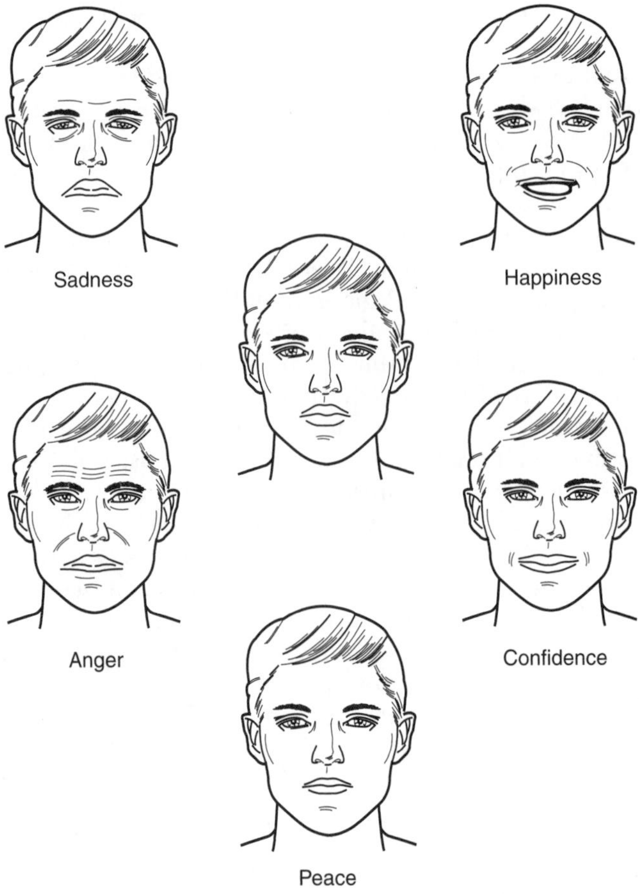

Figure 2–8 Humans Rely Heavily upon Nonverbal Aspects of Communication (e.g., Facial Expressions).

fine-tune our perceptions and be observant of mixed messages whether they are blatant or only somewhat apparent.

The Principle of Communication Inevitability

The idea that communication occurs on both verbal and nonverbal levels brings us to the next important axiom of interpersonal communication: the impossibility of not communicating, or communication inevitability. Watzlawick and colleagues (1967, p. 48) first referred to this idea as a major property of behavior. In other words, there is no such thing as nonbehavior. Putting it in simpler terms, one cannot not behave and one cannot not communicate. If we understand communication as behavior, then we can also say that no matter how much a person tries, he or she cannot not communicate. Drawing from the previous discussion of nonverbal and verbal communication, we find that words or silence, activity or inactivity, all have message potential. They influence others and, therefore, others, too, cannot not respond to these communications. To express this idea in brief: we are always communicating whether we are exchanging words or not. The nurse who looks straight ahead and avoids eye contact when passing by a patient's family, or the physician who reads the patient's chart, moves in front of a nurse to return it, and checks his beeper without acknowledging anyone's presence are both communicating—even though no words are exchanged. The mere absence of talking does not mean communication has not occurred. In both cases, what is communicated is that the providers are busy and do not want to speak to anyone or be spoken to. Family members and staff, respectively, usually get the message and behave, in turn, by leaving them alone. Is this any less of an interchange of information than the most animated conversation?

It is also true that communication may not be intentional. Much of what is communicated is, in fact, unintentional, unplanned, and even unrealized. When we understand that messages are multileveled and include nonverbal behavior, this idea is quite plausible. Consider, for example, that a physician has a particular negative attitude about a nurse. Nothing said can substantiate this suspicion. Nonetheless, it is understood, and if people around them were asked about their relationship, they would confirm this assumption. Still, there are no data, or are there? The data is largely in the nonverbal communication that is exchanged between nurse and physician. Therefore, when we think of communication units, we do not mean simple verbal messages but rather multifaceted occurrences in which several factors are involved—verbal, tonal, postural, and even contextual aspects. Likewise, these factors have varied ways of affecting communication as well as several permutations. Permutations and variance can often be a function of cultural differences. At other times, it is a reflection of the mental or emotional stability of the sender. Some of these permutations appear in behaviors of the mentally ill or functionally impaired. A case in point is an emotionally disturbed patient who is mute and whose withdrawal and immobility express anger at those around him. Some people intentionally avoid verbal exchanges to sever commitment. A sequence of avoidance behaviors may also be interlaced with willingness to communicate. Because human relationships are complex, the explicit and implicit use of communication, which includes both verbal and nonverbal dimensions, is also very complex. Many impasses in communication relate to the complexity of relationships and the involvement of communication channels.

The Principle of Punctuation

The complexity of human relationships is also reflected in the cause-and-effect patterns that communicants claim exist. This notion is especially observed in communications in which conflict exists. The principle of *punctuation* and sequence of events, although not a major communication principle, is relevant to our understanding of the circularity of communications. When we ask two or more people to report on the patterns of their communication, we may get two very discrepant stories. Looking in from the outside, we would say that the communication we observe, from A to B to C and to D, is an uninterrupted series of exchanges. However, to those participating in the dialogue, there is a beginning, a middle, and an end. The participants see a cause-and-effect relationship and behave as though this were reality. They may punctuate their remarks at any one time in the series to depict their believed status or their desired status. These perceived beginnings, middles, and ends depict a pattern of responses that communicates something about how one communicant sees herself in relation to another, such as on issues of power, control, and intimacy. This process of sequencing responses is inherent in all humans and is neither bad nor good. It serves the purpose of organizing behavioral events and is vital to ongoing relationships. Tendencies to organize interactions can display the specific rules of a culture. For example, if males were dominant decision makers and females predominantly followers, the interpretation of a sequence of events A–D would illustrate this cultural prerequisite. That is, we would judge, and others would confirm, that the interaction begins with A directing B to do something; it would not be concluded that B decided to do something and A simply reiterated the objective of the action after it was first initiated.

Interpretations of the inner workings of arguments further illustrate this point. With a couple who argues, who starts the argument? And, does party A withdraw because party B insults A, or is party B critical because party A withdraws? Who initiates and who reacts—party A or party B? Depending on what patterns these communicants see in their relationship, the reported sequence of events will be different. Both parties may be guilty of distorting reality, and this further complicates the situation. Finally, depending on the cultural orientations of the participants, the beginning, middle, and end may be very different from what we perceive as outside observers or even what each party thinks is occurring. It is clear then that the nature of a relationship is played out in the perceived punctuation of the segments of communication.

The Principle of Symmetrical or Complementary Communication

A final axiom of interpersonal communication that is key in understanding human communication is that communication (in relationships) is either *symmetrical* or *complementary*. People take either symmetrical or complementary roles in relationships, and this is evident in their communications (Arnold & Boggs, 1995). In the first case (symmetry), communicants tend to mirror each other's behavior. In the second instance (complementary), one party's behavior complements the other's. In the first case, differences between the respondents is minimized; both parties pull toward their common base. In the second type, maximizing differences is important. If we studied the pattern of communication among and across multiple dyadic relationships, we would come to realize that these patterns are decidedly one or the other. The classic examples of complementary communication are the parent–child, boss–employee, and leader–follower dyads. Usually these dyads participate in socially defined ways to depict superior–inferior and primary–secondary roles. Distinctively different are dyads that interact as if both parties were equal. This may be seen in colleague relationships. What is obvious is that communication that depicts these arrangements will generally hold true regardless of the contexts or circumstances. Boss–employee interactions, for example, will reflect superior–inferior status, even if the parties interact outside their professional roles.

CONCLUSION

In summary, human communication is indeed complex. The neurological, biochemical processes by which we receive information and the neural activity by which we process the information we receive is fascinating. Our abilities to utilize communication in patterned ways to initiate, modify, and maintain relationships distinguishes us from all other species. These processes are put forward in this chapter as axioms or principles substantiated by evidence and scientific observation. In translating science to pragmatics, we run the risk of overgeneralizing or minimizing details. It is not the intention of this chapter to synthesize all scientific data. Rather, the objective is to discuss key principles from both the biologic and behavioral sciences on the subject of human communication. The chapters to follow build on the evidence accrued through time. Indeed, the evidence about the nature and mechanisms of communication continues to expand. Much of this ongoing research can be translated into clinical practice, and there is important new evidence to demonstrate its utility. An example of this is advances in the science of rejuvenating memory and improving sensory awareness among our aging and impaired populations.

CHAPTER 3

The Nature of Therapeutic Communications

Therapeutic communication is an activity which is probably as old as human language. As a matter of fact, one can state, without exaggeration, that whenever a priest, nurse, doctor, or lay person helps another human being, some elements of therapeutic communication are used, regardless of the external situation.

—Jurgen Ruesch

CHAPTER OBJECTIVES

- Define functional and dysfunctional interpersonal communication.
- Compare and contrast these modes of communicating.
- Discuss disturbances in perception, processing, and expression.
- Identify therapeutic interviewing skills.
- Differentiate nontherapeutic from therapeutic interviewing skills.
- Describe the interpersonal context of a therapeutic encounter.
- Discuss the advisability of training programs in interpersonal communications for healthcare providers.
- List guides to nondefensive communication that inevitably lead to functional and therapeutic encounters.
- Complete the personal inventory for nontherapeutic interviewing.

The idea that provider communication can be more or less helpful is not a new idea. Providers' abilities to create therapeutic effects through communication have been at least partially addressed in all the healthcare professions. The idea is often put forth in idealistic terms, where meanings of *good* and *bad* are ascribed to various provider–patient encounters. Thus, we determine whether interaction is *therapeutic* or, conversely, *nontherapeutic*.

This chapter discusses several important assumptions of therapeutic communication—some that can be substantiated, others that reflect biases about communication and the nature of the helper–helpee relationship that need further investigation. The overall premise is that providers need to make communication the central component of care delivery and structure it in a patient-centered manner.

THERAPEUTIC COMMUNICATION DEFINED

Therapeutic communication is interpersonal exchange, using verbal and nonverbal messages, that culminates in someone's being helped. Healthcare providers need to be able to elicit responses from patients and families that are in some way beneficial to them. Therapeutic communication is communication that expresses support, provides information and feedback, corrects distortions, and provides hope. If we consider that humans have an inherent need to be heard and understood, we can conclude that any interchange that permits this activity is, at some level, therapeutic because it provides for a basic human need. Underlying this phenomena is the assumption that humans, to some degree, crave effective communication exchange. Self-expression, for example, is therapeutic; when self-expression provokes acknowledgment and understanding by another person, a tremendously therapeutic event has occurred. The basic need to express oneself and to be heard and understood has been met.

The first and most important assumption is that therapeutic communication is a skill practiced exclusively by healthcare professionals. This is a narrow application of the phenomena. In actuality, therapeutic communication can be practiced by anyone. Whether informal spontaneous interchanges between friends or purposeful interaction such as between provider and patient, it is assumed that one communicant is more able or ready to respond in a helpful manner and that this occurs over a series of exchanges of messages. It is true that providers care much about the impact of their communication on patients. It is also true that the average person may care and is also capable of being therapeutic. The average person may communicate therapeutically toward others for long periods without realizing it. The recipients may gain much from the dialogue, also without knowing it. Sad feelings may be abated, perceptions corrected, and knowledge gained; these outcomes do not require a "healer" and "healee." Therapeutic encounters are events. It can also be said that therapeutic communication occurs spontaneously. The issue for the provider is to harness this potential and make these naturally occurring encounters occur more frequently.

In summary, therapeutic communication can be practiced by many, not just by providers in very specific circumstances. It can be very spontaneous and occur under ordinary circumstances without much forethought or planning. Understanding this ubiquitous nature of therapeutic communication can provide us with optimism about the human potential as well as the natural helping resources that are available.

What differentiates the provider who practices therapeutic communication and the average person who does the same? There are some distinct differences.

1. The provider consciously intends to influence the patient in a therapeutic manner.
2. With this intention, the provider usually has a professional aim in mind; he or she is not using this approach to achieve personal gain. In other circumstances, this is not the case; for example, politicians say helpful things to gain votes and salespersons make people feel good in order to increase sales. Providers have the intention of helping the patient for the patient's sake. The patient's well-being, not the provider's personal gains, are the driving force behind the words used and how they are expressed.
3. The provider will perceive deficits in the patient's perception, processing, or expression of ideas and attempt to correct these deficits. Providers will focus on ill-expressed thoughts and feelings, breakdowns in expression, and distortions in perception. It is not by chance that

deficits in perception, processing, or expression will be addressed. Rather, providers purposefully attempt to improve the communication capabilities of patients (see Table 3–1).

Functional and Dysfunctional Patterns

While some providers will be engaged in restoring patients' abilities to communicate, such as by medications, treatments, or surgical intervention, all providers manage patients' ongoing communication capabilities. In the counseling professions, this responsiveness to communicative behavior is focused in-depth on the form and content of patients' communications. Functional communication is believed to be a sign of health, while dysfunctional patterns of communication are believed to be a sign of disturbance.

Not all individuals are accustomed to expressing thoughts and feelings through expressive language. At a very minimum, persons need capabilities in (1) perceiving appropriately; (2) learning the language and symbolic and meta-communication systems that prevail in their community; (3) acquiring and correcting information in order to maintain an appropriate view of self and the world; (4) integrating experiences into a comprehensive whole and the resolution of contradictions; (5) learning by imitation or experience the means by which one can achieve desires and influence others; and (6) sorting out and eliminating interferences on the part of internal and external noise, including factors in the environment. Depending on the age, health status, educational, cultural, and socioeconomic characteristics of the individual, a command over these abilities may not be possible. When we say that patients have deficits in these capabilities, we are not only judging their stage of growth and development, we are referring to many other factors that are affecting their communication behavior (see Exhibit 3–1).

Disturbed Communication

Patients may not only be impaired in their communication capabilities, they may exhibit patterns of disturbed communication. The concept of *disturbed*

Table 3–1 Differences in Provider and Layperson Use of Therapeutic Communication

Provider
- Conscious intention to achieve a therapeutic purpose.
- Professional aim or goal underscores messages.
- Making people "feel better" or "get better" is the desired outcome.
- Attempts to correct deficits in others' communications through asking questions or seeking clarity.

Layperson
- Spontaneous, sometimes thoughtless responses.
- No particular therapeutic purpose known nor intended.
- Making people "feel good" may be secondary to achieving another purpose (e.g., winning an argument).
- Improving others' capabilities to communicate may or may not be the intention.

Exhibit 3–1 Prerequisites to Functional Communication

- Perceives appropriately.
- Learns the prevailing language and symbolic systems.
- Acquires and corrects information when necessary.
- Integrates experiences into a comprehensive whole, resolving contradictions when and where they occur.
- Sorts out and eliminates interference from internal and external environmental "noise."

---

communication was first addressed in the classic work of Jurgen Ruesch (1961). Subsequent to its earlier uses, disturbed communication has come to be used to describe a wide range of problems: pathology in families, pathological communication in persons with thought disorders (e.g., schizophrenia), and general problems in information exchange through communication channels of the brain (e.g., those related to cognitive decline).

Disturbed communication can occur episodically or be a more stable phenomena. Unlike those individuals whose capabilities have not yet been fully developed due to, for example, learning a new language, people with disturbed communication could have regressed in their usual ability to communicate effectively. Changes in abilities can come on quickly (e.g., in the case of a stroke) or slowly (as in the case of acquired impaired vision or hearing loss).

The reasons for the patient exhibiting disturbed communication are many, including injury and trauma, emotional disturbance and poor self-concept, poor health status, learning disability, and relational stress. Dysfunctional communication is diagnosable through the observations of verbal and nonverbal behavior. When we "diagnose" disturbed communication we are interested in "why" and what needs to be restored or enhanced. It must be said that disturbed communication may also be a function of the environment and the patient, as in the case of intensive acute unit psychosis. This is a phenomena that has been observed, particularly in older persons, among patients in the medical or surgical ICUs. It does not reflect a more substantial psychiatric disorder but is a temporary shift in cognitive capacity. In acute care psychosis, the patient usually shows significant disorientation or irritability and may even have auditory and/or visual hallucinations. It is a form of acute brain failure or delirium frequently associated with dehydration, low blood oxygen, and infectious states. It is thought to occur in many patients whose stay in the ICU exceed five days.

One form of disturbed communication is *incongruence*. Communication is more or less congruent or incongruent. Much interest has been directed at the importance of congruence and our ability to recognize and learn from congruent versus incongruent messages both as children and adults. When one thinks of *congruent communication*, what is usually meant is that the verbal statement is consistent with behaviors associated with the verbal content. For example, when patients are speaking about the uncertainty of their diagnosis, they demonstrate worry in their tone of voice and physical gestures. They may appear tense or agitated or confused. These nonverbal components are generally consistent with being anxious, uncertain, and worried about one's diagnosis. Sometimes patients will exhibit these behaviors but express confidence or denial about the uncertainty of their diagnosis. When this occurs, their communication is incongruent because their verbal message is inconsistent with their nonverbal responses. Similarly, providers can communicate with incongruence. Say for example, you as a provider are delivering some very bad news and simultaneously smile. Your nonverbal communication is not congruent with the message you are giving. Even if the smile is a nervous response, it is confusing to the patient.

Do providers always identify incongruent communication in their patients? In part, this depends on their level of emotional intelligence or their ability to perceive the emotional impact a conversation might have on a patient or the patient's family. Rather than employing emotional intelligence, many providers use the patient's spoken message to understand what the patient is saying. It is possible to gleam some evidence from how the messages of the patient come across. In very basic terms, patients' messages might be too long, too short, or ill-placed. If this is the case, the patient's capacity to communicate effectively is hampered, and this may be either a temporary situation (as in the case of extreme stress) or more permanently disturbed (as in the case of injury or trauma). Other clues that the patient is having difficulty can be picked up from a single aspect of the patient's communication, such as the character of the patient's nonverbal responsiveness. A patient's nonverbal behavior can depict problems that the patient is having in perceiving and processing information adequately. The acoustic dimensions of the patient's voice (e.g., the intensity of speech, punctuation or emphasis, intonation, and speed) can depict disturbed states as well.

What is a *healthy voice*? Can we establish this? We know that people who are under stress speak differently. Actual changes in muscle contraction as well as in the rhythmical patterns of breathing and in the functions of the vocal cords occur when individuals are stressed. Therefore, a healthy voice might be one that displays harmonious tones; smooth transitions; and calm, composed rhythms. But, we might also argue that some people disguise their emotional state and mimic these characteristics to convince others that they are OK when in fact they are not functioning up to par. There is a way to differentiate between feigned functional communication and actual healthy communication. First, look for the general patterns. A sense of well-being may be initially expressed, but within minutes the patient's true level of functioning will emerge. Also, observations of inconsistencies in verbal and nonverbal messages is another way to determine how well the patient is doing.

Another way to conceptualize and diagnose disturbed communication is to take each functional aspect of communication behavior and determine the system that is most defective. Disturbed communication can occur in the realms of perception, evaluation or processing, and expression (see Exhibit 3–2). These systems overlap, and it is extremely important to understand how disturbances are both independently and interdependently manifested. If we take a total-system approach, we will understand that even though these elements (perception, evaluation, processing, and expression) can be separated out, they are highly interdependent. That is, a malfunction or disruption in one (e.g., in perception), will have implications for the other func-

Exhibit 3–2 Disturbed Communication

- Disturbance in perception of stimuli/messages.
- Disturbance in processing stimuli/messages received.
- Disturbance in expression of messages.

---

tions. A disturbance in perception will most likely have implications for how one processes and evaluates input. This, in turn, may affect expression—at least, the appropriateness of the expression. When, for example, perception is distorted, judgments about input will be faulty. Faulty judgment, in turn, has implications for the appropriateness of expression. Finally, if expression is faulty, then a disruption may occur in further evaluative and perceptive functioning. Thus, problems in any one dimension will result in problems in another. The relationship between these systems or channels is complex, and while the principle of interrelationships applies, there is probably more to the interaction than what can be deduced in a causal inference or even from the standpoint of a feedback loop. The human brain and how it interprets the senses is exceedingly complex.

We could, for example, say that the patient pulls away from the physician's hand because he or she fears pain or discomfort. The physician is not there to induce pain, so we could call this a distortion of reality, and we know that the brain is capable of making its own reality. We know that individuals are affected by both internal and external stimuli; what seems illogical to us is very logical to the patient. Former memories of pain come to bear on the patient's current perceptions. A complex array of stimuli impact the patient from a variety of sources, including the data derived from the process of evaluation and expression. If we were to pinpoint the primary system that is disturbed, we would also have to recognize that this is only part of the larger picture.

Disturbed Perception

Disturbances in *perception* or perception as the primary source of pathology are studied by many professional disciplines. The neurobehavioral, psychosocial, neuropsychiatric, and neurophysiological sciences study the exactitudes of human perception and many of these scientific principles have been alluded to in Chapter 2 of this text. The problems of selective inattention, sensory deprivation, sensory distortion, and the inability to balance between sensory input (from internal and external sources) are examples of problems in perception. The classical example of selective inattention occurs when we ignore significant details of events, perhaps to avoid unpleasant feelings, but in doing so, we negate important details. A former common practice of treating people who experienced hysterical blindness was to shock them (e.g., by slapping them in the face). This jolted the patient's awareness and restored the patient's full vision. It was thought that the blunt directedness of this action forced the patient to reconstitute his or her line of vision and to respond to a greater number and/or kind of stimuli.

Can you imagine such practice in health care today? What has evolved as current practice is much different from those primitive methods. With chronic cases of selective inattention, the technique of confrontation is preferred. A provider can awaken the patient to a wider scope of stimuli by observing astutely (nonverbal and verbal communication) and mirroring back or confronting the patient with those facts that he or she has selectively ignored. This does not require the jolt of a slap.

Sensory distortion can occur in other ways akin to selective inattention. *Selective inattention* refers to the blocking out of stimuli and results in distortions of perception. Certain other behaviors also contribute to perceptual distortion. For example, some people misinterpret others' communications because they apply stereotypic interpretations, or they generally experience things differently. They may even have an intolerance for the ideas or behaviors of others. They may also be unaware of the specific social or cultural context of their interpersonal situations. Sometimes, they are so highly adapted and trained at picking up some stimuli that they fail to see others. These are all examples of selective inattention.

Sensory distortion also occurs because of the idiosyncratic strengths of individuals. Consider the fact, for example, that some people are extremely oblivious to inner cues. Emotional feelings—fear, sadness, anger—may be out of their range of awareness; or physical sensations—pressure, tension, and even pain—are not perceptible. These individuals may, however, be very proficient at perceiving stimuli outside themselves from environmental clues or subtle shifts in the moods and behaviors of others. To some extent, healthcare providers fit into this latter category. They are very good at perceiving others' needs but much less aware when it comes to sensing their own needs. These introceptively handicapped persons, in the instance of providers, have transformed their natural tendency into a skill, and the consequences can be dysfunctional perceptivity.

The extrospectively limited individual perceives mostly internal stimuli, neglecting signals and signs from the external world. To some extent, young children fit this category. They are attuned to internal feelings of hunger, pain, and fear, but they will misjudge external stimuli. They may purposefully disregard external clues, or because they are ill equipped, they just do not attend to external stimuli. A major role of adults in our society is to protect children from their underdeveloped abilities to perceive and judge external stimuli. Whether or not individuals are strong at picking up internal, or external, clues, the imbalance is important. To help these individuals, we must strengthen the stimulus capacity that is weakest.

Sensory defects is yet another category of perceptual dysfunction and can be of several kinds. The most commonly witnessed sensory defects are those of vision and hearing. They may be congenital and permanent, or temporary, requiring no significant long-term adaptation. Defects in vision will affect expressive behavior. For example, many blind people do not speak with punctuation or intensity. Their speech tends to be bland, due in part to the fact they cannot perceive and therefore react to the nonverbal expressions of the other person. Likewise, disturbances in hearing will affect the development of speech. Other disturbances in sensory awareness include equilibrium and tactile capabilities. These disturbances also impede individuals' perceptions.

Disturbed Processing

Disturbances in processing and evaluation are many, and they include the capacities to cognitively and emotionally deal with stimuli. Decision making and memory are frequent outcomes of the capacity to process and evaluate the perceived stimuli. If we say that someone is having difficulties in decision making, for example, we are suspicious of some deficit in the area of cognitive and emotional processing. Is this a state condition (dependent on current circumstances) or trait condition (a more lasting characteristic)?

Methods of codification and the ability to assess probabilities are part of the decision-making process. To evaluate by using probabilities ensures individuals of safe and proper actions. When we do not assess events with a notion of probability or when we cannot remember what happened to apply a probability model, we are at risk for evaluating stimuli inadequately. This problem may be more or less serious. Take, for example, the dieter who chooses to have just one bite of chocolate cake. Having been at the mercy of his or her passion for chocolate cake in the past, this is a risky behavior. One bite can lead to a piece, one piece to a second piece, and so on. If we cannot remember what it was like to be seduced by the chocolate cake, or we cannot assign probabilities to the chance of eating more than we should, our processing of data is defective.

Moods, feelings, and attitudes also influence judgment and decision making. As a matter of fact, these factors have a great deal to do with our decisions. We could, for example, conclude that the reason we fell into the just-have-another-bite situation was that feelings or moods influenced our desires to apply probability theory. Having determined that "good sense" would mean we should avoid even the aroma of chocolate, we short-circuit good sense to get to the pleasure. There is no better way to do this than to default on applying probability principles. Our abilities to make decisions also depend on our ability to scan information that we hold in our memories, to consider this information, to modify our considerations, and to act.

The result of acting requires us to make a choice and to regulate our behavior based on our choice. This process can be affected by our abilities to scan, to arrange experiences in an orderly way, and to draw on stored information. Our strengths and abilities in these areas are influenced by many circumstances. Aging has an effect on memory, but it also transforms our abilities to scan for relevant information and establish risks. Some memory disturbances occur when individuals remember experiences but cannot apply what they have experienced and learned to new situations. Each time that they are presented with the problem, they approach it as if they had never experienced it. They carry out the same problem-solving steps that they did when they first encountered the problem. Disturbances in processing information are indeed important, despite the emphasis placed on abilities to perceive and express.

Disturbed Expression

The overriding function of our ability to express ourselves is the opportunity it affords us to participate in interpersonal relationships. Without the ability to express ourselves, and this involves many aspects that affect our central or peripheral nervous systems, including various motor capabilities, we simply cannot relate to others or get confirmation or acknowledgment of our ideas or actions. In short, we have limited ability to make an impact on others. This condition affects not only our enjoyment of relationships but also our self-concept and self-esteem. People who have speech impairments, for example, will exaggerate their associated facial expressions and postural responses. The purpose is to establish enough meaning in their messages to trigger a definitive response from others—a response that they desire. Disturbances of expression can include absent, inhibited, or exaggerated expression. There are also motor defects that can affect our abilities to express ourselves.

Because communication is highly influenced by the interpersonal context we find ourselves in, communicants who display an absence of speech or inhibited or exaggerated expression may be reflecting their perceptions of the interpersonal dynamics in which the encounter occurs. We could say that an adolescent is speechless not because he has a permanent disability but because he is reacting to some stimulus in his interpersonal encounter. Is this the case when the teen cannot clearly tell his parents the results of his exam? For fear that he may disappoint his parents, he may be ambiguous in an attempt to avoid a complete lie. Problems of expression can either be biologically induced or reflect interpersonal relationship dynamics—at least the individual's views of the relationship and what might damage this relationship.

Many of us have seen several cases in which there are defects in expression that are a result of motor impairment. People with nerve lesions, muscular disorders, or other impairments of the peripheral nervous system suffer expressive deficits. This group also includes patients whose expressions are complicated by the involuntary movements of tremors and tics. Essentially, the specific defect alters the character of the person's expression. These deficits are usually permanent, and individuals learn to compensate for the defect. If we carefully apprise the condition we can also identify in our encounters: (1) the immediate effect of the defect on speech, (2) the individual's compensatory response to the defect, and (3) the individual's response to his or her perceptions of the reactions others will have.

In summary then, disturbances in communication run the gamut of perceptual, processing, and expressive functions. They may be temporary and contextual, or they may reflect a longer-standing motor deficit. The exact origin and nature of the problem is important but not always critical to our understanding of how to communicate effectively with these individuals. The most important aspect is that we are able to recognize the systems of communication that exhibit the pathology and persist in our attempts to understand the basis of the symptoms.

It is not the purpose of this chapter to address at length the medical conditions that affect communication, which are numerous and include specific neurophysiologic and neurochemical deficiencies that are found in a variety of patient populations. They include the variety of language and speech disorders, developmental delays, and specific motor deficits. These conditions are extremely important to the study of disturbed communication, but the exact medical explanations are not a topic for this general review.

Before leaving the topic of disturbed communication, it is important to address the phenomena of *dysfunctional* communication. While disturbed communication connotes a specific defect, dysfunctional communication suggests a process that is highly linked to the interpersonal context of relationships. For example, when family therapists describe dysfunctional communication behaviors in family members, they are usually suggesting that patterns of dysfunctional communication are associated with larger-scale family dynamics and difficulties. Therefore, they attempt to change interpersonal or family dysfunctional communication patterns with a variety of approaches, depending on their training and theoretical persuasion.

Some theorists have clarified problematic communication by differentiating dysfunctional communication from the functional type. For example, expressive communication that is too much or too little, too early or too late, or tangential (in the wrong place) is said to reflect dysfunction. Dysfunction, here, not only refers to the explicit communication behavior but to the nature of the encounter as a whole.

Perhaps the most important understanding of dysfunctional communication patterns is found in the historical work of certain theorists' studies of family dynamics (Satir, 1967; Watzlawick, Weakland, & Fisch, 1974; Watzlawick, Beavin, & Jackson, 1967). Satir (1967), for example, explicitly defined the characteristics of a dysfunctional communicator. According to Satir, dysfunctional communicators overgeneralize; assume that others share their feelings, thoughts, and perceptions; assume that their perceptions or evaluations are complete; and assume that what they perceive or evaluate will not change. These individuals assume there are only two possible alternatives (they tend to dichotomize or think in terms of black or white): that what they attribute to things or people are actually a part of those things or people and that they can get inside the skin of the other person (not only to act as a spokesperson for that person, but also that others can do the same with them).

Individuals who exhibit functional communication, as opposed to dysfunctional, are more likely to use qualification and clarification. These individuals tend to clearly state their case, are ready to clarify or qualify their remarks, and ask for feedback. They are also receptive to feedback when they receive it.

Providers who establish effective communication with patients will not only exhibit functional communication, they will also be model communicators. They exemplify clear communication and also teach patients how to achieve it. To do this, they must spell out the rules for communicating accurately, emphasizing checking out the meanings of messages and correcting invalid assumptions. Providers need to be very clear in their own messages, showing a willingness to repeat, restate, and carefully explain how they reached conclusions. It is hoped that through both the providers' modeling and their capacity to interrupt dysfunctional communication that the patient will be encouraged to move toward more effective communication styles.

Therapeutic communications with patients require many knowledge and skill sets. Among these are the abilities to engage the patient in therapeutic interviewing, to assist the patient to communicate more effectively, and to avoid the traps of dysfunctional communication.

THERAPEUTIC INTERVIEWING SKILLS

Much has been written about the principles of therapeutic interviewing. In this text, techniques of therapeutic communication and therapeutic interviewing (referred to as critical competencies) are described in detail, one at a time, in Part II. The purpose of this discussion of therapeutic interviewing is to lay some general groundwork for the most salient principles.

Therapeutic interviewing has certain objectives. Generally, *therapeutic interviewing* is established to accomplish one or more of these aims:

- Elicit full descriptions from patients about their healthcare condition and concerns.
- Create an interpersonally safe place for patients to talk about themselves and be able to explore their problems in detail.
- Reduce any acute emotional distress associated with the patient's immediate condition.
- Offer support and reassurance.
- Establish an expanded list of patients' primary and secondary healthcare problems.
- Engage the patient in a problem-solving process that demonstrates the collaborative aspects of the provider–patient relationship.
- Prepare the patient for self-management of his or her health and illness.

Therapeutic Communications

The specific types of questions and responses that the provider can use are many. With regard to even one therapeutic response, that response can be used again, can be modified, or can be discontinued. For example, the provider can use a question, can re-ask the same question, can refer back to it later, or can even use an inappropriately worded question to open up the patient's expression on an important related topic (see Exhibit 3–3). Therapeutic response modes include but are not limited to:

- Using silence.
- Offering acceptance.
- Acknowledging and giving recognition (e.g., verbalizing the unspoken but implied message).
- Offering broad openings.
- Making and offering observations and summarizing.
- Reflecting one's own perception of the patient's thoughts, feelings, and reactions.
- Focusing the patient, and at other times, prompting exploration.
- Translating thoughts into feelings and feelings into thoughts.
- Encouraging evaluation or appraisal.
- Validating the patient's perceptions and/or beliefs.

There are many responses that achieve the overall aim of the therapeutic encounter. In chapters to follow, specific therapeutic response modes are discussed in detail.

Nontherapeutic Communications

Just as there are various recommended responses in therapeutic encounters, there are also those that need to be avoided. Exhibit 3–4 is provided so

Exhibit 3–3 Therapeutic Response Modes

- Using silence.
- Offering acceptance.
- Acknowledging and giving recognition.
- Offering broad openings.
- Making and offering observations.
- Reflecting on another's thoughts, feelings, and reactions.
- Focusing discourse, promoting exploration.
- Translating thoughts into feelings.
- Encouraging mutual evaluation or appraisal.
- Validating the client's perceptions and/or beliefs.

---

that you can test yourself in this area. Nontherapeutic phrases and gestures are to be avoided because they tend to limit patients' verbal expressions, they cause negative reactions, or they threaten patients. These include the following 14 items:

1. Moralizing—inferring that patients are wrong or not okay. This tends to inhibit expression.
2. False reassurance—stating that the patient will be better when he will not. False reassurance can cut off the patient's exploration of his concerns.
3. Closed-ended questions—asking questions that can be answered in one to three words.
4. Summarizing—summarizing may help the patient but also shut the patient down if it is offered too early.
5. Stereotypic responses—using phrases like "that's bad" (meaning "good") to express understanding or attempt to impress patients. The use of stereotypic responses may appear phony and backfire on the provider.
6. Belittling responses—making replies to patients that diminish the significance of their experience is belittling. Saying to a depressed patient, for example, as she reveals the desire to die, "Oh, those are common feelings of people in your position," tends to devalue the individual's experience.
7. Interrupting responses—introducing an unrelated topic breaks the flow of the patient's conversation before he or she can complete thoughts or ideas.
8. Denial of problems—treating patients' concerns in a cavalier manner.
9. Giving approval or disapproval—communicating approval or disapproval explicitly or subtly limits patients' feelings of freedom to say things.
10. Disagreeing—responding like this puts the provider in opposition to the patient. It can make patients defensive about their own ideas and feelings.

Exhibit 3–4 Personal Inventory for Nontherapeutic Interviewing Skills

On a scale of: 1 (all the time) to 8 (none of the time), how frequently do you do the following when interviewing patients?

I. Switch off problem-centered data by talking about:
- Unrelated focus
- Incidental material

II. Maintain superficial discussion by:
- Avoiding elaboration
- Switching to unrelated superficial focus; denying significance of the patient's stated problems
- Asking closed-ended questions

III. Intervene personally by:
- Giving opinion to life situation of patient without exploring
- Giving unsolicited personal comment or opinion
- Giving personal information or socializing responses
- Expressing approval or disapproval
- Moralizing, belittling, or challenging
- Seeking agreement from the patient/disagreeing with the patient

IV. Close off exploration by:
- Prematurely giving an interpretation
- Prematurely advising solutions
- Prematurely giving reassurance
- Prematurely closing topic
- Using judgmental stereotypical responses
- Interruptive responses
- Excessive probing

V. Introduce or follow illogical content by:
- Changing key words without validating change
- Following vague content or referent as if understood
- Introducing vague content or referent
- Questioning on different topics or levels without awaiting reply
- Speaking to question or statement of patient in conflicting ways
- Ignoring question of patient

Frequency of use: Pattern I. ____________________

Pattern II. ____________________

Pattern III. ____________________

Pattern IV. ____________________

Pattern V. ____________________

Use of the tool: (1) Identify each provider response; (2) Mark NP = nonproblematic or P = problematic; (3) Total P responses using tool.

11. Advising—advice-giving is not always helpful. Although a great deal of what providers do is to offer patients advice, it can have the effect of making the patient feel incapable of being self-directed.
12. Probing—probing too much may make patients feel like objects.
13. Challenging—challenging is a clear and present danger to the patients' expression. This tends to make patients feel that they have to prove what they say; they generally become defensive.
14. Socializing responses—engaging in chitchat or revealing personal data is nontherapeutic. It generally calls for equal time for the provider to self-disclose. This decreases the patients' time to self-disclose.

These responses are usually nontherapeutic, but not always. There are appropriate ways and times to use advice, probe, and even confront patients. However, for beginning providers, it is helpful to know that most of the responses are problematic, can lead them astray, and result in negative outcomes.

The Context of Therapeutic Encounters

The context of the therapeutic interview is extremely important; this context influences the quality of the patient's communicative capabilities and the interviewing environment.

Patients, as is suggested many places in this text, may exhibit dysfunctional communication. Their dysfunctional communication could be a result of a transient state (e.g., stress), or it may be longstanding, resulting from defects. Frequently exhibited disturbances in perception, processing, and expression are:

- Verbalizing too much or too little.
- Verbalizing inappropriately to the context of the events.
- Using incomplete sentences or thoughts.
- Behaving as if they have communicated clearly when they have not.
- Misperceiving environmental stimuli.
- Exaggerating certain meanings of a message, ignoring other aspects, or attributing different connotations to an event than what is intended.
- Overgeneralizing or undergeneralizing and failing to access stored information.

Because patients experience difficulties in communicating, part of the role of the provider is to correct for these deficits. This context of therapeutic interview is extremely important; it includes the social and environmental context for the provider's communication with the patient.

The purpose of therapeutic interviewing is to build or maintain a patient–provider relationship and to assess the patient through the patient's disclosure of thoughts, feelings, behaviors, and experiences. Because interviews require patients to communicate something personal, and even threatening, the interviewer must establish rapport and trust with the patient. This includes creating a safe place for the patient to disclose. A place that is protected from intrusions and interruptions is important for two reasons. First, a protected environment is likely to make patients feel comfortable. Second, in order to collect data adequately—this includes the multiple levels of patient communication (verbal, nonverbal, and meta-messages)—the provider must have a "noise-free" environment.

The data from an interview reflects the context of the interview. It is important to understand how patients communicate based on the context of the interview. We know, for example, that patients react differently to different interviewers. Who you are and what you are like may influence what the patient does or does not tell you. Patients also react to the particular situations in which they are asked questions. They may be rather close-mouthed if the atmosphere is threatening or there is little privacy. Patients also react to their most immediate life circumstances, crisis, and symptom status. Finally, patients react to the provider's approach—the specific way in which the provider formulates questions. All successful interviewers take these elements into account.

One's style of interviewing and choice of questions should be influenced by the perceptual, ethnic-cultural, and educational characteristics of the patient. The adage, "Begin where the patient is," is a good one. Basically, we can never push patients further than they can go, nor expect them to adapt to our stylistic peculiarities. It is inappropriate to use complex medical jargon with patients who are incapable of understanding the meaning of even the simplest medical phrase. It is also inappropriate to require patients to endure lengthy interviews of two hours if their anxiety levels or attention spans cannot meet the challenge. Sometimes knowing and using the jargon or language of the specific ethnic or cultural group is likely to increase patients' desires to communicate problems.

Regardless of the circumstances, providers must always demonstrate respect and concern for patients. Showing interest, concern, and understanding indicate that the provider regards the patient as worthy. The affective tone that the provider uses with the patient is extremely important and can make or break the interview no matter how sophisticated the provider is in using techniques.

AVOIDING THE TRAPS OF DYSFUNCTIONAL COMMUNICATION

Avoiding the traps of dysfunctional communication is certainly possible, but this requires knowledge, skill, and practice. We need to be able to communicate effectively and therapeutically with our patients. This seems so straightforward that it is frequently ignored. However, the techniques of effective communications are being taught everywhere, and people, once trained in effective communication, must go back for booster shots. That we can always improve our communications is a maxim the business and consulting industry knows well. Billions of dollars are poured into (and are made) helping people communicate with each other.

Training in Interpersonal Communications

Training in interpersonal communications is helpful to health providers because it improves their ability to communicate as well as their ability to help others. The purpose of good interpersonal communication is to help others learn about themselves and make decisions based on this knowledge.

Another purpose of good communication is so people can learn about themselves by sharing with others and by monitoring their own words and actions.

One of the biggest entanglements that a provider can experience is the trap of defensive communication. Defensive communication in the provider is generally indicative of a perceived threat and its corresponding feelings of anxiety, fear, and guilt. The consequence of defensive communication is generally that messages will be misunderstood and that communication will reach a standstill. This event in a patient–provider encounter is to be avoided at all costs because a disruption in communication is tantamount to a disruption in care.

Defensive communication tends to be obvious. It has specific elements. The following is a list of behaviors that are generally indicative of a defensive posture:

- Labeling.
- Interrupting.
- Judging.
- Using tunnel vision.
- Advice giving.
- Preparing rebuttals.

While there are many other indicators of defensive communication, these are among the most common. People who are communicating defensively usually use more than one of these responses. So it is not only the specific response that is important, it is the cluster of responses that is used and the impact of this cluster on others. Consider, for example, someone who is reacting very emotionally. They may label or blame, interpret others' behaviors, judge others, and develop rebuttals. When this defensive posture is executed with high intensity, it can be likened to a "machine gun." This machine-gun approach has one result—everybody gets out of the way. No one wants to get caught in the cross-fire, so observers are also likely to exit the encounter. The end result is that no one fully understands, and the communicants have a decidedly negative view about the prospects of being heard and understood.

The alternative, nondefensive communication, enhances the possibility that not only our needs for information but also those of the patient for support and counseling will be met. It is exceedingly more aesthetically pleasing. Nondefensive behaviors observe and report, share information, and engage others in mutual problem-solving processes. They generally produce an increased mutual understanding and encourage communicants to continue their dialogue.

From a diagnostic standpoint, all patient–provider interviews can be judged. Establishing the degree to which one uses nontherapeutic interviewing with a single patient or a group of patients can be determined if one analyzes patient encounters and establishes potential problem areas. Personal inventories help providers establish which, if any, of the common nontherapeutic responses they are using (see Exhibit 3–4). The assumption of this self-inventory is that nonproblematic provider responses are those that maintain focus and guide both the provider and the patient's learning, while problematic responses short circuit the therapeutic process.

Assessing one's therapeutic and nontherapeutic communication responses to patients is only the first step. It is, however, an extremely important step because no real change can occur until such an assessment is completed. These assessments can occur formally, for example, through feedback from coursework, supervisors, or peers. Much of this assessment, conducted on a continuous basis, must be carried out through individuals' personal self-assessments. Self-assessments include, but are not limited to, an analysis of encounters that turned out poorly, especially those that produced conflict and tension. Changing communication patterns is not always easy, but if providers believe in the importance of functional and therapeutic communications, they will understand the need for self-examination and continual improvement.

CONCLUSION

Therapeutic communication is not altogether confined to providers; others less well trained in medical care can communicate therapeutically. Providers differ, however, in that they deliberately employ therapeutic communication skills and knowledge. The therapeutic provider communicates with patients whose communications are potentially dysfunctional. Patients' communications can be dysfunctional for many reasons and have both transitory and permanent causes. As providers, we not only model functional communication, we modify the dysfunctional patterns of others' communication. Therapeutic interviewing is clearly within the domain of every provider's role. Therapeutic interviewing skills tend to focus the patient and increase learning; whereas nontherapeutic communication tends to inhibit communication, especially the processes of feedback, clarification, and qualification. Practicing therapeutic communications requires the provider to conduct ongoing self-assessments in which patient–provider encounters are analyzed on the basis of therapeutic–nontherapeutic dimensions. While formal, peers' and/or superiors' evaluations are critical, providers' personal commitment to conduct self-assessments and gather feedback from their patients is essential to maintaining a therapeutic approach.

CHAPTER 4

Cultural Similarities and Differences and Communication

In addressing mental health service delivery: A major problem is found in the continuing reliance on Western European tradition and practices in the treatment of low-income and minority patients. The "Anglo" approach to serving "people of color" has lost its credibility: It is in direct conflict with Hispanic, Asian, American Indian, and Black culture. There is a commonality of harsh experiences that low-income and minority patients encounter as service users.
—Frank X. Acosta, Joe Jamamoto, and Leonard A. Evans

CHAPTER OBJECTIVES

- Describe the current occurrence of healthcare disparities in the United States and potential contributions of provider–patient communications in creating or resolving disparities.
- Discuss the inevitability of communicating in a multicultural environment where there are both similarities and differences.
- Discuss and define the concepts of culture, cultural differences, acculturation, and culturally competent health care.
- Describe how cultural affiliation influences the meaning of expressed thought.
- Discuss the concepts of majority and minority groups.
- Discuss the influence of subgrouping on communication.
- Describe the hypothetical continuum—cultural destructiveness to cultural proficiency.
- With at least one other individual, discuss your own cultural programming.
- Acknowledge similarities and differences between your cultural programming and that of others.

There is evidence that all people are influenced by cultural programming. While *culture* is an ambiguous term, it generally refers to values, beliefs, knowledge, art, morals, laws, and customs acquired by individuals and groups. According to Page (2005), this definition suggests that individuals acquire patterned ideas and behaviors while residing with others. Cultural programming, a sort of built-in "software," influences our perceptions, ways of processing and interpreting data, and our expression of ideas and feelings. Once we recognize what our own cultural programming is, we have the capacity to explore more fully the communications of others.

In the practice of health care, both our personal and professional culture affect how we perform our roles with our patients. Providing culturally appropriate education and self-awareness training is critical in improving care and eliminating health disparities. It is essential to understand the role of the patient–provider communication interchange in such important outcomes as health disparities. It is appropriate to launch this chapter with some background on culture and factors that influence access to health care among groups. Following this discussion is a review of basic tenets of culture awareness.

DISPARITIES IN HEALTH CARE AND THE ROLE OF PROVIDER–PATIENT COMMUNICATIONS

In 2002 an important document built on a convincing review of existing literature was published: *Unequal Treatment: Confronting Racial and Ethnic Disparities in Health Care* (IOM, 2002a). Wide dissemination of this report raising awareness of the magnitude of the problem in the United States resulted in several healthcare initiatives and subsequent literature representing many areas of medical practice that called for action to reduce these disparities (American Pain Association, 2004; Ervin, 2004; Lavizzo-Mourey & Jung, 2005; Diette & Rand, 2007). The IOM report examines the extent to which certain racial and ethnic minorities receive lower-quality of health care than nonminorities. Among the many reasons given for these disparities were patient stereotyping, culturally related communication barriers, and provider biases. Patient stereotyping can affect quality of communication, especially if perceived as distancing and as a lack of respect. Culturally related communication barriers can result in some groups refusing diagnostic tests and treatment because of fear, confusion about the healthcare system, and beliefs about harm that are not grounded in fact. An increase in the proportion of providers coming from underrepresented minorities and effective training of all providers in the tenets of cultural competence will help alleviate these concerns.

Communication barriers between healthcare providers and patients are often of a sociocultural nature. These barriers can be due to differences in culture, language, race or ethnicity, gender, and social class, or they can be due to generational differences among individuals within the same culture. Providers are often most aware of the power of sociocultural diversity when they are confronted with adapting a medical regimen to the patient's unique personal circumstances. In communicating with patients, it is critical that clinicians understand the cultural patterns that influence patients' perceptions of their problems, the usual ways they cope with health concerns, and their acceptance of the treatment they will be asked to follow.

It is hardly ever simple to interact with patients and patients' families when value systems and cultural backgrounds are unfamiliar. The situation becomes even more complicated when language barriers between providers and patients also exist. Differences in values and the inability to understand the communications of others are important because they can produce social distancing. Social distancing in patient–provider relationships is not conducive to trust and empathy. In these instances, the therapeutic relationship is at risk. Perceived social distancing can affect whether a patient will accept or even return for treatment.

Perhaps nowhere is it more crucial to be able to understand and speak another's language than in the health services arena. Whether in an outpatient or inpatient setting, and across all levels of illness, the patients' and families' ability to express needs and feelings and to know that they have been understood is important. Within health settings, uncertainty and fear are naturally occurring responses to an actual or perceived threat of illness and injury. These fears are accentuated by the awareness that no matter how hard one tries, the provider may not really understand the patients' expressed thoughts and feelings and care for them in the way they need to be cared for.

CULTURE AND THE INFLUENCE OF CULTURE ON COMMUNICATION

Definition of Culture

Despite the fact that the concept of culture has existed for more than 250 years (Page, 2005), the concept remains somewhat ambiguous. Essentially, the literature describes *culture* as identifiable integrated patterns of human behavior that include customs, beliefs, values, behaviors, and communications. Culture is said to be passed from one generation to another and can be observed in racial, ethnic, religious, and social groups. The term *cultural identity* refers to the extent to which individuals subscribe to a given culture. The term *cultural diversity*, then, is the extent to which one's group identities (reflective of individuals' age, gender, ethnic, and social group) differ from another's. Everyone is said to have a cultural identity; more often than not, individuals have several cultural identities—due, in part, to the fact that one's cultural heritage is rich. Current social affiliations as well as religious and ethnic alliances depict an individual's unique programming. Each person is a unique cultural being (Giger & Davidhizar, 2002). Therefore, a patient's religious affiliation, ethnicity, age, and gender can all give clues to a patient's perception of health and illness.

Cultural Affiliations and the Meaning of Expressed Thoughts

Patients may have many affiliations that influence their cultural identity and behavior. For example, a patient (James) is a 60-year-old male, married with six children and four grandchildren; has a college education; is a member of the Mormon religion; is African American; and is employed part-time as a public school teacher making $50,000 a year and part-time as a tennis instructor. His place of birth is Boise, Idaho. This patient's cultural heritage and programming is rich. Predictions about his responses to health care services and communications with providers would best be made with all these facts in mind. Until we know what aspects of his cultural programming are most influential in the context of the interaction, we may not fully understand his communication. Added to this picture is that he is also in the place of accepting the patient role.

Assume that this same patient is hospitalized for surgery to correct a deviated nasal septum. On the day of admission, he engages his physician in the following conversation:

Patient: "Play any tennis lately?"
Physician: "I was in a doubles match Saturday!"

Patient: "Oh, how did you do?"
Physician: "James, I need to get you set up here. You remember what I told you in my office?"
Patient: "Yes."
Physician: "Good, I'm going to order your pre-op medications. I'll be back later."
Patient: "Okay, Doc—you're the boss, boss!"

From the content of his communication, we would say that James's affiliation with tennis is a dominant aspect of his programming. Still, when we examine this interchange at the meta-communication level, we observe that equity is an issue, and deference to the surgeon is an aspect of this interaction. While James attempts to relate to his surgeon as one tennis player to another, his surgeon shifts to a professional doctor–patient relationship. Further, James reinforces the hierarchy by in effect replying: "You're the doctor, I'm the patient—I'm here to follow your orders (boss)." While the physician may have good intentions about establishing a participative and collaborative patient–physician relationship, the outcome of this transaction may be interpersonal distance: "Let's stay within (the boundaries) our roles."

However, there are numerous reasons for James's response, and they are worthy of consideration. One possibility is that James is responding to differences in social status as a function of role differences. Another possibility is that he is sensitive to racial differences and is suggesting that African Americans (historically) are considered inferior in the eyes of this white surgeon. What enables the provider to better understand James's communication is his choice of words and the intonation of those words. Still, without knowledge of his specific cultural programming, judgments about his responses are, at best, tentative.

Social distancing displayed in transactions where minority and majority status exist have long been the subject of social scientists. Pinderhughes (1989) discusses the role of power in the dynamics of cross-cultural communication within the clinical setting. It is clear that the character of clinical interactions can be significantly affected by ethnic diversity in both patients and providers (see Exhibit 4–1).

Exhibit 4–1 Principles of Cultural Identity

- All people are influenced by cultural programming; this programming influences not only our behavior and attitudes, but also when, what, how, and to whom we communicate.
- Once we recognize what our cultural programming is, we have the capacity to explore more fully the communication of others.
- It is safe to say that what was *mainstream* culture a decade ago may not be so today.
- The usefulness of describing *mainstream* culture in today's world is questionable.
- To fully understand an individual or family, an individualized assessment of cultural uniqueness is advisable.

DEFINITIONS OF MINORITY AND MAJORITY

It is safe to say that what prevailed as mainstream culture in the United States decades ago may not prevail today. In fact, the usefulness of describing *majority* (mainstream) culture in today's world is questionable.

While our notions of what is and is not mainstream have changed, the concept of a minority group (or subgroup) still has relevance. We know, for example, that Cambodians are a subgroup within the Asian community. In some geographical regions, Cambodians are minorities within a dominant Asian culture. The critical point about minorities or subgroups is that persons from subgroups may not share the values and perceptions of the dominant (majority) culture. While there are similarities between majority and minority groups within the same geographical region, members of minority groups can feel suspicious and fearful of providers representing the majority group. They may view them as powerful; and because they are from another ethnic-racial group, view them as lacking in the ability to put their interests first. Members of minority groups frequently exhibit, at least initially, suspicion and fear. One must keep in mind that these fears may be realistic based historically on the relationships between both groups. They may respond as if they are in a subservient position. They may perceive the dominant group as authoritative, powerful, and unsympathetic.

Beliefs about Minority and Majority Groups

Providers frequently harbor attitudes or beliefs about both minority and majority groups with whom they come in contact, especially groups that have been underserved in the healthcare system. There is no question that they sometimes have stereotypic views. For example, Asians are regarded as "stoic"; Latinos are seen as "emotional." Patients can have equally firm views of providers. Caucasian patients may view Caucasian surgeons as superior, African American dentists as undereducated, and Asian doctors as "unfeeling." Like many generalizations, these are inaccurate. The key issue in relationships with patients from different cultures is to focus on effective communication based on respect, understanding, and openness—with a caution not to hold onto false assumptions.

Subgroups Shape Communication

It is understood that communication may differ across cultural groups. It is also true that communication differs across subgroups within a given culture. The following example depicts differences within an ethnic category—Asian culture. In the Vietnamese culture, talking is customary. Silence may be uncomfortable, and unless one party is angry or upset, long silences are unusual. Likewise, in the Filipino culture, talking is enjoyed and silence is uncomfortable. The only time that talking is not approved is when an elder is speaking; then it is a sign of disrespect to talk. These patterns run counter to other Asian groups, where silence is considered a sign of wisdom, and speech may be regarded as frivolous.

When healthcare providers intentionally shape their verbal and nonverbal behavior to be respectful of the patient's background, they are practicing with intentions to be culturally competent. This commitment is a step toward removing cross-cultural barriers.

CULTURAL COMPETENCE—A DEVELOPMENTAL PROCESS

In our multicultural society, we are all exposed in varying degrees to diversity. Just how much attention we pay to these differences depends on our values, biases, type of exposure, and the attitudes of our reference groups. If we value individuals as unique in their own right, hold few fixed judgments about a group, and have multiple exposures (especially quality exposures) to the differences of others, and if our own reference groups value cultural differences, we are more likely to be culturally competent in dealing with others. Within the healthcare setting, this means a heightened awareness and appreciation for patients' differences in self-disclosing, in interacting in the provider–patient relationship, and in perceptions of illness and risk of disease.

Issues of cultural competency cross many segments of patient care, including end-of-life care (Curtis, Engelberg, Nielsen, Au, & Patrick, 2004). Tong and Spicer (1994) described the basis for frustration between Eastern patients and Western caregivers, noting two distinct characteristics of which Western caregivers are unfamiliar. The first pertains to the fact that the family assumes the major role of decision maker on behalf of the patient. The second relates to the Eastern belief of silence surrounding the discussion of dying (and impending death) versus the Western orientation, which advocates openness and honesty. By gaining a greater understanding of these cultural traditions and practices, we can deliver more culturally competent health care.

As Bilu and Witztum (1994) suggest, patients often hold divergent explanatory models in regard to their symptoms. The universal structure of symbolic healing stresses the importance of provider (therapist)–patient compatibility for therapeutic success. To reach this compatibility, strategic therapists seek to join the patients' explanatory models and employ metaphors and symbols derived from their cultural world. These interventions bring provider and patient closer together despite cultural differences.

To better understand where one is in the process of becoming culturally competent, it is helpful to consider all the possible ways of responding to cultural differences. According to the classical theory of cultural competence put forth by Cross, Bazron, Dennis, and Isaacs (1989) it is possible to plot competence on a continuum where cultural destructiveness is at one end and cultural proficiency is at the other. But, between these two points on the continuum, there are many possibilities. In applying this theory, it is important to keep in mind that individuals are not easily typed and are capable of a variety of responses, depending on the context of the situation and the persons involved. Some providers may display cultural competence in some contexts but not in all. Therefore, it is more useful and accurate to think about selected behavioral responses than it is to categorize individuals. Having made this point, we can clarify the various terms used to describe level-of-competence and behavioral responses within complex contexts of interpersonal interaction.

Cultural Destructiveness

Way at one end of the continuum and representing an extremely negative position is "cultural destructiveness" (Cross et al., 1989). Attitudes, practices, and communications that are destructive to cultures and, therefore, to the individuals who come from these cultures are represented at this point on the continuum. Individuals and groups of individuals who participate in cultural genocide (targeted at minorities) have been described throughout history. Boarding schools that removed Indian children from their homes, laws that restricted Asians from bringing their spouses to the United States, and the targeted assault on African Americans by the Ku Klux Klan have been blatant attempts to deny people of color their basic human rights. In the healthcare arena, services that have denied people of color their natural healers, removed children from their families based on ethnic bias, or purposely risked the well-being of people of color through medical experiments without their knowledge and consent are examples of culturally destructive clinical practices.

Systems can also deny cultural differences by severely curbing individuals' rights to communicate in their native language. Demands that English must be spoken in major institutions (hospitals, clinics, schools, judicial departments) may not deny individuals their basic rights. Still, one could make the case that without choices, and with multiple demands to relinquish one's native language, cultural destructiveness is occurring. Individuals who adhere to this extremely negative position generally believe that there is a majority culture, that the majority culture is superior, and that subcultures are inferior. Bigotry translates into vast power differences that allow the dominant cultural group to control, exploit, and disenfranchise others. While not many examples are found in the healthcare system today, it is important to be aware that practices that disenfranchise subgroups may have been implemented and may be historically grounded in policy.

At a much more subtle level, there are aspects of culture that are not obvious but may be prohibited. These include nonverbal communication, body motion, and use of space. When these practices (what is considered to be primary-level culture) are controlled, the unique aspects of the culture erode.

Cultural Incapacity

Not as extreme, but still potentially lethal to a multicultural society, is the position of "cultural incapacity" (Cross et al., 1989). Cultural incapacity is influenced by beliefs of supremacy of one group but, unlike cultural destructiveness, is not characterized by intentional behaviors to eradicate minority cultures.

Rather than by blatant intentional acts to control minorities, individuals who are practicing from cultural incapacity lack the capacity to be effective due to their paternal and/or maternal posture toward minorities. Their attitudes are frequently fueled by subtle racial biases. The following clinical example describes how cultural incapacity may occur even though the provider is operating with good intentions.

Ramona H., a 24-year-old Latina, unmarried mother came to the dental clinic with her 6-year-old son, Alton. Her son needed to be seen for a dental checkup. While she was there, she asked the dental assistant whether she could have her older sons, Javier (10 years old) and Juan (11 years old), seen as well. The dental assistant ushering Alton (of mixed African American and Latino races) to the examining room thought to herself: "Why does this mother keep having babies out of wedlock? She's had so many boyfriends; doesn't she care about these children? She is a typical welfare abuser. They (Juan and Javier) look OK—I'm not going to let her 'use the system.' She'll just have to wait three months for their next regular visit."

In turn, Ramona may notice the assistant's disapproval and think to herself: "That woman is treating me like dirt! She thinks I'm a bad person. I need to talk to someone else because she won't help me."

The assistant's view that Latinas "use the system" and do not care about their children is a bias that, while not communicated verbally, is communicated nonverbally to this mother and will no doubt cause some conflict between providers and the patient. By maintaining stereotypes, service in this setting will remain unhelpful. At the heart of the problem is a moderate amount of ignorance and unrealistic fear that probably permeates the facility and results in subtle messages that Latinas are not always welcomed and are generally expected to be poor healthcare investments.

Cultural Blindness

Providers who experience *cultural blindness* also suffer from a lack of information (Cross et al., 1989). Unlike those in the former category, these individuals usually take pride in being unbiased. The problem, however, is that they are blind to their own cultural influences and do not perceive the influence of culture in others' responses. Midpoint on the continuum, these individuals profess that all people are the same, and culture or ethnicity makes no difference. They are participating in cultural blurring. Providers in this category believe that approaches used to provide healthcare services to people of the traditionally dominant culture suffice for all groups. In this instance, culture is invalidated by omission, and this problem is often compounded because services are not coordinated. Patients may be left to negotiate service delivery with more than one provider, in a language they may not fully understand. While the service-delivery philosophy is liberal and unbiased, it has the tendency to make services so stereotypical and rigid that they are ineffective for all but the most assimilated subgroups.

An example of this tendency would be the application of family therapy for all groups whose family members have a serious mental illness. Despite this good intention and the fairness that seems to characterize program planners, the model of care reflects a middle-class, nonminority existence. These services and providers ignore differences in views of health and illness and the tendency for some families to keep problems contained and private. To expect some women to express open dissatisfaction toward their husbands in couple's therapy ignores the cultural tenets regarding traditional male–female roles. Culturally blind providers ignore cultural differences and encourage assimilation.

Cultural Precompetence

Unlike individuals who are culturally blind and disregard both the effects of their own and others' cultural heritages, *culturally precompetent* persons realize the limitations they have in providing culturally sensitive responses (Cross et al., 1989). They also attempt to improve their services to one or more subgroups. People in this group are growing and moving in their capabilities. They may learn the languages, try culturally sensitive interventions, consult others from the culture, and initiate training for themselves and colleagues. They may recruit minority individuals to serve on boards of directors or to develop an adequate needs assessment. Precompetent providers are clearly committed to delivering quality care through culturally sensitive programs.

Cultural Competence

Toward the positive end of the cultural competence continuum is *cultural competence*, which refers to the capacity to accept and respect differences (Cross et al., 1989). This requires continuing self-assessment, careful attention to the dynamics of differences, and continuous expansion of cultural knowledge. A variety of responses are used to adapt healthcare practices for the specific needs of persons from minority cultures.

Giger and Davidhizar (2002) explain that cultural competence development is a dynamic, fluid, and continuous process. Culturally competent providers are highly perceptive. They view minority groups as distinctly different from one another and distinctly separate from traditional majority groups. They understand that within a given minority group there are numerous subgroups, each with important cultural characteristics. Providers in this category seek to hire minority staff who are committed to change and who are capable of negotiating a bicultural perspective. They are concerned that they and their colleagues will become proficient in cross-cultural situations.

Cultural Proficiency

A goal for all providers is to become culturally proficient in a multicultural society. Is anyone ever proficient? This goal is not easily reached and requires a great deal of self-assessment, knowledge building, and consultation with others. Individuals at this end of the continuum hold cultures in very high esteem. These individuals seek to research and develop culturally sensitive practices. As such, they will be regarded by others as experts or specialists and they will be called on to restructure healthcare services (Cross et al., 1989).

At each level in the culturally competent continuum, certain principles can be applied. Movement on the continuum relies on (1) valuing differences, (2) awareness and self-assessment, (3) understanding cross-cultural dynamics, (4) building cultural knowledge, and (5) adapting practice to reflect the patient's cultural context.

The early work of Wilson (1982) was instrumental in identifying the attributes of cultural competence. He identified 24 attributes, knowledge areas, and skills that are essential to the development of cultural or ethnic competence. These three categories apply to the communication of culturally sensitive healthcare providers. A modified list of the original themes of Wilson is provided here.

Personal Attributes

Personal attributes include:

- Personal qualities that reflect a capacity to respond flexibly to a range of possible solutions (openness and nonjudgmental attitudes).
- Acceptance of cultural, racial, and ethnic differences among people.
- A willingness to work with clients of different minority groups.
- Articulation and clarification of the workers' personal values, stereotypes, and biases about their own and others' ethnicity and social class and ways in which these may accommodate or conflict with the needs of patients.
- A personal ongoing commitment to change bias, racism, and prejudice.
- Resolution of feelings about one's professional image in a field that has systematically excluded people of different racial and ethnic groups.

Knowledge

Knowledge includes:

- Knowledge of the culture (history, traditions, values, family systems, artistic expressions) of patients and their families.
- Awareness of the impact of class and ethnicity on behavior, attitudes, and values.
- Knowledge of the wide variations in help-seeking behaviors of patients, families, and communities.
- Knowledge of the role of language, speech patterns, and communication styles in ethnically distinct subgroups and communities.
- Knowledge of the impact of social service policies on patients and their families.
- Knowledge of the resources (agencies, persons, informal helping networks, and research) that patients typically use and that can be utilized on behalf of patients and families across groups.
- Recognition of the ways and extent to which professional values may conflict with, or accommodate, the needs of ethnic minority patients and families.
- Knowledge of socioeconomic political power relationships within the community, agency, or institution and their impact on ethnic minority communities.

Skills

Skills include:

- Techniques for learning the cultures of patient groups and their families.
- Abilities to communicate accurate information to ethnic minority patients, families, and communities.
- Skill to openly discuss racial and ethnic differences and issues and to respond to culturally based cues.

- Abilities to assess the meaning that ethnicity has for individual patients and their families.
- Abilities to identify stress and conflict arising from the current social political structure.
- Techniques of interviewing that are reflective of strength in understanding of the role of language in the client's culture.
- Abilities to utilize the concepts of empowerment on behalf of ethnic minority patients, families, and communities.
- Capabilities of using resources on behalf of patients, families, and their communities.
- Abilities to recognize and address racism, racial stereotypes, and myths in individuals and in institutions that impede delivery of quality care to all.
- Abilities to evaluate new techniques, research, and knowledge as to their validity and applicability in working with ethnically diverse and underserved minority patients, families, and communities.

Cultural competence, skills, and knowledge can be gained through training and experience. Providers must avail themselves of opportunities to build their knowledge and skill. Exposure to the positive aspects of different cultures and even negative experiences in helping relationships will facilitate their learning.

UNDERSTANDING YOUR OWN CULTURAL PROGRAMMING

The culturally competent practitioner has the capacity for cultural self-assessment. This means that providers should be able to assess themselves, their relationships, and communications and develop a sense of their own cultural uniqueness. The premise is that as providers are able to understand how their own culture shapes their life views, beliefs, and communications, it will be easier for them to establish how they may need to adapt in interacting effectively with individuals from other cultures. Individuals who are self-aware can anticipate barriers and minimize the negative effects of cross-cultural differences.

To appreciate cultural similarities and differences, providers must recognize the influence of their own culture on how they think and act. In part, bias and stereotyping behaviors occur on an unconscious level. The unconscious responses toward patients may even be inconsistent with one's conscious beliefs and values (Burgess, van Ryn, Dovidio, & Saha, 2007). Thus, a purposeful self-examination of one's own cultural influences can lead to a better understanding of oneself and the impact of culture on others.

Very simple differences can result in major misunderstandings. For example, when anticipating family teaching needs for patients' care at home, the provider must know what "family" and "family involvement" mean to the patient and the family. To the provider, family involvement means working exclusively with the spouse to perform care giving. To the patient, involvement could mean ignoring the spouse and involving the extended family (e.g., the patient's older siblings). Knowing one's own cultural biases can minimize the effects of cross-cultural misunderstanding.

Self-Recognition of Personal Programming

Understanding one's personal cultural programming is best arrived at by questions, provided the questioning mirrors back to providers their personal programming. Sometimes questions administered in small groups of diverse people have a higher yield. The group discussion tends to stimulate one's own recall and recognition, and, at the same time, each member who hears another's self-analysis is learning something about cultural similarities and differences. Exhibit 4–2 provides a list of general questions aimed at stimulating self-recognition of cultural programming.

Many providers do not recognize how their own cultural values have shaped their day-to-day experiences and how day-to-day behaviors have been reinforced by their family, peers, and social affiliations. For those who are still somewhat doubtful of the ability of culture to determine behavior, specific and detailed cultural analysis will reveal just how persuasive culture is. Remember aspects of culture include (1) one's set of values and norms; (2) shared beliefs and attitudes; (3) relationship patterns; (4) communication and language patterns; and (5) prescribed daily activities, including dress and appearance, food preferences, and time consciousness.

Acknowledging Differences

Taking each one of these more global aspects of culture, it is possible to generate a specific list of the ways in which cultures influence individuals. That which is accepted in one culture may be considered inappropriate in another. The mainstream Anglo culture, for example, has been said to be characterized by individualism, self-reliance, action, and a sense of control over one's environment. In contrast, Buddhist teachings project a fatalistic view of life. Life is suffering, and

---

Exhibit 4–2 Recognizing Your Cultural Programming

- Identify your cultural heritage by acknowledging your place of birth, current affiliations, and religious and ethnic alliances. For example, are you from the United States or outside the United States? A small town or large city?
- What reactions/curiosities do you have about your own cultural programming?
- Does any aspect of your cultural identity come in conflict with other aspects? For example, do you see yourself as assertive, but your culture does not support this behavior?
- What is the most influential part of your cultural programming?
- How does your cultural programming affect your communication? For example, are there things that you would share only with close family members?
- What do you know about the cultural programming of others (patients, peers, etc.)? How can you learn more? Does their communication give you clues about their cultural programming?

suffering is caused by desire. In this context, suffering in pain may be considered to be simply a fact of life rather than a health emergency. Many Asians prescribe to the theory of three possible causes of disease—the physical, the supernatural, and balances (yin-yang). They rely heavily on forms of self-care that include offerings to spirits, dermabrasion, and hot-cold and herbal remedies.

There are 21 Spanish-speaking countries in the world whose people are called *Latino*. Latinos, however, are not monolithic. While it is not possible to generalize and be absolutely accurate, it has been observed that Latino communities value a present-time orientation, the extended family, the interdependence of family members, differentiation of sex roles, unconditional respect for adults, and deference to authority. Although all Latinos have similar values, there may be a great deal of differences among them. Communication styles among groups differ. Some Latinos are more formal in language and style; South Americans, for example, are said to be more formal than are Latinos from the Caribbean. Characteristics (e.g., immigration status, history, religious affiliation, social makeup, and reasons for migration) all play a role in the cultural programming of Latinos. In Latino communities, the main barrier to health care is usually economic, but in addition there exists a general distrust of modern medicine. Many Latinos believe in folk medicine and have great faith in their *courandaro.* They feel that the courandaro (or neighborhood healer) always knows exactly what is wrong with a patient, while a physician does not. The Latino observes the doctor asking many questions before offering a diagnosis, while the courandaro seems to recognize the problem immediately and knows how to deal with it.

There are other reasons patient–provider relationships with some Latinos might inhibit effective communications. Latinos generally show a good deal of deference for persons in authority, including the healthcare providers they see. Van Servellen and colleagues (2003) noted the importance of considering this cultural phenomena in building medication adherence intervention programs. Deference to providers may, in fact, prohibit full disclosure of what is actually occurring in the patients' response to the treatment regimen. Are patients likely to say everything is "fine" in order to please the provider?

Knowing that a patient's culture may judge certain behaviors or interactions more acceptable than others will assist providers in communicating more effectively. Aspects of culture that influence healthcare encounters are multiple. Values and norms, beliefs and attitudes, relationship patterns, communication and language, and daily activities are influenced by one's culture. Essentially, when aspects of culture are operationalized, the link between culture and patients' responses becomes clear. In the helping-healing process, awareness of the other's culture and the differences that exist between the patient and provider will enable the provider to anticipate misunderstandings and further sensitize providers in their interactions with patients.

While the first task is to raise one's consciousness, this is not sufficient to establish cultural competence. One must go beyond. Going beyond requires acknowledging cultural differences between yourself and the patient. Operating on the basis of differences is as important, or more so, than acting on similarities in establishing an effective healthcare system. Furthermore, the ability to analyze interactions in which cultural differences exist is an important skill that is not easy but may be a long term goal and commitment.

Exhibit 4–3 presents each of five previously identified cultural aspects and compares and contrasts a hypothetical patient and provider. Differences in values and norms, beliefs and attitudes, relational patterns, communication and language, as well as usual daily activities illustrate that differences that exist between provider and patient may be significant and may potentially cause opposition and conflict. For example, the value placed on direct communication (provider) and indirect communication (patient) has the potential to generate conflict, misunderstanding, and mistrust. If cultural and medical practices are not in sync, there is a strong possibility that the patient will leave and not come back.

CONCLUSION

By the year 2030, ethnic and racial minority groups in the United States are expected to increase to nearly 40% of the total population (U.S. Census Bureau, 2004). The issue of healthcare disparities in these groups loom over

---

Exhibit 4–3 Analyzing Interactions in Which Cultural Differences Exist

Aspects of Culture

I. Values and norms
II. Beliefs and attitudes
III. Relationship patterns
IV. Communication and language
V. Daily activities

Patient's cultural reference

Formal

Bows, embraces, handshakes, kissing.

Hierarchical destiny predetermined race, class, gender inequality.

Focus on extended family. Loyalty and responsibility to the family of origin. Relational intimacy less important.

Implicit, indirect. Emphasis on context of messages.

Religion may control dress. Eat when hungry. Value on promptness, efficiency.

Your cultural patterns

Informal

Handshakes.

Egalitarian.

Determinism.

Individualized race, gender equality.

Focus on nuclear family; independence from family is valued. Interpersonal intimacy is desired.

Explicit, direct communication. Emphasis on content of message.

Wide range of dress/style accepted. Eat at a social function. Time is relative. Schedules are changed to accommodate relationships.

the health of the nation. A facet of this problem is the contribution of inadequate patient–provider communications.

The cultural backgrounds of providers and patients are composed of learned norms, values, customs, and beliefs that are similar but different. If providers are to be as effective as they can be in providing holistic care to patients of culturally diverse backgrounds, their technical expertise must be complemented by knowledge of and respect for the various cultures they will encounter (Rooda, 1992). This is particularly true for situations in which providers are from cultural and ethnic backgrounds different from the patients for whom they are caring.

Is the current health provider work force ready, willing, and able to provide culturally appropriate care? Sound cross-cultural practice begins with a commitment to provide culturally competent care. At the very heart of this commitment must be an awareness and acceptance of culturally different expressive behaviors and an understanding of the dynamics of difference in the patient–provider relationship.

Culturally competent healthcare providers not only acknowledge cultural differences but also incorporate these differences in planning and implementing care. A culturally competent system of care acknowledges and incorporates—at all levels—the importance of culture, the assessment of cross-cultural relations, vigilance toward the dynamics that result from cultural differences, the expansion of cultural knowledge, and the adaptation of services to meet culturally unique needs. While cultural competence is a concept that can be applied to an entire system of care, it is also a concept useful in assessing one's individual facility in relating in multicultural contexts.

Cultural competence should be viewed as a goal toward which providers can strive. To be realistic, becoming culturally competent is a developmental process. We are all, at some point, on a continuum. Our behaviors and attitudes reflect where we are on the continuum at any one time. It is important for providers to assess their own personal level of cultural competence with the understanding that it may be a long-term investment.

Verbal and nonverbal expressive behaviors are influenced by one's cultural orientation. Above all other circumstances, inattention to obvious and even subtle differences in expressive behavior may serve to alienate patients and their families.

The healthcare provider must be sensitive to differences in cultural perceptions about the role of the sick, the role of the family in health care, the roles of young and old, the roles of women and men, and even the symbolic importance of foods and diet. Helping the patient comply with healthcare regimens requires knowledge about these and other cultural values.

A final word of caution is important. While it is imperative for providers to be culturally sensitive, too much attention to differences can inappropriately distance the provider from the patient. Beginning clinicians may be too willing to acknowledge these differences and act accordingly. Accommodating patients, for example, by offering to get someone else to care for them can be problematic. This offer can be interpreted as a lack of acceptance or even rejection. Where language barriers exist, it is important to get assistance, and if the patient openly requests a different provider, then this request should be honored if possible. Cultural differences are inevitable, and diversity training can equip providers in most situations to deal effectively with cultural nuances.

Several programs offer substantial training in developing cultural competency in health care. For example, Stumpf and Bass (1992) proposed a combination experiential and content course to help providers become more unbiased in their healthcare interactions. The model, "Differences + Discomforts = Discoveries," promotes depth of knowledge about underserved groups as well as personal awareness of prejudicial feelings. As a result, students learn techniques to provide less biased health care to these and other populations. Since 1992, the Cross Cultural Health Care Program has addressed this need, offering interpreter trainings as well.

In practice, respect for diversity is often inadequate and, therefore, the healthcare needs of many cultural groups are not being met (Roberts, 1994). Blackburn (1992) reminds us that caregivers and clients cannot be brought together under the assumption that a harmonious union will occur. Cultural competence does not eliminate all problems in communicating with patients and their families, but it does help reduce cultural conflict as it occurs in healthcare settings. A point well worth noting is that culturally competent care requires an openness on the part of patients and families to resolve the barriers they face. Cultural and language barriers—together or alone—have great potential to lead to mutual misunderstandings between patients and healthcare providers (Joint Commission, 2007). By lessening these barriers, we may be able to make a significant impact on existing health disparities among our ethnic and racial minority groups.

PART II

Professional Skills in Managing Care—Critical Competencies in Therapeutic Communications

Good communication skills are not acquired by osmosis. They must be learned, and in many cases, relearned. Acquiring therapeutic patient-centered communication skills can be time intensive, but these skills are critical elements in effective provider–patient interactions. Patients do and will react to providers' interpersonal skill deficits. They will not necessarily distinguish between personal skill deficits and system barriers that make an otherwise compassionate provider appear cold, distant, and uncaring. Providers need to take their fund of skills and competencies in therapeutic communications seriously.

If the reader completed the personal inventory on nontherapeutic responses (Chapter 3), some understanding of one's personal needs for change has been established. In the chapters that make up this part of the text, important therapeutic response modes are presented and discussed in depth, one at a time.

While attention to technique is important, it is equally essential that providers understand that using techniques is devoid of authentic connection with these approaches. Over the last decade, considerable attention has been given to alternative, less formalized approaches that strengthen patients' ability to shape the encounter. These approaches include talking (Roter & Hall, 1992; Cade, 1993), listening to patient stories (Smith & Hoppe, 1991; Cole-Kelly, 1992), and the conversational interview (Brown, 1995) and have appeared in the literature as alternatives to more formalized clinical interviews. According to Brown (1995), "the conversational interview" is advocated because it is more client focused and is less interpersonally controlling.

Masson (2005) suggests that, as of late, more emphasis is placed on listening to patient stories as a means to provide culturally competent care. Taking time to get to know the patient through stories, preferred language, even photographs can increase our ability to care for culturally diverse individuals and underserved groups. This alternative, more than the structured interview, is felt to produce an accurate shared understanding of the patient's health status. As indicated by Roter and Hall (1992), *talk* is the main ingredient of health (medical) care. It is the fundamental way in which the provider–patient relationship takes form and the fundamental instrument by which therapeutic goals are achieved. While providers use a number of other tools and tests, talk is what organizes the patients' history, symptoms, and experiences. Several positive changes are advanced and are summarized in seven communication-transforming principles (Roter & Hall 1992). Communication:

1. Serves patients' needs to tell the story of their illnesses and the provider's need to hear it.
2. Reflects the special expertise and insight that patients have into their physical state and well-being.

3. Respects the relationship between patients' mental states and their physical experiences of illness.
4. Maximizes the usefulness of providers' expertise.
5. Acknowledges and attends to emotional content.
6. Respects the principle of reciprocity, in which the fulfillment of expectations is negotiated.
7. Overcomes stereotyped roles and expectations so that both patient and provider gain a sense of power and the freedom to change within the encounter.

Interactions between patients and providers vary in structure and intensity. The therapeutic response modes discussed in this section are relevant regardless of the mode in which provider–patient talk occurs.

Chapter 5, The Pervasive Role of Confirmation and Empathy, discusses the importance of a major element in helping relationships. The ability to discern the experience of others and reflect this sensitivity in helping encounters is critical. The process of formulating and delivering effective therapeutic empathic responses is discussed. Another concept, confirmation, which is associated with empathic communication, is presented and discussed.

Chapter 6, Communications That Contribute to Trust and Mistrust of Providers, addresses the basic role of trust in the process of assessing and helping patients. Without trust in providers, patients will not easily disclose their fears and concerns. Because trust is also critical in promoting change in patients, it is vital to the helping process. Mistrust can derail therapeutic interventions. Trust, once established, can be broken. Understanding conditions under which trust is cultivated and mistrust avoided arms the provider with capacities to achieve and sustain meaningful in-depth relationships.

In Chapter 7, The Art and Skillful Use of Questions, questions as therapeutic response modes are discussed. One of the most prevalent forms of communication in the healthcare professions involves the use of questions. In part, this is due to the diagnostic orientation of providers. In short, questions are the primary means by which providers gather data. The format of questions itself provokes different responses. Therefore, it is important to understand the types of questions available to us.

Sometimes questions fail to produce in-depth disclosure. Silence is a therapeutic response mode that is examined for its power to establish a comprehensive, in-depth gestalt. Chapter 8, Therapeutic Use of Silence and Pauses, details ways in which this response mode enhances empathy, respect, and understanding. Because silence and pauses can also be used in destructive ways, it is important to understand the power of silence as it is used in helpful and unhelpful ways. Silence also has specific meaning in various cultural contexts. Silence responses may be respectful or punitive; the actual interpretations are dependent on a multitude of interpersonal factors.

In addition to questions and silence, providers can use self-disclosure to facilitate the aims of helping relationships. Chapter 9, The Impact and Limitations of Self-Disclosure, discusses this important nondirective approach. Self-disclosure by providers frequently begets self-disclosure by the patient. This is because provider self-disclosure communicates authenticity, genuineness, and empathy that encourages, in turn, self-exploration and self-disclosure. The key to provider self-disclosure, as is the case for many other response modes, is appropriateness. Appropriately delivered, self-disclosures will be met with matching responses. Inappropriately offered self-disclosures, such as those that are ill-timed, will lead to confusion. Guidelines for the formulation and delivery of self-disclosures are discussed in detail.

Up to this point, the therapeutic response modes addressed are considered to be facilitative and foundational. There is yet another set of response modes that involve being evaluative. In Chapter 10, The Proper Placement of Advisement, the skill of advice-giving is discussed. Providers issue advice on a regular basis; this mode is somewhat reflexive. The provider assesses or diagnoses a problem and follows with a solution. While advice-giving is commonplace, it is a poorly understood phenomena in interpersonal communication. Advice-giving usually contains evaluative and judgmental components. Like other modes, advice-giving works best when a strong relationship has been built through repeated use of facilitative dimensions like warmth, respect, and empathy.

If advice-giving does not provoke action, other approaches may. Chapter 11, Reflections and Interpretations, examines how these distinctively different strategies produce self-awareness and change. While reflections merely paraphrase patients' expressions, interpretations provide additional information. Interpretations can be mild, moderate, or intense; the level of interpretation frequently designates the degree of threat that may result when an interpretation is offered.

The maximum level of demand in health professionals' communications comes from the use of confrontations, orders, and commands. These modes are not comfortable for many providers, especially those who want to facilitate, not dominate, the patient's course of action. Were it a perfect world, we could settle for less judgmental, nonevaluative forms of communicating. But the fact of the matter is, it is not a perfect world; these response modes are necessary and cannot be supplanted by facilitative, nondirective approaches. In the final chapter of this section of the text, Chapter 12, The Judicious Use of Confrontations, Orders, and Commands, these approaches are addressed. Providers who utilize these response modes risk being evaluative, judgmental, and conditional. This risk is minimal if these strategies are employed when a strong relational bond exists between patient and provider. The probability of action toward problem resolution is frequently highest when patients are exposed to these strategies. Yet, like many of the other evaluative, judgmental modes, these response modes are most successful when a strong therapeutic alliance has been formed.

In therapeutic relationships, healers must try to understand what health and illness means to the patient and create a therapeutic sense of connection in the patient–provider relationship. Several interviewing techniques can enhance such an outcome: rapport setting, silencing internal talk, accessing unconscious processes, and communicating understanding can help providers enhance their sensitivity to subtle clues on which issues of meaning and connection often depend (Matthews, Suchman, & Branch, 1993). Therapeutic response modes are skills, and like all skills, they are to be practiced. Providers will need to exercise patience in the acquisition and perfection of these skills. It may surprise the reader to learn that the ultimate objective is to learn the skill but then to forget it. The mark of a seasoned clinician is knowing the skills but blending the skills with his or her own unique interpersonal style. In large part, it is providers who heal, not the enumerable strategies and skills they have at their disposal.

CHAPTER 5

The Pervasive Role of Confirmation and Empathy

A world with emotions, yet without empathy would be absurd. It would be a world of musicians without hearing . . . without the capacity to empathize with feelings of another, we would be just bodies located physically in space alongside one another—no interhuman connection would exist at all.
—*L. Agosta*

CHAPTER OBJECTIVES

- Distinguish between empathy and sympathy.
- Discuss how empathy is "emotional knowing."
- Discuss how empathy is achieved through active listening.
- Identify how interpersonal confirmation leads to the experience of empathy.
- Discuss two outcomes that cause empathy to be a therapeutic response.
- Identify the steps that providers can use to arrive at an empathic position.
- Discuss several barriers to being empathic with a patient or developing the capacity for empathy; discuss client, provider, and environmental barriers.

Empathetic listening is central to modern thought on listening in patient–provider relationships. Understanding the unique ways health status or a health condition affects individuals legitimizes patients' illness and suffering and contributes to feelings of connection with others. Carl Rogers, on the topic of empathy, stresses that with listening and empathetic responses, health providers assist patients in feeling less alone and isolated for the moment; at least the patient is feeling "a connected part of the human race . . ." (1980, p. 150). Sherman and Cramer (2005, p. 338) clarify that empathy is not only the ability of the provider to understand a patient's experiences and feelings, but "the capability of communicating this understanding."

The intellectual, clinical knowledge of a patient is understood to be insufficient. Empathy in the patient–provider relationship builds hope and trust. The provider, then, must know the patient beyond the clinical data immediately available. That is, one cannot truly grasp subtle and complicated feelings and experience except by emotionally knowing the patient. Current educational programs in the health professions stress the importance of empathy in order for providers to give care while sensing what it must be like to be the patient. And yet many providers seem to disregard the relevance of this experience, or they take empathy for granted. Travaline, Ruchinskas, and D'Alonzo (2005) warn that providers should not ignore or minimize patients' feelings (e.g., with a redirected line of inquiry focused on symptoms).

It is the purpose of this chapter to define and describe empathy and the nature of empathic responses. Second, the therapeutic value of empathy is described, and steps to achieve empathy are identified. Nonverbal aspects of communication as well as reflective statements and silence are discussed as they enhance empathic communications in the provider–patient relationship. Finally, common barriers to empathic understanding are identified, and ways to overcome these barriers are addressed.

Evidence about the impact of empathy in patient–provider relationships suggests a number of important contributions to health outcomes. The literature reports that there may be associations between empathy, empathetic interviewing, and empathetic response and (1) patients' views that the provider really cares, patient satisfaction, and trust (Suchman, Roter, Green, & Lipkin, 1993); (2) greater treatment adherence (Frankel, 1995); (3) more accurate diagnoses of patients' conditions, patients' abilities to process negative information about their diagnoses and treatment, and ability of the provider to shift patients' negative responses to some level of therapeutic value (Halpern, 2003); and (4) less probability of medical malpractice claims (Levinson, 1994; Frankel, 1995).

DEFINITIONS OF EMPATHY AND EMPATHIC RESPONSE

The word *empathy* was originally coined "Einfrehlung" by German psychologist Teodor Lipps who, in 1887, used this term to refer to the experience of losing one's self-awareness and fusing with an object. Today, empathy is described as an objective awareness of and insight into the thoughts, feelings, and behavior of another (including their meaning and significance). It has also been discussed in the context of *emotional intelligence*, which is defined as the awareness and management of emotions in self and others. According to Satterfield and Hughes (2007), in the context of the provider interacting with patients, this would include the providers' ability to work with emotions in oneself as well as in the patient for the benefit of both provider and patient.

Empathy, or the capacity for "emotional knowing," is a behavioral attribute thought to contribute to the humane qualities of social interaction (Clark, 1980). For those who study empathy phenomenologically, empathy is a complex process describing a holistic experience of the patient. It involves a synthesis of human dimensions: conscious and preconscious awareness, subjective and objective views, and closeness but distance from the patient's experience. Physical, psychological, emotional, and cognitive processes—occurring simultaneously—achieve an empathic response.

As indicated, interdisciplinary literature on empathy is vast. Empathy, like creativity, is a complex phenomena not easily measured. While there are surveys to measure empathy, it is difficult to observe in its totality. Rather, an aspect of empathy is observed. According to Davis (1990), empathy is a commonly used but poorly understood concept. It may be confused with related concepts such as sympathy, pity, and identification. Empirical studies of empathy emerged clearly in the middle of the 20th century because of the influence of Sullivan (1953) and subsequently as a product of the efforts of Carl Rogers (1957; 1961). In recent times, the increased interest in empathy is found to be contextually relevant. Satterfield and Hughes (2007) summarized the state of affairs in health care. Essentially, providers are under increased pressure to see more patients, within no additional time periods and with less administrative support. As a result, patients frequently feel rushed, unsupported, disconnected, devalued, resentful, and distrustful (Safran, 2003). The consequences, along with provider fatigue and burnout, can be a vicious cycle with the potential of unprofessional behavior and further decline in both patient and provider satisfaction.

Perhaps the most significant work on the concept of empathy and its therapeutic value stems from the early writings of Carl Rogers in the 1950s. Rogers, in his client-centered approach to counseling, conceptualized empathy as a major factor influencing client (patient) growth and change (1957; 1961). Rogers's description of empathy stresses the importance of multiple facets. The empathic way of being with another person, according to Rogers, means entering the private perceptual world of the other and becoming at home in it. Rogers further states that it is a process of being sensitive, moment by moment, to the changing experience of this person, to a multitude of feelings—fear or rage, tenderness or confusion (whatever the person is experiencing). It also means checking with the other person the accuracy of one's sensing and being guided by the replies and responses one receives. Rogers's model and assertions about the influence of empathic understanding stimulated considerable research aimed at measuring empathy and its impact on those seeking counseling. Truax and Carkhuff (1967) designed the first empathy scale, the Truax Accurate Empathy Scale, later revised by Carkhuff (1969). Now we have the Jefferson Scale of Physician Empathy (JSPE), which is used in evaluating empathy in physicians, medical students, residents and dental students (Hojat et al., 2002).

Differences Between Empathy and Sympathy

Perhaps the most confused notion and misunderstood idea is that sympathy is empathy. While sympathy does express feeling "with the patient," it is very different from the expression of empathy, which is the task of mentally putting one in the shoes of another and then verbally conveying that one understands what it must be like. While empathy is a preferred skill, sympathy can be considered risky. The actions of sympathy include the inclination to think or feel like another, but the crucial difference is that sympathy also includes the display of pity or sadness. People who sympathize are unable to separate their own feelings from those of the other. Empathic responses are not the equivalent of feeling sorry for another person; they involve appreciation for another's thoughts and feelings without displaying feelings of pity and sadness. There is the chance that patients and families will react very negatively toward sympathetic responses because, rather than bringing them together, sympathy tends to set patient and provider further apart.

Emotional Knowing

With sympathetic responses, that which is usually missing is the emotional-intellectual connection that guides the provider to articulate a reply. Without the ability to fully understand the perceived experiences and feelings of the patient, an attempt to empathize becomes a self-centered exercise of sympathy. Consider the following dialogue between a nurse and a patient who is hospitalized and whose diagnosis is end-stage cancer. The patient has not seen her small children for two or more weeks. The nurse approaches her to assess her depressed mood and establish a relationship.

Provider: "Hi Mrs. ____. How are you doing today?"
Patient: "Okay—I guess."
Provider: "You know, I've noticed that you have no pictures of your children in your room."
Patient: "No . . . I don't."
Provider: "How would you like it if we called your husband and asked him to bring some in?"
Patient: "Well—yes. That would be good!" (Silence)
Provider: "You know, better yet, we could make it possible to have you do a videotape for them—that way they could actually see you . . . see how you are."
Patient: Looks at nurse, studying her response.
Provider: "What is good about a videotape is that they can keep it forever."
Patient: Begins to cry. "I'm sorry . . . I guess I'm just upset."
Provider: "It's right to feel upset . . . you don't feel that you are going to be around for your children much longer."
Patient: Nods. Silence.

Sometimes providers are not ready to deal with the experience and feelings of the patient. They have feelings; yet their attempts to empathize become exercises in sympathy that actually make the patient feel worse. In the dialogue preceding, the nurse was probably feeling the helplessness that the patient projected in both her state of illness and her emotional response. To recover from her own emotional pain, the nurse responds as if she were trying to make the patient feel better, giving bits of advice on how the patient could establish communications with her children. Believing she had "hit on a good idea," she pursued the idea of videotaping. While videotaping may have been a good idea, what the nurse expressed made the patient feel that the nurse could not handle her feelings nor the tragedy she faced. Thus, the patient apologized for her feelings. Then, in a feeble attempt to make the patient feel better, the nurse follows with a sad commentary: "You don't feel that you are going to be around for your children much longer." While this may be true, it may not be the most salient point for the patient; rather, loneliness and no one to talk to may be. And, while this is a critical issue, the way it is approached tends to be rather cold and distant. Most observers would judge the nurse to be sympathetic. The reader may also judge the interaction as a self-centered gesture on the part of the nurse to find an easy solution, a quick fix. As Stanley L. Olinick (1984) points out, sympathy is rarely a purely altruistic and conflict-free response; rather, it can either serve a defensive or an exploitive function, disguising other feelings that may be inappropriate in the relationship. Frequently, sympathy can mask feelings of relief: "I'm glad I don't have your problem" or feelings of helplessness and powerlessness: "Sorry I can't help you . . . and I don't know who can." Providers may think that their verbal replies do not reveal these conflictual attitudes (let me help you with this; I can't help you); but, the fact is, providers are rarely able to completely disguise their innermost thoughts and feelings.

Unwittingly, providers reveal these attitudes in the choice of their words or nonverbal communication. Merely feeling what the patient is feeling or "suffering with" the patient may not give the provider the objectivity that is needed to fully comprehend the patient's dilemma. In the previous dialogue, the nurse lacked an awareness of herself and her ability to tolerate the patient's expression of pain. This was not immediately revealed in her verbal comments, which appeared accurate but rather, it was more apparent in the direction that her dialogue took—her lack of anticipation of the effects of her statements and her attempts to "fix things." What the patient really wanted was someone to talk to, to listen to her, to be present in her painful situation. When providers establish a high level of empathic responsiveness, feelings of pity and sorrow are irrelevant. Providers are able to sustain a recognition of the patient's pain, maintain separateness, but also prevent unnecessary distancing.

Active Listening and Empathy

An empathic response to patients is facilitated by the process of "active listening." In most descriptions of the process of healing, it is clear that the provider of healing has taken some time and energy to learn about the experience of the sufferer's ailments or difficulties in the process of developing the basis for the plan of care. Further, there has been data to establish that the troubled and the sufferers have yearned for an interested and concerned listener (Jackson, 1992; Fleishman, 1989). Fleishman, recognizing the need for persons to have someone to listen with nurturant attentiveness, grouped such yearnings with the need to be seen, known, responded to, confirmed, appreciated, cared for, mirrored, recognized, and identified. He described this need as a yearning for "witnessed significance." Active listening is different from merely hearing and repeating what was heard. Active listening refers to a sensitive, discerning use of the sense of hearing akin to Theodor Reik's (1951, pp. 144, 146–147, 150) "listening with the third ear." Reik, in describing the skill needed by the psychoanalyst, stated that the analyst needed "to learn how one mind speaks to another beyond words and in silence." This process can reveal not only what the sender is saying but what the sender is thinking and feeling.

Empathic listening is a term, claims Jackson (1992), that is a significant feature of thought on listening within healing contexts. Characteristics of this process involve the clear intentions of the listener to "harken" to the sufferer, to hear but also to know and understand. And, listening within the Rogerian client-centered framework captures both the active aspect of the healer and the increased sensitivity to the world as the patient sees it. It is the healer's role to assume, in so far as he or she can, the internal frame of reference of the patient. It is the healer's role to perceive the situation as the patient sees it and to perceive the patient as the patient sees himself or herself. In doing so, the healer must lay aside all perceptions from the external frame of reference. This process, an active, not passive activity, places the healer at an advantage in fully understanding the patient.

In summary, active listening is a vehicle for empathy. Active listening increases the probability that the provider will focus his or her full attention on the patient. Without active listening, empathy does not occur. With active listening, providers take in data using all communication channels simultaneously—visual, auditory, and kinesthetic—to fully perceive the patient's needs and concerns. Providers who engage in active listening can be distinguished because they exhibit a variety of behaviors indicative of good listening. These behaviors are listed in Exhibit 5–1.

Active listening requires providers not only to hear, but to listen; not only to see, but to perceive; and not only to touch, but to feel. Sensing without integrating data from these major communication channels falls short of understanding the patient. When it comes to integration, the provider must gather personal strength to see the patient's condition no matter how tragic and painful it may be.

Exhibit 5–1 Behavioral Signs of a Good Listener

- **Eye contact.** Good eye contact need not mean that the provider is "glued" to the eyes of the patient. Rather, good eye contact may be given in spontaneous glances that express interest and a desire to communicate. Poor eye contact consists of never looking at the patient, of staring at patients constantly and blankly, or of looking away from patients as soon as they look at you. Cultural differences may also affect the level of eye contact appropriate for a given interaction. In some cultures, to demand eye to eye conversation would be disrespectful.
- **Postural position.** Posture includes both body gestures and facial expressions. Good postural positions include sitting or standing with your body facing the patient, while communicating responsive facial expressions. Rigid body posture can be modified with flexible movements toward the patient, again, indicating a desire to be with and attend to the patient. Being preoccupied and in constant movement not related to the patient generally communicates distrust. No facial expressions (stoicism) or too much inappropriate smiling, nodding, or frowning could, under certain circumstances, communicate a lack of authenticity.
- **Verbal quality.** Good verbal quality is as important as the words that the provider chooses to use. These qualities include a pleasant, interested intonation. The provider's speech is neither too soft nor too loud. It can reflect the context of the contact and reflect back any particular feeling state that is expressed by the patient. Speaking harshly to a patient who is crying is obviously inappropriate; still, expressing concern when there is no reason for concern is confusing. Patients may "read things into" verbal and nonverbal messages.
- **Verbal messages.** Messages to the patient can be worded to reflect the provider's understanding of the patient's experience. This may include choosing culturally relevant terms, the patient's own words for his or her experience, and analogies or paraphrases selected from the patient's description. The provider's interpretation of the patient's message needs to be clearly separated from the provider's own account of what the patient says or feels.

Confirmation and Empathy

There has been a long-standing interest in humanity's basic need to be heard and attended to, relating to an inherent search for confirmation that one is valued. These needs have been described by some to be as important as needs for personal safety. Without a sense of being seen and heard, most individuals will not trust their interpersonal environments. This condition has been described in theories of growth and development, in explanations about viable work settings, in concepts of functional–dysfunctional relationships, and even in paradigms that predict conditions of escalating tension and dispute. Lloyd and Berger (2002) emphasize that there is probably nothing more powerful to individuals than our need to be understood and that our natural tendency to judge or discount patients' feelings and thoughts is counterproductive in the patient–provider relationship. Those who study the process of conflict resolution and mediation realize that the number-one culprit in creating conflict is the absence of communication in which parties are not really listening and paying attention to the messages of one another. It is the mediator's job to restore communication and set the ground rules that will enhance effective attending and listening behaviors in the disputants. It is presumed that this change will not only prepare the parties to negotiate their interests, but will also demonstrate parties' willingness to value one another.

Disconfirming responses are typical in disputes and are usually what anger parties and make resolution of differences next to impossible. Consider the case of two parties who express through their communications that the views, desires, and concerns of the other are not important. The dangerous aspect of this encounter is that these parties interpret the attitudes to mean: you are not important or valuable. Such interpretations fuel attitudes of mutual resentment and tend to fix each individual in a position—usually a position antagonistic to that of the other party. Interpersonal "war" results as each party is certain that the other is not to be trusted under any circumstances because no trustworthy person would deny another's views and, in essence, their existence.

In contrast, consider the situation in which disputants communicate that they understand that each other's point of view is important (at least to them), but they disagree or have interests that seem to contradict those of the other individual. In this situation the parties acknowledge, up-front, that there are other ways to perceive the situation and that the views of one another are equal in importance. These parties acknowledge each other as persons.

Health providers should issue confirmation in their dialogue with patients as if it were a significant healing agent. Confirmation responses have the effect of making the patient feel worthy. Confirmation responses acknowledge the other's unique value as a person.

In the classic work of Northouse and Northouse (1992), five ways in which confirmation occurs is outlined:

1. Direct acknowledgment.
2. Agreement about content.
3. Supportive responses.
4. Attempts to clarify messages.
5. Expression of positive feelings.

These responses make a patient feel valued, and although the provider may not agree with everything the patient says or does, these replies demonstrate responsiveness that is necessary in a supportive patient–provider relationship.

Just as there are specific ways in which providers can confirm patients as individuals, there are certain response patterns that deny a patient's worth and tend to make patients feel less valued. Disconfirming responses are generally inappropriate or irrelevant. Not only do they express a lack of empathy, they generally suggest that empathic responses will not be forthcoming. As Northouse and Northouse (1992) suggest, disconfirming responses can be of several kinds. They include:

- Irrelevant replies.
- Interruptive remarks.
- Tangential comments.
- Impersonal responses.
- Incoherent or incongruent replies.

Most of these responses ignore or disregard the spoken word as well as the intent of the patient, sometimes not allowing the patient full expression of thoughts and feelings. And, while incoherent or incongruent messages may be confusing to the patient, the indirect effect suggests that the provider is not "in tune" with the patient.

Consider the following dialogue between a provider and a patient who is asking to have a prescription filled.

Patient: "Can you fill this, please?"
Provider: "Humm, Pru-Care; George is this thing working now?"
Patient: Appears confused and concerned; is silent.
Provider: Turns to patient: "We've been having problems with this computer."
Patient: Looks expectantly as providers talk behind counter for about 5 minutes.
Provider to Patient: "It will be about 15 minutes."
Patient: "Will it really be 15 minutes?" (Noticing that there is no one else waiting.)
Provider: "I say 15 minutes; it might be less. This way patients don't get upset if I give them a high number and it is ready sooner."

Note that the beginning response to this patient was to offer an irrelevant remark. The patient did not get a direct answer—only a remark that ignored her need to know. Although the issue of the computer's being down was relevant to the provider, it was not relevant, at least initially, to the patient. In fact, it really was not until several minutes had passed that the patient's question was answered directly. Notice that the patient even questioned the response—"15 minutes?"—not totally convinced that the provider knew how long it would take. The provider made a vague reference to wishing to please patients but implied that he was more interested in preventing patients from getting angry than addressing their needs for reassurance that the prescription could be filled and that this would occur in a timely manner.

The following dialogue between a provider and a patient who is anticipating surgery is yet another example of how patients are commonly disconfirmed in dialogues with providers.

Patient: "You know . . . I'm kinda worried . . . It probably is silly to worry. I guess it's a minor surgery—certainly not a liver transplant or anything. (Heh heh!)"

Provider: "There is nothing to worry about—you've got a good surgeon. Before you know it, you'll be in the recovery room." (Irrelevant remark)

Patient: "Yeah, I guess you're right. It's stupid of me to worry about it." (laughs nervously)

Provider: "I'll have the nurse come in and get you ready. In the meantime, try to keep your mind on how you're going to feel when you get out of here." (Irrelevant remark)

Here, again, is an illustration of what appears, on one level at least, to be an innocuous conversation. The provider is not critical—in fact, she comes across as friendly and somewhat helpful. However, the subtle underlying messages tend to negate the patient's thoughts and feelings. The patient's fear of surgery is minimized to the point that even he feels there is something wrong with him for having those feelings. Through irrelevant and somewhat tangential replies, the provider succeeds in avoiding what is bothering the patient. The message—your feelings are not important enough to discuss—will probably have a deleterious effect on further attempts by this provider to communicate effectively with the patient.

In short, as Northouse and Northouse (1992) suggest, it is painful if others respond in a disconfirming manner that neglects the receiver's own experience, and it is rewarding or satisfying if others affirm these experiences. Taken in the context of the patient–provider relationship, such responses can "make or break" the relationship.

THE THERAPEUTIC VALUE OF EMPATHY

When the impact of empathy is put in very simple terms, it can be said that empathy allows the listener to heal. To the extent that providers' communications become the foundation of the relationship, the empathic response is central to more basic issues of trust and self-disclosure. Additionally, in clinical practice, empathy is the skill used by providers to decipher and respond to the thoughts and feelings of the patient in the provider–patient relationship. Empathic understanding and empathic response occur in three phases of every contact: the negotiation phase, the clinical-reasoning phase, and the establishment of therapeutic alliance (Brock & Salinsky, 1993). Empathic providers can be trusted. When patients trust providers, they are more likely to disclose important details about their condition, thoughts, and feelings.

Increasing Connectedness

In part, the impact of empathy is achieved through the patients' feelings of connectedness with the provider (Lloyd & Berger, 2002). Feelings of connectedness are reinforced by confirmation, described earlier as a co-commitant factor in binding the provider and patient together. In Rogers's model of client-centered therapy, empathy, together with unconditional positive regard and congruence, elicits important patient outcomes beyond facilitating the patient–provider relationship. Rogers (1980) stated that through the use of these factors, the client (patient) will feel understood and be better able to cope. Rogers's method is said to build patient's self-esteem due to feelings of being cared for, no matter what (Wade & Tauris, 1990). The provider's support for the patient, according to Rogers, is eventually adopted by the patient, who thus becomes more self-accepting and better able to cope.

Reducing Alienation

Additionally, according to Rogers (1980), empathic responses reduce patients' feelings of alienation. Feelings of alienation can arise in patients for many reasons. Their condition, especially conditions that appear visually distasteful (e.g., scars from severe burns) or that trigger social judgment (such as AIDS), may cause them to be stigmatized. Alienation can be self-imposed as certain patients distance themselves from others either because of their illness (e.g., with schizophrenia) or because of their recovery process (e.g., with grief). Feelings of alienation can provoke loneliness and even separation from reality and can have serious implications for people who need treatment and who need to follow medical regimens. People who feel alienated and socially stigmatized may not always pursue early treatment. Feelings of alienation can cause a patient to feel timid about being seen again, as well as feelings of incompetence in following medical advice. Empathic responses acknowledge patients and make them feel understood and accepted, thus directly countering the effects of alienation. In this way, the patient is helped to seek advice, continue treatment, and endure, for the purpose of getting better.

The therapeutic effects of empathy are most notable in the early phase of the provider–patient relationship. The early work by Carkhuff (1969) describes empathy in early phases of the patient–provider relationship. He states that during the early phase of helping, empathy is critical because, without an empathic basis on which to understand the patient's world, there is no foundation for helping. Attempts to help will be perceived as insincere gestures, and advice will be felt as irrelevant facts that have little to do with how patients see their world and their difficulties. It is clear to the patient that empathy from the provider is an investment of time and effort. Providers who demonstrate their willingness and their ability to be empathic are perceived as trustworthy. They are perceived as potentially capable of helping and as possessing sufficient interest in the patients' state of well-being to handle the task of caring. Under these conditions, the patient feels secure enough to enter into a relationship with the provider with renewed hope.

The following dialogue between a nursing student and a patient demonstrates how empathic responses can create the leverage needed to move the patient beyond initial dysfunctional responses to the illness.

Provider: "Do you remember me?"
Patient: "I think so."
Provider: "How are you doing today?" (Sitting down, maintaining eye contact.)
Patient: "I'm better . . . my leg hurts a lot. It's difficult for me to be in bed all the time."
Provider: "That is very difficult . . . I'm sure. You know, I'm concerned about your pain medication. Is your medication making it (the pain) tolerable?" (Empathic response)
Patient: "Well—I want to be fully awake. I don't like to be 'drugged up'—you can't think straight."
Provider: "You have a valid concern." (Confirmation) "Have you had a past history of bad experiences?"
Patient: "No, not really. Well I've heard what morphine does—the horror stories about being on medications like that."
Provider: "What have you heard?"
Patient: "Oh, of people becoming addicted—being mean and saying things they don't really mean."
Provider: "So you are really concerned that this might happen to you." (Empathic response) "And, I'm thinking that the pain you have now is more than you need to have."
Patient: "There's the emotional pain too."
Provider: "Yes—would you like to talk about that—the emotional pain?" (Confirmation)
Patient: "I have a good husband. People—well they say, 'Oh my God, what happened to you.' I hide my leg. I can't take it when they say those things."
Provider: "Are you afraid I might react the same way?"
Patient: "No . . . "
Provider: "You know you've kept the covers over your legs the whole time. Do you think you could show them to me?"
Patient: "Sure—I get upset with other people—I don't like to watch their faces—I feel like a 'circus act.' My legs are three times the normal size from my knees down."
Provider: "Yes, well I can understand that your legs are very painful to you—in more ways than just one." (Empathic response)

During this somewhat lengthy discussion, the nursing student was able to establish the meaning that "pain" held for the patient. From the provider's initial assessment, physical pain was the issue. How to get the patient to accept more pain medication was the challenge. Yet, a fuller understanding of the patient's experience of her condition leads the provider into the feelings of shame and disgust that the patient experiences and how this is of equal, if not more important, concern to the patient. The empathic responses of the student become the catalyst for discovery and for gaining insight. It is highly likely that the student will now attend to the patient's world as the patient perceives it, integrating in her plan of care ways in which she can help the patient master the emotional pain associated with her disfiguring medical condition. It is also more likely that the patient will regard the relationship as helpful—not tangential. Under these conditions the patient may be more receptive to taking the advice of her physician and nursing staff.

THE EMPATHIC PROCESS—STEPS TO ARRIVING AT EMPATHY AND THE CAPACITY FOR EMPATHY

It is accurate to say that empathy is established through a series of steps that engage the provider's cognitive and affective capabilities. We are not just empathic when we want to be, and it is not an inherent trait that we are born with. Individuals do have different capacities to be sensitive to others, and some people listen more carefully than do others. Still, it is important to remember that empathy is a skill and is a great deal more complex than simply being sensitive to others' thoughts and feelings in the process of listening well. Later in this chapter, when barriers to empathic communication are addressed, it will be clear that empathy cannot always be easily established, and an otherwise empathic provider may not be consistently empathic in all patient–provider encounters.

The process of establishing empathic communication has been described by various authors, some of whom describe verbal and nonverbal components, others of whom attend to cognitive awareness in the provider. Gladstein (1987, p. 178) identified the various nonverbal behaviors that are usually perceived by the patient as empathic. These are face-to-face positioning with direct eye contact and interest and a receptive appearance conveyed with an absence of defensive postures (e.g., crossed arms and/or legs). Various behavioral indicators of active listening are outlined in Exhibit 5–1.

Ehmann (1971), cited in Sundeen, Stuart, Rankin, and Cohen (1994), and Smith (1992), identify steps to be taken in communicating empathically to patients. These recommended procedures attempt to combine cognitive and affective capabilities in providers in order for them to achieve empathy. Satterfield and Hughes (2007), in speaking of emotional intelligence, describe attitudes, knowledge, and skill in using empathetic emotional intelligence in encounters and how these can be taught. Ehmann (1971) described the process of empathy as formulated by Katz (1963). According to Katz, the empathic process is summarized in four basic steps.

Identification

The first condition or step is *identification*, stated as the need for the provider to first comprehend the situation and feelings of the other. This step requires that the provider relax some self-control in order that the other's situation seems real, rather than remote. In the previous example, the provider relinquished her tendency to advise the patient about appropriate dosages of pain medications in order to try to comprehend the patient's view: "Have you had a past history of a bad experience?" This question requires that the provider temporarily refrain from telling the patient what she needs to do. Additionally, it brings the very remote aspects of the patient's experience into better proximity to the provider.

Incorporation

The second step or condition is *incorporation*. The process of incorporation means that the experience of the patient that is now known to the provider is taken into the self of the provider. Although the experience is recognizable as that of the patient, not of the provider, this step helps bring the patient's reality and its underlying meaning to the provider. In the dialogue between the nursing student and patient, the student commented: "So you really are concerned that this might happen to you." This comment is a verbal indication that the provider has allowed the patient's experience to penetrate the provider's awareness of her condition.

Reverberation

Reverberation is the third step. According to Katz, the provider's past experience interacts with that which is known to the provider from the patient. The student's innermost thoughts—the patient is afraid of becoming an addict; know this won't happen; still, the patient feels that it may—is an example of reverberation. This process of reverberation leads to further understanding of the feelings of the patient.

Detachment

Detachment, the final phase in establishing empathy, refers to the provider's return to his or her own frame of reference. The results of the first three steps culminate with other objective knowledge of the patient (e.g., the patient is ashamed of her disfigurement). This information is then fed back to the patient so that more appropriate steps can be taken in responding to the patient and additional approaches can be identified. The student replies: "Yes, well I can understand that your legs are very painful to you—in more ways than just one." It is important to note that this one fact about the patient's experience is the outcome of empathic understanding. And, this one fact will influence from this point on the approach that the provider will take in addressing the patient's pain.

Smith's (1992) identification of steps in communicating empathically can be useful to providers who are struggling with impediments to their abilities to concentrate. Smith first alerts providers to the need to clear distracting thoughts and priorities from one's agenda. Second, providers must focus on the patient, giving the patient full attention and communicating interest. Third, providers must reflect on both the verbal and nonverbal aspects of the patient's communication. With this as a basis, the provider must then pick out the predominate themes of the patient's experience (e.g., the fear of addiction to pain medications, the patient's desire to be cognitively intact, and the shame she experienced from the disfigurement). The fifth step is conveying to the patient an empathic response, reflecting some of the patient's key words to acknowledge her anguish and anxiety (e.g., "the emotional pain" you are feeling). The sixth and final step, according to Smith, is checking to see if the empathic response was effective. Because the purpose of being empathic is to reduce the patient's burden (e.g., her emotional pain about her legs), it would be important to assess whether the patient did feel better after disclosing her concerns.

While the dialogue between the patient and student did not include an appraisal of the results of the conversation, it is easy to suggest what this may have included. The dialogue could have gone like this:

Provider: "I have a much better idea of what you are dealing with."
Patient: "Yes, I didn't know myself . . . I guess my real 'pain' is about how I look. The physical pain is important too—but not as important."
Provider: "Oh."
Patient: "I feel better that I finally talked about this. I thought you would think it is silly—guess you don't."
Provider: "I don't."

If the patient were asked directly what was helpful about the dialogue, she might reply: "feeling that the staff understand me better, knowing myself better, realizing that the staff may not think that my feelings are silly."

These guidelines, identified by both Katz and Smith, are useful to providers who are attempting to acquire or improve on their empathic responses. Still, the context for empathy is multifaceted. And what will become clear in the discussion that follows is that in the context of healthcare delivery, empathy and its necessary conditions must be executed in some instances under considerably negative odds.

BARRIERS TO EMPATHY IN THE PROVIDER–PATIENT RELATIONSHIP

As stated previously, empathy engages providers in multidimensional ways: cognitively, affectively, and behaviorally. Demands in the process of communicating empathically cannot always be met. The reasons are multiple and reflect the provider, the patient, and the environment of the delivery system. The following discussion focuses on barriers originating from each of these three sources.

Provider Barriers

Beyond the simple intellectual barriers—not knowing how and why to use empathy—are the personal characteristics of providers that inhibit their abilities to be empathic. These include various cognitive and affective capabilities. Empathy requires passion, more so than does equanimity, so long cherished by providers (especially physicians). Early on, Spiro (1992) warned that medical students lose some of their empathy as they learn science and detachment, and hospital residents lose the remainder in the burden of overwork and in the isolation of the intensive care units that modern hospitals have become.

As previously desired, providers may have little to no control or distracting situations in their encounters with patients. Some providers are easily distracted by other pressing concerns. There may be pressures to complete a work assignment, to finish paperwork, or to make it to a meeting. Other distractions of a personal nature (e.g., relationship problems, financial strains, minor health problems, and emotional distress) may contribute to the provider's inability to set aside competing concerns and focus on the patient. Some providers lack the ability to concentrate, which tends to be a trait phenomenon, not a state condition reflective of current stress on the provider.

A second provider barrier is the inability to relax personal self-control sufficiently enough to experience the patient's circumstances. A condition also affected by provider stress is the tendency to regard the patient's condition in terms that are familiar to the provider. Sometimes rigidity narrows the provider's focus to the extent that no new information or new insight is allowed in. When this occurs, provider control works at cross purposes to therapeutic patient encounters. Although provider control makes the patient encounter appear manageable, the truth is that nothing much is managed, except the provider's anxiety. Any assumptions about real management of the patient is illusionary.

Empathy also requires providers to incorporate the patient's experience of forming cognitive associations with what they know. Providers who are unable to concentrate will not be able to complete this process. Those providers who can make the associations but cannot maintain objectivity can participate in reverberation, but they fail to remain detached and fail to complete the cycle by offering salient observations. Errors of this kind may not only be the result of provider stress but also be the result of bad habit.

A final comment that pertains to provider barriers is the individual's ability to identify and witness the pain and agony of patients. As previously stated in this chapter, empathy is an emotional knowing of the patient. The sharing of unpleasant and sometimes painful thoughts and feelings can create an urgency in the provider to do something to block this experience in order to alleviate these feelings. Providers vary in their abilities to witness painful thoughts and feelings, which is due to many factors—including personal vulnerability at certain times to certain patients. It is probably not the case that the provider lacks this courage entirely, but that for whatever reasons, one's tolerance waxes and wanes. Obviously, if the provider exhibits a long-standing inability to be in the presence of patient agony, the healthcare field may not be the career for which he or she is best suited.

Before moving to conditions in the patient that inhibit empathy, some mention of the "burnout syndrome" is appropriate. *Burnout*, sometimes referred to as "the professional stress syndrome" (Gardner & Hall, 1981), refers to a cluster of behaviors intended to protect the provider from identifying too closely with patients. In those professionals in which burnout has continued unchecked, emotional exhaustion is followed by depersonalization (Nayeaux et al., 1982). *Depersonalization* refers to the inability of the provider to experience patients as other than objects. The development of a detached, callous, and even dehumanized response is indicative of depersonalization. Professionals may experience burnout more than once in their career. Sometimes it is accompanied by clinical manifestation of anxiety and depression and even somatic problems like headaches, backaches, or functional disturbances (e.g., in sleep and eating patterns).

Patient Barriers

There are inherent conditions in the patient that may inhibit the level and frequency with which providers can achieve empathic understanding.

Not all patients are open to in-depth exploration of their thoughts and feelings. Some groups of patients regard self-disclosing as a sign of weakness or as a betrayal of relationships with significant others. Patients of this type may not be willing to share their experiences on a more intimate level, even if they could be convinced of its merit. Still other patients may want the provider to understand them but fear disclosure. Disclosure for them may raise concerns about being rejected that may be more painful than not being fully understood in the first place. Risking exposure is highly unlikely, and the provider may need to accept a rather cursory level of communication with the patient that may improve over time.

Some patients accept being known more fully but lack the ability to communicate in words what it is that they do experience. This could be due to problems in health literacy, communication deficits due to illness, or language differences between the patient and provider. In these instances, the provider may feel like a "fishing expedition" has begun, but as the patient and provider have established a common frame of reference with language that suits them both, empathy can improve.

Unlike the circumstances previously described, patients who desire empathy but have difficulty expressing thoughts and feelings may not regard empathic responses as an infringement on their privacy. With this type of patient it is appropriate to try to establish grounds for improved empathy despite the obvious barriers that difference in verbal faculties and language present.

Environmental Barriers

Some providers will tell you: "It isn't me, it isn't the patient. It's the system!" That so-called something else usually refers to the administrative and organizational features of the clinical setting. Active listening, for example, requires the absence of distracting noise. Recounting how a patient's experience fits the provider's knowledge of other patients' experiencing the same trauma requires time in order to piece together facts and observations. Identifying unique aspects of the patient's circumstances requires attention to facts and features not easily derived from patient charts. Providers are "behind the eight-ball" because they frequently practice in environments that are full of distractions where time and individual attention to patients are at a premium. And this appears to be worsening as providers are expected to see more patients within the original time frame.

There is no doubt about the fact that providers practice under challenging circumstances that raise stress levels. In part, this is due to the fact that patients and families experience extraordinary distress. Lack of time to attend to detail is extremely stressful under circumstances of maintaining safe care. Unsafe practice environments may exist that place increasing demands on providers to take professional risks that they are not prepared to manage. Beginning clinicians may be least equipped to manage such care complexities. Unsafe environments create high levels of tension and, of course, such situations are less likely to yield empathic responses from providers.

Consider the following circumstance in which a patient is experiencing excruciating pain and the environment is not conducive to empathic responses.

> The child lies screaming in terror as the clinician proceeds to change dressings covering burns on three-quarters of her body. Noise from patients in the next room, the whirlpool, and providers' communications over the intercom compete with the frightening cries of the young patient. Several other clinicians stand by in silence, appearing numbed to the sounds of the young patient. No one speaks to the patient; they hardly speak to one another.

The barriers to empathic response to this patient are more than those coming from within the providers who are witnessing the patient's agony. They come from the patient's inability to express her fear and also from the circumstances. Debridement of wounds, especially burns, is very difficult to witness. Noise, machines, people trying to communicate, and failure to control the patient's distress all inhibit empathic responsiveness. In actuality, it is these circumstances that present tremendous challenges to providers, and ones they are not likely to forget. Left unexpressed, providers' feelings about this patient care event may influence them adversely in the future as they are confronted with situations that are agonizing to them and to their patients. The absence of empathy, regardless of its cause, hinders therapeutic outcomes, which is the ultimate goal of patient–provider interactions.

CONCLUSION

Discussions of empathy appear in our concerns for humanizing patient care. It has been said that computed tomographic (CT) scans offer no compassion and magnetic resonance imaging (MRIs) have no "human face." Only human beings are capable of empathy (Schatz, 1995). This is not a message to discount the value and contribution of our technical advancements; these screening possibilities help us see things we can otherwise not see. However, empathy is another diagnostic tool, and it is an essential part of our roles as caregivers. Schatz (1995) warns that we must enhance this natural emotion that exists in each of us. Discussions of the roots of our need for detachment and equanimity go back to classic writings of Sir William Osler. Lest the pendulum swing too far and recent trends in communication patterns reduce our abilities to "see within" another, we must protect our capacities for forming empathetic relationships.

In successful empathic responses, providers are able to "stand inside the patient's shoes," participating in the world of the patient while maintaining sufficient objectivity. In more recent teachings, the skill of emotional intelligence depicts our need to both assess and control emotional responses in ourselves and our patients. Sympathy tends to be a reactive response, turning attention to the provider and away from the patient. If providers share the very feelings and needs of the patient, it is likely that they will be unable to provide any help in meeting these needs.

Empathy is a complex phenomenon that involves cognitive, affective, and communicative components. The process of observing the world of another, feeling what it must be like to be that person, yet maintaining separateness from that world, is not a simple process. There are guidelines, steps to be completed that demand attention and concentration abilities. Smith and Hoppe (1991) advocate patient-centered interviewing in order to obtain patients' biopsychosocial stories. This actively involves the patient and ensures that patients' perceptions, needs, and concerns are articulated in the provider (physician)–patient interaction. Evans, Stanley, and Burrows (1993) suggest that the traditional format of interview training and the social ethos of medical training and medical practice result in clinical detachment. Empathy is an important skill that providers need to develop. These authors claim that it helps the provider establish effective communication, which is important for accurate patient diagnosis and patient management. The construct of empathy, however, is complex, incorporating a range of complex emotional and behavioral components not easily taught and not easily evaluated.

There are inherent challenges in achieving empathy. Barriers may come from providers themselves (e.g., their inability to witness difficult patient situations), or they may come from patients who are either unwilling or unable to permit the provider an inside view of their condition. And, finally, barriers are inherent in many healthcare environments in which distractions are commonplace and time and attention to the unique aspects of patients are at risk. Satterfield and Hughes (2007) warn that the medical professionalism of our providers is being challenged by growing demands that may significantly erode the patient–provider relationships.

Empathy can be fostered and barriers can be reduced. If providers are willing to use this therapeutic response, there are no limits to one's capacity to heal—an outcome set in motion by active listening and the capacity to acknowledge and affirm the unique experience of the patient.

CHAPTER 6

Communications That Contribute to Trust and Mistrust of Providers

It is probably obvious to most of us that trust is a difficult quality to achieve and sustain in these days. As a society, we do not seem to trust our government, our institutions (public or private), our professions, or even, in many instances, our traditions. Somehow, we must continue to emphasize regaining, sustaining, and fully deserving the unqualified trust of the patients and society we serve.
—Christopher C. Fordham III

CHAPTER OBJECTIVES

- Define trust as a therapeutic element in patient–provider relationships.
- Differentiate between trust and mistrust in provider–patient relationships.
- List at least three phases in the process of trust building in a therapeutic relationship.
- Describe how trust and confirmation are intimately linked.
- Differentiate between confirmation and disconfirmation.
- Describe the confirming-interaction cycle in provider–patient relationships.

While barriers do exist in every patient–provider relationship, one that should not be ignored is a lack of trust. Trust is critical, and a trusting relationship needs time to build. However, research by Ridsdale, Morgan, and Morris (1992) showed time as a necessary, but not sufficient, condition to promote the greater use of communication techniques by providers.

Critical to the feeling dimension in provider–patient encounters is the phenomena of trust, particularly as it manifests between provider and patient. While it is difficult to tease out the impact of any single communication skill because there is a great deal of overlap, establishing trust is felt to be the single most influential factor behind the patient's acceptance of provider opinion and willingness to engage in positive health-related behaviors.

There is unanimous support for the premise patient trust in providers is a critical aspect of the patient–provider relationship (Kao, Green, Davis, Koplan, & Cleary, 1998; Pearson & Raeke, 2000). It has been referred to as "the cornerstone" (Tarn et al., 2005) and "the bedrock" of medical care (Levinson et al., 1999). A relationship predicated on trust allows for many things to happen. Patient disclosure is more likely when trust exists, and this disclosure is also more complete if the patient trusts the provider. Trust, then, is important to successful patient assessments. Trust also potentiates change. Patients are more likely to attempt new health-related actions (e.g., screening) and adhere to their new medical regimen if a climate of trust exists in their relationships with providers (Thom, Hall, & Pawlson, 2004; O'Malley, Sheppard,

Schwartz, & Mandelblatt, 2004). Finally, trust is particularly important to patients with illnesses and/or injuries that make them feel personally vulnerable. Feelings of helplessness, powerlessness, and hopelessness are eased when patients feel that providers can be trusted. Shenolikar, Balkrishnan, and Hall (2004) address this principle in their study of patient–physician encounters with vulnerable populations. In part, the unpredictability and uncertainty surrounding illness and treatment is lessened when providers can be trusted to behave in positive and predictable ways.

DEFINITIONS OF TRUST AND TRUST-BASED RELATIONSHIP

To *trust* is to rely on the veracity and integrity of another individual. People whose trait is to trust others have confident expectations about the benefits to be derived in relating to others. Trust exists when one individual believes that another individual will behave in ways that are beneficial to the relationship, without controlling or directing either the relationship or the individual (Pearce, 1974). Halbert, Armstrong, Gandy, and Shaker (2006), among others, believe that patients experience trust when they believe that their welfare is placed above all other considerations. Northouse and Northouse (1992) add that trust is defined as an individual's expectation that the communication behaviors of others are reliable. Evidence of trust occurs in patients' perception that providers are sincere, honest, benevolent, and credible in what they do (Berry et al., 2008).

Levels of Trust

In their classic work describing relationship potential, Northouse and Northouse (1992) differentiate between two types of trust—general and specific. According to these authors, *general trust* is the trust that individuals have of other people in a global sense. This kind of trust is consistent much like a trait characteristic. People who generally trust others would be categorized as having a high level of general trust. *Specific trust*, the second type of trust, is the trust an individual has of another person in a specific relationship. People who mistrust a particular provider would be categorized as possessing low specific trust. Trust of this kind depends on the state of current affairs, the specific interaction in the here-and-now. This distinction is important because individuals can manifest high global trust and low specific trust simultaneously. They may also exhibit low global trust and high specific trust. Trust is not something that is just absent or present. It is a complex phenomena that is manifested differently in interpersonal relationships and can change when an individual is involved in specific relationships, in particular situations. In provider–patient relationships, trust occurs when two conditions are met:

1. Trust occurs when patients perceive that providers have their best interests in mind.
2. Trust occurs when patients perceive that these same providers are capable and competent to help them.

For patients to truly trust a provider, both criteria must be met. Consider the contrary. If a patient perceives a certain provider to have his best interests in mind but this provider is judged to lack competence, then the patient may withhold trust. Or, if a patient perceives another provider to be technically competent but uncaring about his or her interests or concerns, trust is likely to be withheld. Feelings of trust create the belief that events are predictable and that providers are both sincere and competent. It follows that beliefs to the contrary evoke suspicion or mistrust. A list of patient beliefs that contribute to mistrust of providers is contained in Exhibit 6–1.

Trust, Respect, and Genuineness

Trust encompasses respect. All patient–provider encounters, if they are to be therapeutic, must be based on respect and genuineness. *Respect* means acknowledging the value of patients and accepting their individuality as well as their unique needs and rights. Communications of this type include listening to patients, acknowledging patients' preferences, giving choices where possible, and treating patients with dignity. *Genuineness* refers to a provider's ability to be open and honest with the patient. Providers who are genuine are congruent in their communications. Their verbal statements are congruent with their verbal and nonverbal communications.

Genuineness is often achieved by self-disclosures; providers' self-disclosures can lead to greater closeness with patients. While provider self-disclosure generally encourages greater intimacy, it is a response mode that warrants careful use. Some disclosures can actually create the opposite effect and create distance.

A critical factor affecting patients' trust of providers is the distancing behaviors that communicate disinterest and lack of concern. Providers' nonverbal communications—for example, avoidance of eye contact, lack of expression, physical distancing, and hesitancy to be in a patient's presence for any significant length of time—create feelings of distrust. These behaviors do not send messages about the provider's incompetence; rather, they tell patients that because the provider lacks concern and caring, he or she does not have their best interests in mind. While interpretations about providers are not

---

Exhibit 6–1 Patient Beliefs and Attitudes Contributing to Provider Mistrust

- You won't like me, approve of me, etc.
- You won't be there when I need you.
- You don't really care about me, my condition, my care.
- You are more concerned about making money (from tests, procedures, etc.) than being honestly interested in me and my care.
- To you I am a guinea pig, a burden, unimportant (compared with other patients you see, things you do).
- You won't be able to help me or my condition.
- You may be helpful; but, something will go wrong and I will not get the care I need.
- You can't possibly know or understand how I feel.

always accurate, the behaviors just cited have indelible effects on patients' assessments of providers. Providers who conduct themselves in this manner will not be convincing in their roles as patient advocates. Neither will they easily persuade patients to alter their health habits.

Trust, like many other aspects of interpersonal relationships, is best viewed on a continuum. That is, patients can exhibit a very high level of trust or a very low level of trust. Somewhere in between are those individuals who exhibit a healthy appropriate level of trust. Beck, Rawlins, and Williams (1988) see the continuum of trust and mistrust including pathological elements; that is, *blind trust* is an example of trusting with insufficient reason. *Pathological mistrust* is at the opposite end of the continuum. The place wherein a person lies on the continuum depends on many factors, including a personality predisposition for trust or distrust and an environment and/or relationship that evokes trust.

While it is true that trust is "earned," it is also true that some individuals have difficulty trusting under any circumstances. Patients' personal health and social histories will reveal clues about their level of trust and the likelihood that trust will come easily. Patients who have been traumatized as youth, those who have been abused as children or adults, and those who experience cognitive impairment may be particularly cautious or guarded. They are suspicious and need to question the motives and/or the behaviors of providers.

Just as trust is earned, it can also be broken. Providers who behave in nurturing ways with their patients one day and then neglect them the next day show inconsistency. If trust requires consistency, inconsistency will deter trusting encounters. It is difficult for patients to trust providers if they cannot depend on them. Dentists who promise their patients pain-free extractions and actually cause pain will evoke mistrust. Thus, energy that could or should be directed toward coping with the pain gets confused with the patient's need to assess the provider's true level of caring and trustworthiness.

Sometimes patients will deliberately test the sincerity and trustworthiness of the provider. As long as the provider recognizes this potential and sets appropriate limits, such tests hardly ever result in broken trust.

Trust and Mistrust

Patients who mistrust typically behave differently than those who trust. They might communicate with defensiveness. They might be guarded in their speech or be altogether noncommunicative. They can exhibit suspiciousness and caution. In contrast, patients who have healthy levels of trust are generally more open and responsive. They are likely to communicate hope and faith and are willing to take risks under provider guidance.

The early origins of trust emanate from infancy, where individuals learn trust based on what they see, hear, and experience. Beginning feelings of confidence and faith stem from learning that they will receive or have done what is needed. Parents and caregivers perform these functions early on; but, in time, self-confidence results from perceiving that one is self-reliant.

The process that patients go through in becoming confident in their abilities to render self-care parallel this primary experience. That is, trust in providers is felt, and with it comes a growing trust in one's own abilities to get what is needed. Identification with the provider and the helping relationship enables patients to experiment with and become adept at aspects of self-care. Patients who look back on learning self-care measures (e.g., giving themselves intramuscular injection medications, testing their urine, or caring for their colostomy) may comment that they never thought they would be capable of these tasks. Through trust in the provider, patients learn to cope with their limitations, master skills, and resolve problems and frustrations related to their health conditions.

Thus, positive outcomes arise from trusting relationships. Trust creates a climate of support. It also produces feelings of comfort and security. Additionally, because it reduces defensive communication, it generally yields more complete and honest disclosures. Because of this, the process of establishing trust is taken very seriously.

THE PROCESS OF ESTABLISHING TRUST

Concerns about trust surface in beginning encounters with patients. Patients' trust in providers usually evolves over time as the patient tests both competence and respectfulness of the provider. An important consideration today is whether current delivery systems and realities of health care defer the establishment of trust.

The emotional climate of initial encounters may be guarded. Patients may avoid risking self-disclosure until they observe that providers are acting on their behalf. When we speak of the process of establishing trust, we are referring to the establishment of a good relationship based on mutual trust. Trust specific to a relationship is not arrived at quickly.

The phases of a therapeutic relationship are described in several ways. These phases are usually conceived of in three stages; however, some models contain four or more stages or substages. The model presented here addresses the specific issues of self-disclosure and trust. For a relationship to be therapeutic, respect, honesty, and consistency are critical; but, the essential variable of trust and the beliefs congruent with a trusting relationship are even more essential to provider–patient interactions.

The Initiation Phase

The first phase is termed the *initiation* phase, also referred to as the introductory or orientation phase. This phase consists of the very first contact between provider and patient. Whether through a telephone conversation or an actual face-to-face encounter, this contact sets the tone and climate for the relationship. Initially, the provider's demeanor, attentiveness, and responsiveness give patients an idea of what to expect. But, as Doescher, Saver, Franks, and Fiscella (2000) explain, this is only a rough indicator of how the relationship might evolve as the patient and provider become more acquainted. The essential importance of this initial contact with respect to trust is that the potential for trust is scrutinized. Patients in this phase are likely to project onto the provider attitudes from former relationships that may have been positive, neutral, or, in some cases, negative. The expectations of patients based on previous experience surface and begin to be confirmed or altered. Additionally, providers may have developed preconceptions of the patient, and these impressions are validated and/or revised in this initial phase.

In these initial interactions, it is the provider's obligation to establish a climate that is conducive to trust. This climate includes expressions of respect and caring in a context of genuineness and consistency. These elements, sometimes referred to as a supportive relationship, enhance or foster the possibility that a trusting relationship will result. Any pre-interaction expectations that have negative effects on trust must be changed or revised for the patient.

Some providers develop preconceptions of patients that include expectations that the patient cannot be trusted, will be unreliable in following directives, and will lack faith in the treatment plan. The provider's own preconceptions must be tested in this initial phase.

Initial encounters that display understanding and caring for the patient are important because they help dispel patients' anxieties and fears surrounding their health and any care that they may require. The supportive, nonthreatening aspects of this encounter make it easier for patients to share their fears and concerns. Beliefs patients have that contribute to mistrust must be countered with factual information or sequential experience. As seen in Exhibit 6–1, examples of beliefs specific to the relationship that may create mistrust, or at least present barriers to trust, are listed. Sometimes these beliefs depict patients' overall global perspectives on relationships. Whether they reflect global or specific attitudes, they are potentially destructive to the therapeutic relationship.

Putting the patient at ease is not only achieved by the general tone or climate of the encounter, it is also achieved by specific communication strategies. One very common strategy is the use of "small talk." This would include comments about finding the clinic or office, about the waiting period, or comments about the weather or time of day. Small talk has the potential for putting the patient at ease because it reveals the humanness of the provider—that providers are people and are affected by the same earthly events or conditions that affect patients. Sometimes this small talk includes humor, which also seems to reduce initial tension.

Not all providers are comfortable with small talk. There are some pitfalls in engaging the patient superficially. First, the patient may judge the provider's comments or attempts as superficial and insincere. Even more problematic is the patient's interpretation that the provider is not amenable to serious discussions. For these reasons, small talk is frequently replaced by nonverbal expressions of caring and more direct commentary about how the provider envisions the encounter. Small talk can also be problematic for providers because the shift to more important health issues may be difficult to bridge once this superficial tone has been established.

Trust, then, begins with an initial testing of preconceptions and early attempts to place the patient at ease. These steps are not sufficient, however, either in establishing trust or in completing the initial phase.

Recall that trust is built on the perception that providers are reliable. It follows, then, that an important aspect of creating trust is the task of clarifying the purpose and procedures in a patient encounter. This includes a description of how care is usually rendered and what can be expected at different points in time. While the purpose of contacts is usually clear, the procedure or process to meet the treatment aims is not. For example, patients may understand that the purpose of their visit is a physical exam. The exact steps they must take and when and if they will need X-rays or lab work is not always specified. Additionally, the relationships between these procedures and the original purpose may be unclear. The patient may understand that he is having a follow-up exam but be unclear about how a certain test gives evidence of his recovery.

It is important when communicating the purpose of procedures to give complete information. Partial explanations or incomplete instructions will only serve to increase patients' anxieties. It is always important to give patients sufficient time to ask questions and to obtain enough feedback to put them at ease. Their inability to obtain clarification in a timely manner will serve to be a significant barrier to their trusting providers.

Although this is changing, among many communities, patients think that providers are powerful and know everything. If providers do not elevate the patient's knowledge, then providers are suspect. They are suspected to be uncaring, unable to understand, or, worse yet, incompetent. Any one of these scenarios creates distrust. And, once in place, it is difficult to convince a patient of the contrary. Providers sometimes try to "cover their tracks" with explanations that they are too busy or do not have enough time to provide patients with the necessary factual information. These explanations are generally perceived as weak and inadequate excuses. Refer back to the definition of a trusting relationship: patients want to be convinced that they take priority over other considerations.

Explanations about what to expect and what procedures will occur will provide additional structure to the encounter—structure that gives meaning to the actions that are to follow. Eliciting the patient's willingness to participate, however, is a separate intervention, albeit following naturally as a consequence of the providers' description of the purpose. In many provider–patient contacts, this agreement is taken for granted (i.e., the patient is assumed to accept and be willing to follow the providers' directives). Consider, for example, that patients are generally expected to accept such things as lab work, X-rays, and the taking of vital signs without needing clarification or even without giving their explicit consent. What underlying assumptions operate to suggest that patients have, in fact, agreed? We would say that if patients objected, they could register this objection. However, there is an implied contractual arrangement between provider and patient that is important to understand. Provider and patient roles are, in fact, social roles. Complementary role behavior in most provider–patient interactions consists of the helper (provider) doing something to help the helpee (patient). It is understood that once an encounter has occurred, professional responsibility dictates the performance of role behavior. Appropriate complementary role behavior includes patients' responsibilities to receive the care that is presented to them by providers who are recognized as clinical and professional experts. Unless otherwise cued to be more assertive, they might be hesitant in expressing their objections.

Informal contracts are generally replaced with specific mutually agreed-upon plans of action. In health care, these plans are communicated verbally and in writing in the patient's chart. A mutually agreed-upon plan of action depends on goals that are clear and fully communicated. The mutuality behind goal formulation, by definition, implies that the care plan is not imposed on the patient. Rather, it is based on collaboration between the patient and the provider.

A level of mutually agreed-upon care planning would seem to be impossible without sufficient trust. First, mutual goal-setting requires patient self-disclosure. This level of revelation occurs under conditions of trusting attitudes. Second, for any patient to explicitly agree on a plan of action, he or she must be convinced of the provider's competence and goodwill. Thus, it is safe to say that a provider–patient relationship will falter at the point of a mutually agreed-upon plan if trust has not sufficiently been established beforehand.

There are specific problems in communicating about plans of care that do not enlist patients in the decision-making process. While these problems may not reflect a lack of trust, they will affect the level of trust that will emerge in the provider–patient relationship. First, providers may withhold health data or test results because they believe the patient cannot or is not yet ready to deal openly with the information. Second, providers may move too quickly over descriptions of the plans, leaving the patient with an incomplete and sometimes confusing understanding of what things mean and what will happen next. Patients who express experiences, for example, of not thinking to ask the provider about something during the visit are demonstrating that the communication was rushed or devoid of good feedback exchange. Another example is when the provider spends time communicating but patients are unable to understand the information they are given, perhaps due to low literacy, fear, anxiety, or some other factor (physically or emotionally). Problems of no trust or of inadequate trust in the initial phase have significant implications for the treatment or implementation phase.

The Implementation Phase

Implementation of a course of action whether it is a structure for assessing health or treating disease is ideally grounded in a relationship of mutual trust. During this phase, assuming that trust is in place, the provider and patient are mutually engaged in confronting and working on health problems.

A major role of the provider in the implementation phase is to help patients cope with and master threats to their health. This includes instruction in health-related changes as well as giving provider feedback from clinical assessments that will help evaluate the success of the medical regimen.

As a rule, this phase does not proceed without disruptions and barriers. The first barrier is reluctance. To put a plan into action, the patient must accept the authoritative opinions of the provider. If the patient is not convinced of the provider's competence, then forward movement will not occur, even if the patient expresses commitment to the treatment goals.

A common problem that also relates to patients' faith in their treatment is that the plan of action may not result in expected and desired outcomes. Failed approaches are sometimes interpreted as provider incompetency. Failed plans can also be internalized, and patients may blame themselves for failed attempts. If patients fail to comply and deliberately fail to follow directives, then this cause of personal failure is realistic. However, patient guilt about treatment failures can be irrational much of the time.

Whether the provider's competence or the patient's responsibility is perceived to be at the crux of the problem, failed treatment can severely threaten mutual trust and subsequent therapeutic encounters. It is advisable to discuss the results of interventions fully and completely, pinpointing reasons these actions fell short of expectations. Providers who are trustworthy are willing to discuss failures and successes. Trust, if damaged, can be restored. However, failed treatment can result in patients failure to return and must be addressed openly and honestly.

An important component of trust building and maintenance in this phase is the process of assisting patients to manage the impact that illnesses or the threat of illness may have on them. Providers who not only address disease but also the impact of disease will convince patients of their caring and concern. Appropriate supportive self-management is critical.

Because providers do not customarily address patients' reactions to their illnesses, it is important to explore why this might be the case. One explanation is that providers do not recognize this aspect of a patient's experience as germane to their discipline or as important to the patient. Recent research on patients' quality of life criticizes the preoccupation with a "cure" approach. With an emphasis on patients' quality of life comes a commitment to patients' responses to their illnesses and treatment regimens.

Another explanation for providers ignoring patients' ways of coping with their illnesses and treatments is providers' inability to confidently deal with this aspect of patients' experiences. While this is a possibility, there is also increasing evidence that providers are being encouraged to deal with patients' coping responses in therapeutic ways and are actually promoting patients' abilities to cope more effectively.

Just as in the initial phase, the implementation phase can produce problems that are unique to the level of intimacy expected of provider and patient. One problem is the provider's inability to appropriately deliver advice and directives. Inappropriate advice-giving or too-zealous confrontation can disturb patients and actually cause them to withdraw. Responding in stereotypic or evaluative ways can also negatively influence patients. Trust, once secured in the initial phase, might be at risk. However, in most cases the ongoing experience of the patient in relationship to the provider usually encourages patients to explore concerns, disappointments, or conflicts. At this phase, patients are not likely to abruptly terminate the relationship, even if there has been treatment failures. This is a generality that applies to all patients, although some patients will be more apt to stick it out while others will think nothing of aborting a treatment plan and leaving the provider. These situations are always important and, if not fully explored with the initial provider, should be addressed with the new provider.

The Termination Phase

If all goes well, the helping relationship that is initially established will survive the course of an illness. This includes the vicissitudes of treatment where plans are not always successful and barriers to sustained trust have been dealt with. The termination phase is that point in time when the therapeutic relationship is closed. Closure ideally occurs because goals have been accomplished and there are no further apparent needs for care. It is the case that many patient–provider relationships, however, end abruptly or before care is no longer necessary. Patients may require referrals, may leave the geographical area, or their health may deteriorate to the point that a different level of care is required.

The primary principle behind a successful termination is ample preparation. This means that providers should discuss termination and discharge issues with the client from the start in the initiation phase. One might ask, however, in the current state of healthcare delivery, if lack of continuity in the patient–provider relationship influences how "termination" occurs.

While the major issue is the appropriateness of the closure, the major task when this issue is resolved is to draw the lines of separation. Officially, termination means no longer being responsible for treatment decisions. It is extremely important that the patient fully understands the conditions of this phase.

Patients, particularly those who have learned to trust and value the provider, may have difficulty relinquishing their emotional ties to the provider. This reluctance is an important signal to providers to specify and clarify the meaning of ending the relationship.

One difficulty that may occur and that is potentially very detrimental to patients is the patient's assumption that the provider is still very much in a provider role with them. Sometimes they will incompletely execute a referral because they think, or at least feel, that they can return to discuss their complaints with their original provider. Because of this, providers must clearly indicate how the patient needs to proceed if certain symptoms or needs surface. This plan may include returning to the original provider, but if it does not, patients need to be given clear directives about the appropriate means of getting the care that they feel they need.

Using final encounters with which to review the care plan and course of treatment, including discussions of successes and failures, will not only provide the patient with perspective but also reaffirm the professional aspects of the relationship. Terminations of treatment are always accompanied by written documentation to the patient, with copies to the medical record, regardless of whether closure occurred in a face-to-face encounter or not.

Problems associated with terminating care include:

- Providers failing to communicate clearly and fully the conditions of closure.
- Providers failing to handle the patients' emotional responses to terminating the relationship.
- Providers inappropriately continuing relationships despite the advisability of closing treatment.

In summary, each one of the several phases of the provider–patient relationship is affected by patient trust in providers. Therapeutic alliances are believed to proceed through these phases. Trust is a factor that can sufficiently affect the speed and quality of progression, and without trust, chances for a therapeutic alliance can be seriously derailed. Progress, whether it includes gathering patient data for a comprehensive assessment or persuading patients to change health-related behaviors, will not be possible.

TRUST AND CONFIRMATION: AN IMPORTANT CONNECTION

As previously indicated, one dimension of trust is patients' observations that providers have their best interests in mind. It was also suggested that without satisfying this element, trust would not occur. Provider competence is only one part of the picture. A bias toward a patient's best interests is communicated to patients through various behaviors. A listing of provider-based behaviors and specific communications that can evoke trusting responses are found in Exhibit 6–2. Several of these confirm the patient's value as an individual and were previously addressed in Chapter 5. Acknowledging the value of patients is a necessary part of conveying concern for their best interests. However, confirmation is a distinct way of communicating acknowledgment and acceptance. It plays a unique role in patient–provider communication.

Confirmation Response Modes

As indicated in the classic writings of Northouse and Northouse (1992), *confirmation* refers to specific verbal and nonverbal responses that acknowledge and display acceptance of the patient. Trust is intimately linked with providers' communications that confirm patients.

The origins of the belief that confirmation can be helpful are embedded in existentialism. Buber (1957) believed that all individuals want to be confirmed and accepted for what they are and what they can become. Laing (1967) was also interested in the implications of confirmation but focused on the consequences of disconfirming communications. Laing described the opposite of confirmation to be those attempts to constrain another, forcing actions with ultimate lack of concern and indifference to the other.

Further understanding of confirmation was also an outcome of studies by Sieburg (1969) of small-group interaction. In analyzing ways of responding

---

Exhibit 6–2 Provider Behaviors That Evoke Trust

Global behaviors
- Honesty.
- Consistency.
- Respect and caring, openness, and genuineness.
- Reliability, adequate follow-up, and follow-through.
- Congruence between verbal and nonverbal communication.

Specific communications
- Direct acknowledgment, appreciation of patient's uniqueness.
- Informing about and clarifying expectations.
- Continued supportive responsiveness.
- Verbal expressions of positive regard, including respect, warmth, and caring.
- Active listening.
- Nonverbal expressions of positive regard—smiling, appropriate eye contact, warmth in tone of voice, and approachable body posture.

and peoples' preferences in interactions, two distinct factors were isolated through factor analysis. One was a set of responses that confirmed the person and that were largely supportive and expressed positive feelings. The other set ignored and/or mistreated the unique contributions of the person. The first factor was labeled *confirmation*; the second, *disconfirmation*.

According to Sieburg (1969) confirming responses can validate an individual in three ways:

1. Confirming responses acknowledge the presence of another and decrease a person's fears of depersonalization. This obvious but extremely important step in patient–provider encounters includes such things as acknowledging the physical presence of the patient and attending directly to what the patient is saying or doing to avoid patients feeling like inanimate objects.
2. Confirming responses validate the individual's own way of experiencing events; thus relieving fears of blame or rejection when those experiences differed from others' perceptions of events. In patient–provider encounters, this component is conveyed in responses that reinforce or support what the patient is saying and in expressions of understanding and reassurance.
3. Confirming responses also reduce feelings of isolation and alienation because they create clear messages of being in relationship with another. In patient–provider encounters, responses that ask for further information and encourage patients' expressions of concern in greater detail not only make patients' thoughts, feelings, and concerns more understandable, they communicate the relational aspects of the contact where mutual understanding is important.

Disconfirming Responses

If confirming responses make persons feel valued and acknowledged as unique individuals, *disconfirming responses* do the opposite. Disconfirming responses value the person less and may cause the person to devalue himself. In health care, disconfirming responses deny the existence of patients.

In the early work of Sieburg (1969), several examples of disconfirming responses from actual interpersonal interaction were identified. These behaviors included five specific responses: impervious, interruptive, irrelevant or tangential, impersonal, and incoherent. They are defined here:

1. *Impervious* responses ignore or disregard the other person's attempt to communicate, such as offering no verbal response to what the other has said.
2. *Interruptive* responses cut the other person off before a feeling, thought, or idea is fully communicated.
3. *Irrelevant* or *tangential* responses react in unrelated ways to what the other person has communicated. These comments may also be tangential if they take the conversation in another direction than the initial focus.
4. *Impersonal* responses genuinely communicate distance; they may intellectualize or communicate separateness such as by using the third person.

5. *Incoherent* responses are those that are incomplete or otherwise misunderstandable. They may contain long, rambling explanations. Incongruous responses or acts reveal discrepancies between what one says and what one really means.

Confirming-Interaction Cycle

Confirmation is needed by both patient and provider. Northouse and Northouse (1992) stressed that confirmation is mutually distributed in the patient–provider relationship and that providers are also in need of confirmation from patients. It is difficult, for example, to confirm a patient when the patient responds in a disconfirming manner. Additionally, providers who are disconfirming in their approach are likely to get disconfirmed.

There is some evidence that confirmation is a cyclic phenomena. Patients may feel that they are not valued, but so may providers. The interaction between patient and provider can either worsen or lessen the feelings of being unimportant or insignificant. Further, providers may treat each other in disconfirming ways, and this may affect their feelings about themselves and their abilities to give confirmation to others. While the continuum may be viewed at any point, the idea is that one person will feel disconfirmed or confirmed and respond in turn to another person in a disconfirming or confirming manner.

One would hypothesize that patients who receive confirming responses may feel differently from those who receive disconfirming responses. In all likelihood, patients who are dissatisfied with their care are probably those patients who have been treated in disconfirming ways. Additionally, patients who receive more confirming than disconfirming responses may experience greater confidence in their ability to deal successfully with the demands of their illness or the threat of illness. As indicated earlier, patients who get embroiled in the relational aspects of their care lack energy to cope with their illness. Because their energy is siphoned off, they may also have less energy to participate in self-care measures.

The cycle becomes evident. The provider may be feeling disconfirmed, either unimportant or even disenfranchised from the helping process. This provider enters into a contract with the patient but lacks the emotional energy to affirm and acknowledge the patient. Consequently, the patient—already vulnerable to threats of isolation and alienation—may increase the prospect for disconfirming responses by being argumentative or resistant to the provider. We would expect then that patients' disconfirming responses would make the provider feel more unappreciated and unsuccessful. This chain of responses could be broken by either the patient, an outside person, or a provider, or it could continue for a period of time.

An example of disconfirmation can be observed in the following situation. First, the provider enters the encounter with good intentions to help the patient to take his medication appropriately. Second, the patient takes it upon himself to do as he sees necessary which includes deviating from the prescribed directions. Third, the provider senses that something like this is occurring and recognizes that she really doesn't know how the patient is taking his medication. In this situation, the provider feels mistrusted and disconfirmed and consequently develops concerns about treating the patient. The patient might perceive some hesitancy on the part of the provider and question the degree to which the relationship can help him. What might occur here is an abrupt termination. Clearly, the cycle of disconfirmation was set in motion with both the patient and provider falling victim to the process.

Interruption of the cycle requires a realization of the dynamic factors that are involved in producing hurtful feelings. Interacting at the peer level to obtain provider mutual respect can alter the initial sensitivity that providers have. Assessing the chainlike quality in the interaction with the patient is important in the continued assessment of patient–provider interactions. Finally, providers' conscious and deliberate efforts to confirm patients, even if they are still feeling somewhat disconfirmed, potentially relieve the tension between patient and provider and reconstruct encounters to be more confirming.

As previously emphasized, confirming interactions build trust. Disconfirming encounters present barriers to trust building. It is important that providers evaluate this dimension of the relationship if they are to build and sustain trusting relationships with their patients and patients' families.

CONCLUSION

The purpose of therapeutic patient–provider contacts is not only to obtain information needed to assess patients but also to establish a relationship that serves as the context for a working alliance between the patient and the provider. Provider–patient encounters are effective to the degree to which important data can be obtained and health behaviors negotiated.

Trust is so basic to provider–patient relationships that it is often taken for granted. We know that trust, defined here as confidence in provider competence and perceptions that providers have one's best interests in mind, is critical to therapeutic alliances. Trust in providers helps patients deal with the fears and uncertainties surrounding their care and conditions. Patients are simply unable to do many of the things providers do, and in many ways are forced to depend on providers. Patients need to see professionals as competent and caring individuals. Providers who want to foster trust will seek to build their professional-clinical credibility as well as their reputations to be interpersonally trustworthy.

Patients may have generalized global trust of most things and people or they may be inherently suspicious and guarded. They may also display a range of trust with specific providers and in specific contexts. Sometimes patients are generally trusting individuals but have a specific mistrust of healthcare providers or healthcare delivery systems. Patients' reactions to hospitals is a case in point; most patients (and many providers) mistrust what occurs or could occur in hospitals. This mistrust can originate from previous negative or traumatic experience or from a lack of information. Each time a patient encounters a new provider and/or new system, trust must be negotiated, or renegotiated.

The ability to create trust in the patient–provider relationship is dependent on certain individual predispositions as well as specific communication strategies. Approaches that demonstrate honesty, genuineness, comfort and caring, competence, encouraging, explaining, and asking questions contribute to faith in providers (Thom, 2001). Without the ingredient of trust, the therapeutic alliance will be vacuous.

Trust can be enhanced through individual- and system-level factors. Provider training in trust building is critical. Also, institutional commitment to building trust in their patient populations through securing quality care is important. Providers might lament that there are too many demands on their time during this era of managed care to build trust in their relationships with patients. Still very vulnerable patients in acute care settings who do not have the luxury of long, continuous processes to build sound relationships are expected to put their trust in providers (Axelrod & Gould, 2000). No matter how forced or fragile, patients will develop expectations of beneficence, even in emergency and surgical situations. While the building of trust does take time, it is a task that cannot be neglected even under the most challenging situations and in this era of greater demands on provider time. Thom, Hall, and Pawlson (2004) optimistically summarize the potential of trusting patient–provider relationships by explaining that lower levels of trust can be changed and improved trust might reduce disparities, increase access to care, and improve health outcomes. It is not that we cannot afford to build trust; rather, we cannot afford not to build trust. Learning communication skills help providers attain and preserve patient–provider relationships.

CHAPTER 7

The Art and Skillful Use of Questions

What you want to know is not in the answer to your question—
but, I'll answer it anyway.
—Anonymous Patient (1994)

CHAPTER OBJECTIVES

- Describe different ways in which questions can be used therapeutically.
- Differentiate between the therapeutic use of questions and the nontherapeutic use of questions.
- List ways in which questions can be used with deleterious consequences.
- List and describe three suggested formats for questions.
- Explain how the choice of question format can significantly lessen or increase the client's response burden.

Asking an answerable question is one of the most important skills to be learned. Pawar (2005) maintains that perhaps the most critical skill in uncovering the needs of a patient is that of inquiry. Patients' answers to our questions are part of the database around which we collaboratively determine and evaluate their care. Health histories and the majority of the patient's physical assessment are the direct result of the skillful use of questions on the part of the provider. Thus, a primary goal of patient interviews is essentially to elicit information from patients about their condition. For this process to occur effectively, the provider must have knowledge of, as well as skill and judgment in, the art of questioning. This chapter will review basic principles behind the use of questions.

THERAPEUTIC USE OF QUESTIONS

One of the most common modes of human communication involves the use of questions. These questions are generally formatted as who, when, where, what, and why questions. Questions are customarily the primary tool for healthcare providers because providers are diagnostically driven and are continually seeking to assess patients. In fact, the provider role is characterized by the privilege, expectation, or habit of asking questions. For the most part, providers engage the patient in an interpersonal context through the use of questions (Tongue, Epps, & Forese, 2005). Familiar openings include: "What brings you here today?", "How are you feeling?", and "What seems to be the problem?" Tongue and colleagues suggest that we should be careful with the use of some questions that place the patient in the awkward position of answering, "Fine." Although typical salutations are common, other ways of engaging the patient are preferable.

Questions yield data; data provide information needed to begin our assessment. There has been much evidence to suggest that when information exchange is weakened, the quality of health care, including costs of care also suffer. Incomplete information inhibits our ability to distinguish the best care and can lead to unnecessary tests and referrals. Providers use several types of questions to obtain, clarify, and specify information about the condition of the patient. According to Nunnolly and Moy (1989), questions allow the provider to follow, focus in depth, and redirect if necessary.

Collecting Information

As previously indicated, the most basic use of questions is merely to begin the dialogue. From there, a provider becomes focused and moves more quickly into specific questions. When the patient provides ambiguous or unclear statements, the provider is challenged to alter the question format to meet the specific challenges of communicating with the patient.

Questions can be likened to "an invitation" to patients to collaborate in identifying problems and creating solutions. In this sense, questions are lead-ins for the patient to begin talking. Information collected from a patient may involve health history data (e.g., previous diseases, surgeries, hospitalizations, and medications). It will also include sociocultural data dealing with age, income, race, ethnicity, years of education, marital status, and number of dependents. Although this information appears to be straightforward and easy to extract, this is not the case. For example, unless the patient has made a point of bringing a list of concerns and questions and an outline of her health history, she may not know or remember her health histories. Data about primary language, literacy, and cultural background may be sensitive, and patients may be suspicious about why providers are interested. Yet, to be seen in a diabetic clinic or for hypertension, for example, it is helpful to understand a patient's background and perception of health issues. Information about their sociocultural background (e.g., immigration status), religious affiliation, and even marital status can be sensitive topics, and patients are not readily convinced that responding to these kinds of questions is a good idea. Some questions can elicit shame, fear, guilt, and embarrassment. For this reason, the skillful use of questions may make the difference between incompleteness and completeness and accuracy of data collected. Giving the patient choices about the amount of data disclosed (if it is not directly related to his condition) and the context in which the data are provided (privately) are always important principles to keep in mind.

Clarifying and Specifying

Because patients are not usually able to assemble information in ways that are meaningful to healthcare providers, a second function of the use of questions is to clarify and specify the information provided by the patient. In this case, the provider begins to focus on relevant areas as the conversation unfolds.

For example, when a patient complains of abdominal pain, the clinician wants to know the location, character, and severity of the pain. This assessment requires assisting the patient to clarify and specify features of her experience of the pain. Is it a dull or sharp pain? A radiating pain or localized pain? Is it low grade or very severe? These data are needed from the patient and require providers to focus their questions to elicit specificity. While exploratory questions are generally useful, a carefully worded question that seeks clarification or specificity of patients' accounts of their experience is critical in this appraisal process.

When patients are having difficulty describing their experience due to immediate distress, language deficits, or some other barrier, the provider must thoughtfully sort through those phrases or words that will prompt clarification. Using the patients' own terms or phrases can be quite useful. If patients refer to their pain as "pressure," then providers can seek to clarify this "pressure." The provider uses the patients' terms to engage them further in the collaborative effort to define their problem.

In conducting a health history, performing a physical exam, or delivering care, it is very important that the provider become specific in the data required. For example, when changing dressings, the provider will need to know exactly which moves are extraordinarily painful and which are less painful. Questions that are focused help to specify the experience and reduce distress from the procedure. Carefully chosen questions direct and focus the interview or assessment in productive ways.

Ruling Out/Ruling In

Ruling out and ruling in is a way of gaining specificity on patients' concerns. Ruling-out questions include questions that seek clarity and are generally more direct (e.g., "Does the pain extend to your left shoulder?"). They also can require the patient to observe a phenomena, compare the experience, and choose a response that fits the choices that the provider has given (e.g., "If I press here, do you feel the pain as sharply as you do now in your left shoulder?").

Some ruling-out and ruling-in questions require patients to recall past experiences and compare them with present experience. For example, the provider might ask: "Does this medication cause you to feel nauseated if you take it before a meal?" And, "Is the nausea you feel different from what you always feel?" In this dialogue, the provider is seeking to pinpoint and rule out various possibilities and might have certain hypotheses about what the problem is.

In summary, while questions seem to have very specific information gathering purposes in the clinical interview, they also have a more subtle secondary effect of providing reassurance. Sometimes questions are used in a slow-moving encounter as a filler. An occasional question lets the patient know that the provider is listening and attentive to the patient's concerns and needs. Pawar (2005) reminds providers to "think dialogue, not monologue" by asking questions, exploring concerns, and making connections. Rather than hearing concerns and responding with an immediate solution, all dialogue with patients require digging deeper.

NONTHERAPEUTIC USE OF QUESTIONS

Questions are the primary vehicle for therapeutic communication with the patient. While they provide the basis for effective interviewing they can also be misused. Thus, questions can be used therapeutically or nontherapeutically. The following discussion highlights various ways in which questions can be inappropriately positioned in provider–patient interactions.

Interpretative Purposes

Sometimes providers pose questions as interpretations. Interpretative questions are not used to collect data; they are used to give information. An example would be: "If you choose not to let your daughter have braces, wouldn't that make you an irresponsible parent?" The point is that the provider is not interested in whether the parent shares this opinion or needs to be further engaged in dialogue to come to this solution herself. The provider appears to be more interested in the mother knowing that if she refuses having braces for her daughter, she is neglecting the health of her child. While this interaction focuses around a question, no new information is sought. Under the guise of this question, the provider delivers an opinion and an interpretation of the parent's behavior. In some sense, it is a disguised accusation.

Self-Disclosure Purpose

A second type of question used to give, not request, information is the self-disclosure question. An example would be: "Do you know that your rolling back on the bed (after I got you in position) is making it hard on me?" In this scenario, the provider wants to tell the patient not to do something; instead of being direct and clear, the provider uses a question instead. The question is another form of a telling response. It tells what the provider is experiencing (i.e., difficulty and hardship). The underlying message might be missed. Several patients might be confused by this comment. However, the patient might also get the point that the provider is irritated while the message, "Don't move," is missed.

Advisement Purpose

A third type of question that tells and does not ask is one that gives advice. Consider the following question: "Don't you think that if you take a little juice first, that pill will be easier to swallow?" Behind this question is a piece of advice: "It will be easier to take your pill if you drink some juice first." Usually when providers put advice in the form of a question, they are attempting to soften their advice and appear less authoritative and paternalistic. They may actually believe that they will have greater success in changing the patient's behavior if this advice is indirect because direct advice is offensive and might elicit negative, resistant behaviors.

Telling questions, presented as self-disclosures, interpretations, or advisements, are used when direct telling is seen to be too harsh or in some other way ill advised. The provider may think that directness is too disrespectful. Telling questions may be viewed as more tactful and sometimes kinder ways of making observations or stating opinions. However, they are problematic. The major problem is that telling questions can be confusing. It is not always wise to be more tactful with advice when it is absolutely essential that the advice be followed. The repeated use of telling questions can also be distracting and annoying to patients. Some patients mistrust the manipulative quality of this form of communication. Because trust is the cornerstone of effective self-disclosure on the part of the patient, using telling questions carries a risk. A good rule of thumb is to use as few telling questions as possible. Even though one might use them to vary the structure and pace of the dialogue, if questions that honestly gather information are to be believed, questions that tell should be avoided. Interpretation, self-disclosure, and advice are more appropriately delivered directly.

Questions, whether telling or authentically data-gathering, can be used defensively. Using questions defensively is also inappropriate. Questions are used defensively to evade the spotlight. Beginning practitioners, when confronted with patients who ask direct and personal questions of them, might answer a question with a question. Being asked, for example, if they are married may be something the provider finds inappropriate. Furthermore, the process of being asked a number of personal and direct questions by the patient may be disconcerting because it is the provider who needs to be doing the questioning. The provider responds defensively to evade the spotlight and to avoid the anxiety of the moment.

Indirect questions are often used in place of other stronger response modes. Consider this question used by the provider to inquire about the patient's mood: "You seem angry today. Are you angry about something?" Such a question is less blunt than using the reflective statement, "You're angry." The former question simply requests the patient's verbal response; it does not challenge the patient as the reflective statement, "You're angry," seems to.

Deleterious Use of the Direct Question

Perhaps the most frequently misused question format is the use of endless direct questions. Examples of direct questions would include: "Are you taking your medicine?", "Are you following the diet and exercise plan I gave you?", and "Did you use the ice packs every 2 to 4 hours?" There is no formula about how many direct questions can be asked within a particular period of time. However, asking direct questions in machine-gun-like fashion is inappropriate. Repeated direct questions may have several negative effects on the patient–provider relationship (Gazda, Childers, & Walters, 1982). In their earlier work, Gazda and colleagues identified several undesirable outcomes that may occur if direct questions are misused. A number of these are described here.

The first problem they cite is the creation of a dependent relationship. The use of multiple direct questions can give the effect of provider "takeover"; the respondent learns to expect that important outcomes are a result of provider dominance.

A second deleterious effect, related to the first, is that direct questions can put the responsibility for problem solving on the helper. The provider, assuming the role of expert by asking many direct questions, conveys to the patient that a solution is forthcoming. The provider's solution, however, is not always one the patient can use. Although prescriptive actions are appropriate, much more of medical practice is the result of collaborative patient–provider problem solving.

Responding passively to direct questions prevents patients from actively modifying solutions so that the solutions work uniquely for them.

Patients who take a less active role in formulating solutions are also less likely to accept responsibility for their behavior. Overreliance on experts primes the patient to hold the provider responsible for success or failure of the treatment plan. Again, use of direct questions by the provider might have the impact of lessening the willingness of patients to be active participants in designing and evaluating their care.

Another important deleterious effect of direct questions is their tendency to result in information that might not be altogether valid. Almost every direct question has within it the preferred answer (Gazda et al., 1982). Consider the following direct questions:

- "Are you ready for your bath?"
- "Would you like help getting out of your chair?"
- "Would you like to be discharged tomorrow morning?"

In every case, the patient can read between the lines; their answers should be affirmative because that is what the provider expects. Most patients want to be agreeable, approved of, and liked by providers. Conversely, they may fear that if they disagree, their care will suffer. If this is the case, they are more likely to answer as they assume the provider wants them to. The agreement elicited merely reflects the patient's obligatory response to the provider. The fact that a patient is not really ready to have his bath or that he wants to go home but he thinks his family is not ready to care for him yet goes unexpressed. Thus, the brief response to the question, whether yes or no, may not be the true picture of the patient's preference and gives incomplete information about the patient's circumstances.

An additional critical attitudinal problem can arise from the misuse of direct questions. The overuse of direct questions by providers can lead to resentment in the patient. Sometimes questions appear to relentlessly probe for hidden motivations, thus causing resentment (Collins, 1977). Additionally, relying on direct questions too much can make the provider inattentive to the entire patient. The first problem relates to the fact that sometimes providers' questions are asked out of curiosity rather than because they are relevant. Many questions asked at one time can be irritating if they are not interspersed with reflective thought on the part of both provider and patient.

The following dialogue reveals how useless, probing questions can make the patient resentful.

Provider: "Did you see your doctor this morning?"
Patient: "Not yet."
Provider: "When did he say he'd be here?"
Patient: "He really didn't say."
Provider: "When did he come yesterday?"
Patient: "In the morning."
Provider: "Probably between 10:00 and 11:00 o'clock, right?"
Patient: (Angry tone of voice) "Probably; why?"

This series of direct questions can be irritating and confusing to patients. It appears that the provider is interested in the patient's need to see the doctor. However, the specificity and line of questioning suggests that the provider may have other reasons for wanting to know the doctor's schedule. Had the provider explained why more exact information was important, the patient might have been less irritated and confused.

Questions usually carry demands; too many questions increase the demand aspect in the patient–provider encounter. The patient may feel pushed and pulled in ways that are uncomfortable, especially if the line of inquiry lacks warmth, respect, and empathy. The consequence could also be replies that are hostile and superficial. Sometimes providers ask too many questions because they are feeling pressure to keep the conversation going or because they are uncomfortable with silence. Providers who have what appears to be an endless list of questions to ask are better off allowing for silence between what the patient says and what they say. This will also enable the provider to reformulate additional questions that are meaningful and to the point.

The inattentive provider is in serious jeopardy. This provider will rely on direct questions and miss the numerous cues that come from the patient's nonverbal communication. The provider may pay little attention to the person in the patient and be "out of touch" in attempts to understand how and what help is needed. In some respects, the greater the number of direct questions that result in minimal data, the less likely it is that patients will be helped in meaningful ways. This principle is important to remember both in applying questions and in choosing the appropriate format for questions. The reason that many direct questions impose great limitations on the helping process is that they severely curb the quality of listening that occurs. It is listening, not good questions, that enables providers to render compassionate quality care.

Asking "leading" or "loaded" questions is another type to avoid. These questions, usually closed-ended in format, restrict or influence the patient's response because the wording suggests an appropriate answer. Actual data collection is blocked due to the fact that response options are limited. An example might be: "This doesn't hurt, does it?" This type of questioning is usually used because the provider's needs or goals are paramount. The patient may respond out of deference to the provider and give the desired response, such as, "No-o-o." Still, this answer could be invalid. The patient might deny feeling pain or the intensity when she is feeling more than a moderate amount of pain. There is the possibility that the patient will minimize the pain by describing the experience as a "little ache," for example. In either case, patients feel need to alter their responses out of deference or even intimidation.

A final type of question that should be avoided is the double-barreled question. This format allows only one answer, when really two or more separate questions are asked. An example would be: "Would you like the chair lowered, a glass of water to rinse out your mouth, a magazine while you're waiting?" While this particular double-barreled question seems acceptable, it can be annoying. More than one double-barreled question may anger the patient. These questions are disrespectful because they rush the patient to compare these alternatives and give a quick response.

While using questions properly may seem simple, there are many dos and don'ts associated with the therapeutic use of questions. The next section of this chapter focuses on formats for therapeutic questioning and the effects of different types of questions. Question formats allow providers options in meeting data collection objectives. Each type of question elicits a certain type of answer. Collecting information, clarifying and specifying, and ruling out/ruling in are the major purposes for using questions. Different question formats perform these functions.

TYPES OF QUESTION FORMATS

When we think of questions that we want to ask the patient, our intent is usually to utilize the most efficient approach to arrive at the maximum information. Patients' potential reactions to questions are important to consider because we are not only interested in the approach that will provide the most information, we are also concerned that what we ask and how we ask it builds on the therapeutic relationship we have achieved and want to maintain. Questions can be framed in a variety of ways to elicit information. The following discussion outlines the types of questions available for use.

Closed-Ended Question Format

The most common category of questions is closed, sometimes referred to as convergent, questions (Riccardi & Kurtz, 1983). These questions require short, one- or two-word responses. Usually the responses are simply one-word replies: yes or no. Providers frequently ask: "Do you have any questions?" This is a commonly used question to close out a patient visit. What do you expect the answer will be 9 times out of 10?

Closed-ended questions have the effect of restricting the patient's range of response. Because of this, the patient is not encouraged and helped to express his or her true thoughts, concerns, or feelings (Hames & Joseph, 1986). Closed-ended questions ask for specific data and provide limited possibilities for response; thus, the information that is gathered is frequently incomplete.

The following example illustrates this possibility.

Provider: "Are you having much pain?" (Closed-ended question)
Patient: "Yes."
Provider: "Is it about the same?" (Closed-ended question)
Patient: "I think it's worse."

Observe that the provider's questions call for brief responses from the patient. The patient is not encouraged to describe the pain or give any details concerning the character of the pain. Important information may be missed because the patient does not expand on the information that he provides. In the example cited, the patient could have given important information about his tolerance for the pain. Because the patient receives a second closed-ended question asking him to compare this current pain with the pain he was previously experiencing, full exploration is again blocked. Although the additional information, comparing the current pain with former pain, is relevant, the information may add much to our assessment about how the patient is tolerating the pain or whether and how this pain is different.

The patient may also feel that there is a chance that the provider will not understand the nature and experience of pain he is having. Asking closed-ended questions when the patient needs to talk openly about his pain can cause him to forget important information.

Closed-ended questions are not always inadvisable, however. When closed-ended questions are asked after patients give their own account of their experience, they help focus, clarify, and specify certain essential details. Closed-ended questions, placed judiciously in the conversation, do not hinder communication. Thus, the characteristics of closed-ended questions that can hamper therapeutic communications are those that can be useful. Say, for example, that this same patient is in an emergency situation and it is difficult for him to verbalize his experience of pain. Vital information must be collected quickly, and closed-ended questions are very useful in cases where, for example, the level and location of pain must be rapidly assessed (Cournoyer, 1991).

Open-Ended Question Format

Open (divergent) questions, according to Riccardi and Kurtz (1983), are underused in health care. By their very nature, they cannot be answered with a single word. Tongue and colleagues (2005) explain that open-ended questions allow patients to define the conversation, both in content and direction of the interview. They also suggest that while it might be hard to do, providers should also wait until the patient is finished; it takes two minutes for patients to tell their story and explain why they need attention. However, the average physician might interrupt in the first 18 to 23 seconds.

Open-ended questions are powerful because they invite full disclosure. "What keeps you from following your diet? taking your pills? calling for an appointment?" are questions that ask the patient to tell more. They are effectively used as lead-ins and ways to gain the patient's perspective on an event, issue, or condition. Open-ended questions not only invite a range of responses, they tend to elicit critical thinking and active participation on the part of the patient (Gazda et al., 1982).

Open-ended questions work very well at the start of an interview because they identify unrecognized needs for information. First, the patient is not only encouraged to provide information but also to establish an open, collaborative relationship with the provider. Responses to these questions also reveal what the patient does and does not know, which may be the target of providers' teaching plan. Generally, open-ended questions have more of a tendency to convey caring and concern when compared with the closed-ended format.

Consider, for example, the time and individual attention generated in this provider's use of open-ended questions.

Provider: "Hi, Kristina."
Patient: "Hi."
Provider: "I'm Dr. Landon's nurse, Julie. He wanted me to speak with you for a few moments before he comes in to talk with you. I understand this may possibly be your fifth surgery."
Patient: "Yeah . . . yeah." (Nodding head)

Provider: "Can you tell me how you're feeling about the possibility of having a fifth surgery?" (Open lead-in)

Patient: "Um, I'm getting really frustrated because when they did the reconstruction last September, they told me that was it. I could go to college, play my volleyball, and do whatever I want. Now it's giving out on me (sounding exasperated). I don't feel happy at all . . . not that I'd feel happy about my knee giving out. But it's just that when they tell you that you should be OK, and that you'll be a normal young person again, and then you're not allowed to and they can't do anything about it, it's hard. I know I'm gonna be here. I'm gonna probably go to surgery so they can look and see what happened. But, I mean, I can't even walk down a hill because it was giving out on me. I'd have to be carried down the hill, and it was really humiliating, especially when, you know, you've gone through a surgery. After that surgery you're supposed to be fine, and you go through a year of physical therapy. And you're supposed to be fine. And then it gives out; you just don't trust anything anymore."

Provider: "What has the doctor told you about your problem?" (Open-ended question)

Patient: "Oh, well, he . . . well, ya know, he reconstructed the anterior cruciate ligament which, um, I don't know what the problem is right now. Because finally I'm walking on regular land, and I'm walking uphill—it's just the downhill part. He didn't tell me what the possibilities were for the surgery. He didn't tell me if it was, uh, if it was the cartilage, or if the meniscus was torn, or what. So, I don't know. Maybe I could talk to him about that."

Provider: "Yeah, maybe you could talk to him about that, so you can get a better picture for yourself; so you can have a better understanding of this next surgery. How did you feel about your last surgery?" (Open-ended question)

Patient: "That was OK. That was the reconstruction. It was OK because I went in there really hopeful, ya know, because I hadn't played volleyball in four years. I skipped my entire high school career of volleyball. And I figured, not that I'm planning on playing in any big way when I get to college or anything . . . but I want to be able to go outside and play and have a good time. I haven't been able to run, or dance, or swim, or anything. The reconstruction was just a really big hopeful thing for me."

Notice that the nurse started the interview with a brief introduction followed by a broad lead-in. Although the lead-in was not a "what" or "how" phrase, the result was effective. It led to open exploration of how the patient viewed surgery and the prospects of functional recovery. Because the lead-in was broad, the patient was able to elaborate on some feelings and concerns that she had had throughout the past year, giving the provider an overall appraisal and attitude about the patient's condition. A point worth noting here is that the provider could have reflected upon and validated the patient's feelings of frustration and helplessness in order to communicate an empathetic presence, but the open-ended method of inquiry provided the patient maximum freedom to explore the relevant issues. The patient's care then can be individualized.

As Northouse and Northouse (1985) point out, open-ended questions allow patients to give unlimited answers. While the patient feels free to express herself, the provider gains essential knowledge on which to build a better understanding of the care that the patient needs. Also, open-ended questions usually evoke more self-exploration by the patient, increasing the probability of further collaborative problem solving.

As with closed-ended questions, open-ended questions have limitations. First, because these questions are broad in scope, they result in a certain amount of unpredictability in the direction of the dialogue, and it is frequently the case that some very relevant information or facts might not be included. Open-ended questions then are rarely completely effective if not interspersed with other types of questions that focus patients and direct them along the lines of an in-depth exploration of a specific topic. Sometimes it is very important to limit and focus patients' responses. Patients in crisis or those unable to carry on extended dialogue are examples of situations in which open-ended questions may not be the format of choice.

In summary, effective use of open-ended questions requires careful wording of the questions to give some, but minimal, direction. The provider's conscious effort to actively listen to the patient responses and then willingness and ability to interject when needed to keep the patient focused on the topic is important. Open-ended questions should never be without structure and direction, even though they invite many possible responses. Still, the open-ended question format (e.g., "What questions do you have?") is more productive than closed-ended formatted questions ("Do you have any questions?"). Clearly, expertise in asking open-ended questions is a skill that needs to be developed and maintained in clinical practice.

Multiple-Choice Question Format

A third question format is the multiple-choice question. Typically, this question offers a number of alternative topics or decision routes, and the patient is expected to choose among the options provided.

Consider the following dialogue between a nurse's aide and a patient.

Provider: "Good morning, Miss Wilson."
Patient: "Good morning."
Provider: "Miss Wilson, in what order would you like me to help you with your morning care? Would you like to brush your teeth, wash up a little, or eat breakfast first?" (Multiple-choice question format)
Patient: "Brushing my teeth first, then eating my breakfast."
Provider: "OK. Now, the doctor recommended that you walk twice a day for 15 minutes. Do you want to take a nap before you walk or take a shower?" (Multiple-choice question format)

Patient: "Let me take a nap because I was not able to sleep last night. Then we can walk."

In view of the dialogue presented, the patient was clearly given a choice, was able to assess the options, and was able to select among them. This process can be extremely helpful to patients who feel as if control has been taken away from them and who feel as if they are mere objects in care-delivery activities. When patients are given the opportunity to choose and prioritize aspects of care, some of the dependence feelings based on these experiences may be lessened.

The multiple-choice format is helpful when the provider is attempting to sort issues and prioritize concerns but needs the patient's cooperation to fully explore these areas. For example, physicians may want to know whether the patient is concerned about postsurgical recovery but also needs to discuss the type of anesthesia and the expected surgical outcomes. The physician can decide, independently of patient input, what topics will come first or give the patient some choice. It is not that the physician presents a menu of topics from which the patient selects; rather, the patient is informed of all the issues that the physician feels need to be addressed and the patient selects areas in sequential order based on his or her readiness to explore the topics that are presented.

The multiple-choice question format works well with patients who are withdrawn, anxious, depressed, and indecisive. This approach also works well with children and adolescents because it provides security in structure, while at the same time engaging their active participation.

The major drawback of multiple-choice questions is that they are frequently complicated. They can be experienced in much the same way as double-barreled questions, where two or more questions are posed at the same time. If patients are not cognitively able to separate, sort, and evaluate options, the result may be frustration. Like double-barreled questions, multiple-choice questions can also cause the patient to feel rushed and confused.

CHOICE OF QUESTION FORMAT AND RESPONSE BURDEN

In considering which question format will be best, providers might use a variety of criteria. These include the purpose of the data-collection activity, details about the patient's condition, and the nature of the provider–patient relationship.

Factors about the patient that determine which question format is best includes the patient's present level of physical and emotional distress, the patient's actual and potential responses to the subject matter, and the patient's knowledge and experience. All of these factors significantly affect patients' abilities to communicate verbally and meet the demands of the question–answer task. These elements comprise the response burden. As indicated earlier, types of question formats have certain response burdens. When using a question format, it is always important to consider not only what type of information this format elicits but also the nature of the response burden on the patient.

Open-ended questions allow the patient to verbalize without restriction. They require a minimum amount of sorting and processing. Decisions about what is appropriate or inappropriate are not imposed on the patient. Patients who respond positively to open-ended questions are usually those who need to talk, like to express themselves verbally, and have the energy to engage in extended conversations. They usually have moderate levels of trust and positive attitudes toward providers. Certain other patients are not amenable to data collection with the open-ended format. These patients are those who are less comfortable verbalizing, or they may not have the energy or freedom from symptom distress to engage in lengthy conversations. They might also have language deficits or have fairly low literacy levels and feel inadequate in gathering out this type of conversation. Even when offered a broad open-ended leading question (e.g., "How are you doing today?"), they are likely to be parsimonious in their response ("Not so good" or "OK"). While the response burden of open-ended questions, at first glance, seems to be negligible, there are many situations in which open-ended questions tax the patient's ability to respond.

Closed-ended question formats impose a different response burden. With closed-ended questions, responses are brief. Those patients in pain or distress usually respond better to this type of question. However, it is important to understand what is required of the patient. When a provider asks, "Do you feel pain?", several requirements are made of the patient. First, the patient must decode the provider's terms (e.g., *pain*). Patients must discern what is meant by these terms and why the provider is asking for this information. Additionally, patients must identify their experience as pain or perhaps something else. Patients must be able to focus, decode, and encode their experience and, at the same time, be brief. While not much is required in terms of verbal explanation, more is required in terms of decoding and encoding the communication between the provider and the patient.

Questions worded in the multiple-choice format are like closed-ended questions because they require further data-processing and decision-making capabilities on the patient's part. As indicated previously, this format is usually used to pinpoint (i.e., to rule in or rule out) different possibilities.

If the provider asks the patient, "Are you having pain here, here, how about here—and, where is the pain worse? here or here?", certain patient skills are needed. As with closed-ended questions, the patient must be able to focus and decode the provider's language and encode his own. However, what is also required with this format is the ability to compare and contrast, cross-referencing different experiences of pain or pressures. For some patients, this requirement is beyond their capability. They may have problems in encoding and decoding and also have problems with comparative analysis. While it would seem that the multiple-choice question mode leads to efficiency in data collection, the provider may get very little accurate data. Language barriers, present distress, and cognitive deficits can all contribute to patients' inabilities to use this question format.

CONCLUSION

As indicated in this chapter, the provider–patient relationship is characterized by the privilege and expectation of asking questions of the patient. The primary therapeutic motive for asking questions is to derive complete and accurate data on which to provide care to patients. Secondary to this purpose is the opportunity questions afford in building a therapeutic connection. Providers should encourage the full expression of agenda, concerns, and expectations (Lang & McCord, 1999).

Questions help open dialogue, direct the interview, command attention in a given area, and clarify. In our society, people experience questions of all types. Many questions seem irrelevant. Still, within the patient–provider relationship, questions are more deliberate than accidental or capricious. Providers are diagnostically oriented, and this orientation is based on thoughtful selection of the appropriate context and the appropriate format for questions.

The appropriate use of questions includes gathering data, seeking clarification and qualification, and pinpointing or ruling in or out possible conditions. Question formats—closed, open, or multiple choice—are options in the provider's exploration of the patient's condition and experience. Different question formats elicit different responses, and it is important to understand the strengths and limitations of each of these formats. In truth, one format alone will not suffice. Rather, providers need to be able to draw on each format discriminately.

Questions are not always used in therapeutic ways. Clearly, they can be misused. Several examples were provided in this chapter. Questions can mask interpretations and advice. In these cases, while questions are used to soften the impact and directness of other response modes, the provider runs the risk of confusing the patient. Direct questions are particularly problematic, because too many ill-placed direct questions can make patients confused and defensive and can defeat the essential purposes for which they were designed. Questions should always allow reply without intimidation or defensiveness.

Questions, whether open, closed, or multiple choice in format, are providers' primary means of gathering information from patients and families. The art of questioning and the skill of asking an answerable question is central to conversing therapeutically.

CHAPTER 8

Therapeutic Use of Silence and Pauses

To learn how one mind speaks to another and in silence; one must listen with "the third ear."
—Theodor Reik

CHAPTER OBJECTIVES

- Define silence as a therapeutic response mode.
- Discuss what occurs in the absence of silence.
- List several therapeutic purposes for the use of silence and pauses in the patient–provider relationship.
- Analyze the meaning of silence in patients' responses and reactions.
- Describe how one might intervene with defensive silences.
- Identify certain negative effects of silence and pauses.

In some cultures *talk* is valued, and *silence* is considered a deficit in social skills and/or a lack of knowledge. An unwillingness to converse is perceived as an attitude of unfriendliness; silence is interpreted as impolite, unkind, or arrogant (Barbara, 1958). Talkativeness, on the other hand, exemplifies intellect and social poise. This is not the case in all cultural groupings, however. For example, among certain Asian groups, silence is regarded as a sign of wisdom. People who are talkative are generally perceived as lacking an awareness of the natural order of things. These mixed cultural interpretations of silence influence how comfortable we as providers will be in employing silence as a therapeutic technique. For those providers whose culture values talkativeness, silence may be uncomfortable, and for those who come from cultures that value silence, talkativeness may be uncomfortable. Thus, for this group, spacing remarks with silent periods is not difficult.

Silence has received positive and negative acclaim: "silence is golden" and the notion that silence is to be "overcome." Silence can mean fear, anger, depression, disinterest, withdrawal, confusion, and inability to express one's thoughts or feelings. In therapeutic encounters, silence on the part of the provider can be received with warmth and understanding or seen as withholding. Patients can feel threatened and confused about why the provider is remaining silent. Lane, Koetting, and Bishop (2002), describing the use of silence in psychotherapy, remark that if not skillfully done, this technique can be perceived as therapist's distancing, disinterest, and disengagement.

Silence is a type of interaction that can increase both the patient's and the provider's anxiety. High levels of anxiety can result from too much silence. The reason is not only the value that a given culture places on talking. There are other reasons. In some groups, silent responses are used as punishment.

Reactions to silence are, in part, triggered from very early uses of silence. When children are bad, they are told to be "quiet." Adults punish one another by withholding thoughts and feelings. The reasons behind silence are not always clear; to the extent that an individual's silence is unclear or possibly punitive, these quiet periods can evoke anxiety and increase social distance. For some providers, the measure of a successful interview is the extent to which silence is kept at a minimum. For others, it is the provision of silent periods to help the patient take stock of his or her situation and feel accepted in an understanding, supportive, and safe environment (Lane et al., 2002).

As with all therapeutic responses, silence can be underused or overused. This chapter emphasizes the need to become comfortable with silences, to understand their meaning when it is the patient who is silent and to draw on them in the therapeutic interview to enhance the productivity of patient–provider encounters.

DEFINITIONS OF SILENCE

Silence is the absence of speech. According to Hein (1980), it is that period in the therapeutic relationship during which the provider waits, without interruption for the patient to begin or resume speaking. Further, when used therapeutically, silence can be interspersed with encouragements, e.g., "humm" or "uh-huh" since these sounds do not interrupt the patient (Norton & Miller, 1986).

In actuality, there are two types of silence in the therapeutic relationship. The first is when the patient stops speaking and there is absence of speech before the provider starts speaking, or when the provider stops speaking and there is absence of speech before the patient speaks. The implicit understanding behind conversation is that patient and provider verbalize in the pattern of first one, then the other. A second type of silence refers to that absence of speech that occurs when either patient or provider stops speaking and then the same person resumes speaking. In either case, the silent space may be long or very short, such as in a pause (see Exhibit 8–1). A *pause* is said to be a natural rest in the melody of speech; whereas silence is longer. Usually absence of speech beyond three to four seconds is considered a silent period, not just a brief interruption in the course of conversation.

Another way to perceive silence is as an *interpersonal space*. The psychosocial space between two individuals is referred to as interpersonal space, which continually changes for the duration of the dialogue. This space can be expanded or reduced, depending on either or both individuals. Applying this principle to our daily experiences, it is obvious that increases or decreases in silent periods do occur and reflect the nature of our moods and the characteristics of our relationships. Experimenting with the effects of changing the length of silences enables us to measure the different ways in which we relate to others. Changes, even small ones, in how interpersonal space is used can make a difference in the quality of our interactions.

The following interaction illustrates the impact these changes can have on personal distancing in this physician's first visit with a new patient.

Provider: "What we should do is take a blood test, increase your Theophylline. Also, I think we should add . . . "

Exhibit 8–1 Summation of Basic Principles Underlying Silence as a Therapeutic Response Mode

- There is a relationship between interviewer and respondent use of silence; the more silent the interviewer, the more likely the respondent will follow with silence.
- The speech–silence behavior of any given individual in the context of an interview is highly consistent, despite large individual differences in the characteristics of interviewers.
- Unfilled pausing times (silences) are associated with more concise expressions; those filled with pauses (e.g., "uh huh," "er," and "um") might yield inferior responses (e.g., long-windedness).
- In some cultures, silence means wisdom; in others, silence might be viewed as withholding, defensiveness, insecurity, and dullness.

Patient: (forcefully) "I don't want to have the blood test."
Provider: "You're not going to get significant results if your dose is not at therapeutic level." (Silence)
Patient: "I go to an allergist. He told me what I need to do. I just want an antibiotic for my bronchitis. (Pause) I don't think a blood test is necessary!"
Provider: (Silence)
Patient: "You think I should increase my medicine? And, I should probably increase my inhaler, right?"
Provider: "Yes, that's right." (Pause) "And, if you're not feeling better in a week, come back and see me."
Patient: "OK."

In this case, silence by the provider shifted the apparent "power struggle" in this relationship. The patient was openly resisting the provider's advice, even the idea of doing much more than getting an antibiotic was out of the question. This provider, through the use of silence, moved the patient from a position of resistance to one of considering the physician's advice. Although the physician did not persuade the patient to take the blood test, agreement about increasing the patient's routine medications was established. There may be other reasons the patient refused a blood test. These reasons could reflect noncompliance on routine medications, which would be apparent with the blood test. In this case, the patient would not risk discovery. There are other less directive approaches the physician could have used; still, the use of silence seemed to reduce the patient's blatant resistance in following the physician's orders.

IN THE ABSENCE OF SILENCE

To understand silence, it is important to question what occurs during silence. There are three basic aspects of silence that are worthy of attention:

(1) interresponse time, (2) the interruption response, and (3) the over-talk response.

Interresponse Time

Interresponse time refers to the number of seconds or minutes in a silence period. A typical social conversation contains many interresponse times that are less than a second long. This feature of conversation, many short silences, tends to characterize social interaction. It would be peculiar to engage in longer silences when speaking with casual acquaintances, yet it is expected in psychotherapy sessions.

In some cultures, shorter response times are typical. However, there are some cultures that abide by longer response times. This and the slowness of their speech are typical. For example, inhabitants of Maine, the Appalachians, and parts of the South and Southwest may speak slower and use interresponse times that are more than a second in length. These communities can be contrasted with residents of New York; where fast-paced speech is common. Crowded speech in these individuals might contain many examples of interresponse times that are much less than a second. These distinct tendencies become even more obvious when situational or environmental situations affect their speech. For example, the city dweller on a camping vacation in the mountains or on a sailing excursion may feel out of sorts but adapt to the slower pace of everyday life. In turn, those slower-speaking individuals may find it very irritating to stand in line at Kennedy Airport or hail a cab on Fifth Avenue (New York). Over time they might adapt and view it as exciting.

Patients' conditions frequently affect the speed of their speech and their tendency to use short or long durations between phrases. For example, patients who are suffering pain, fatigue, or lethargy, or who are depressed, will tend to exhibit longer interresponse times. The elderly usually require added time to assemble their ideas due to physical and mental processes as do people with limited literacy or developmental delays. Patients who are anxious, excitable, agitated, or manic are likely to exhibit more rapid speech that allows for fewer interruptions.

Interresponse times of three or four seconds or more are more than brief pauses between expressed ideas. They are frequently used as space to think something about something new or to think over a previously expressed thought. These times are distinct and do not resemble pauses wherein little thinking is occurring. In a fast-paced conversation, however, two-second interresponse times may be enough to provide additional thinking and feeling experiences and, thus, are not merely pauses. In a helping relationship or therapeutic dialogue, silences can last up to 10 seconds. Also, a change in dialogue, where one or two seconds of silence are added, may communicate allowance to think and feel and assists patients to regroup thoughts or develop a new slant on the feelings they have expressed.

One study of physicians and adult patients revealed that the use of silence (reaction-time latency) between speakers contributed to patients' satisfaction (Rowland-Morin & Carroll, 1990). Patients were more satisfied not only when silence occurred in interviews but also when physicians utilized words that the patient used and interrupted with reflections.

Interruptions

Just as adding a mere two seconds to silence can provide patients interpersonal space, taking one or two seconds from the silent pattern can create a feeling of being crowded or rushed.

Consider the following dialogue and the effect of changing interresponse time in periods of silence. This is a dialogue between a nurse and a patient, where the patient is describing his headaches.

Provider: "Did the medication help you?"
Patient: "Yup—but it was hard . . . "
Provider: "Do you have any ideas about what you can do?" (Interruption)
Patient: (Looking at nurse) "No—I feel frustrated!"
Provider: (Silence, four seconds).
Patient: "I really don't know what I'm going to do about this stuff the doctor gave me. If I take it, I'm worthless as far as working goes and actually everything else, and so I just get further and further behind. If I don't take it, I can't see straight and I don't get much more done. God, I feel frustrated!"
Provider: "Yes . . . " (Silence, two seconds)
Patient: "Actually, I wonder what would happen if I only took half the pill? Maybe I'll run that by the doctor and see what he thinks. Or, I could call him and see if there is anything else he could give me."

Notice that in the beginning of this conversation the nurse crowded the patient, even interrupted him in mid-thought. Providing extended interpersonal space, the patient was able to gather his thoughts and decrease his frustration by coming up with a plan. He constructed two potential solutions to the dilemma he was facing. By altering the interresponse time between statements, the nurse was able to alter feelings of pressure generated from the frustration and create a climate for problem solving.

Interruptions have a significant impact on conversation. *Interruptions* are disruptions of another individual's speech and generally have the impact of cutting short the expression of the person's ideas. Interruptions can occur in the middle of a statement or in the brief lull that occurs between expressed thoughts and feelings. The circumstance in which both parties begin speaking simultaneously is called over-talk.

Over-talk

Conversation can be filled with interruptions. If this is the case, *over-talk* is usually a significant impasse in the productive expressions of both individuals. There are specific instances in which most people will engage in over-talk. For example, when either or both parties are feeling threatened, over-talk may be a defense against any distress they may be experiencing. Over-talk essentially communicates the message: cease or stop this. What might occur is the opposite, an escalation of comments, which may be accusations.

Some people habitually interrupt. This style of communicating influences the way these people work with others and the way others feel about them. Patients of this type may feel exceedingly threatened. Because they crowd out others in their communication, they are prone to fear rejection. Interruptions can also reflect boredom, the need to dominate others, reactions to redundancy, or reactions to freshly stimulated thoughts and feelings. Providers can over-talk because the patient is not quickly providing the information needed. In this way, the provider is saying: "Don't finish, listen to me!" Or "I can guess what you are going to say—let me say it." Conversations with many interruptions and a good deal of over-talk are filled with incomplete messages. If one individual does not back off for three or four seconds, over-talk fills the space, and significant interpersonal crowding sets in.

In sum, over-talk and interruptions are important aspects of interresponse boundaries when there is no silence. As previously explained, over-talk and interruptions crowd conversation. Silence allows for thoughtful reflection and the development of understanding and insight, which is the primary objective in provider–patient relationships. Hence, silence in helping relationships can extend to 10 seconds or even longer. Crowding can actually reduce the tendency for patients to disclose. With crowding, patients will experience being misunderstood, frustrated, and dissatisfied. Patients who are recipients of crowding might fear that their needs to be understood will go unmet.

A final point is that like all other response modes, there is a tendency to respond with silence, interruptions, or over-talk. Providers can actually elicit these responses from patients by using them first. Additionally, if they did not initiate these response patterns, they might mirror them back to the patient almost unconsciously, matching the pace and character of the patient's over-talk or interruptions. The results are two frustrated and dissatisfied individuals. In the event that this happens, the primary corrective measure is the provider's conscious and deliberate use of silence to alter the nature of the encounter. Providers can use silence to slow down the pace and change any tendency to interrupt and over-talk.

THERAPEUTIC PURPOSES OF SILENCE IN THE PROVIDER–PATIENT RELATIONSHIP

There are several important purposes for using silence in therapeutic dialogues with patients. These include (1) providing space for assessing and analyzing the patient's condition and (2) communicating empathy. However, the primary purpose in providing interpersonal space is to encourage patients to take the initiative to communicate their experiences verbally.

Encouraging Patients to Speak

As previously indicated, silence can cause patients to speak, especially if the provider shows interest and expectation. This kind of silence indicates to patients that the provider expects them to speak—to initiate the topic that they feel is most pressing or important. Silent interludes give patients the opportunity to collect and organize their thoughts and think through what they want to say next. Using silence can also reduce the pace of the interview, creating more interpersonal space in the dialogue. This strategy can cause the patient to delve more deeply, weigh a decision, or consider alternative actions—in essence, be more participatory in planning and evaluating their care.

These therapeutic effects of silence were illustrated in the earlier dialogue between the nurse and patient. By providing the patient with silent interludes, the nurse prompted the patient to delve more deeply into his dilemma; as a result, he generated a new course of action. By not asking pointless questions, the provider gave the patient room to be spontaneous and to move from simple to more complex analyses of his dilemma. Rather than remaining confused and upset about the medication he was prescribed, he decided to talk to his doctor and request a change in dosage or a new drug with the same effects. While the nurse could have cut short this decision process by merely advising the patient what to do, the real value of this interchange was that the patient came to his own decision; this process emphasized both his responsibility to communicate with his physician and his right to receive more appropriate care.

Communicating Empathy

Silent periods have been noted for their ability to touch emotions (Martyres, 1995). Emotions are experiential and complex, having origins in personal history. Sometimes words that are used to describe emotions are inadequate and simplistic. According to Martyres (1995), silence is a useful experiential medium in which to identify and work with emotions. It is important to recognize what is being communicated by silence during each silent period.

Communicating empathy in a therapeutic interview is facilitated with the use of silence. Silence conveys *active listening*. To successfully achieve active listening, the provider must display interest. As active listening, silence communicates that providers have a willingness to hear what patients have to say—to enter the world of the patient and understand it more fully. It conveys an interest in the patient's well-being beyond that demonstrated by specific gestures that "do" something. The power in silence is that it provides an unhurried atmosphere in which patients can reflect on their experiences in the presence of their provider. Providers, in their own hurried states, are usually perceived as incapable of full understanding. When they relinquish their distractions and focus in silence on the patient, they are conveying not only the willingness to understand the patient but also the capability to do so. While it would appear that the provider is doing nothing in these moments of silence, in actuality much is going on. During these interludes, the provider is observing what patients do, hearing what patients say and how they say it, feeling how patients feel, and sensing what patients have not said but may want to say. Silence often communicates caring when words are superfluous.

Assessment of Patient Condition

In addition to encouraging patients to verbalize and to convey empathetic understanding, silent interludes are critical to more fully assessing patients. This idea goes beyond the obvious point that to obtain clinical data, providers will lapse into silent periods as they listen for chest sounds, palpate a pulse, or examine a severe overbite. During silences, providers have opportunities to observe verbal and nonverbal behaviors. They also have opportunities to look for incongruencies in how patients feel about their condition or the prescribed plan of care. To be aware of incongruencies, providers must understand the full range of nonverbal expression of effect: fear, anxiety, hostility, sadness, depression, relief, happiness, and excitement. Because silences provide open-ended opportunities to observe, clinicians may need to organize their points of focus: use verbal and nonverbal messages of thoughts and feelings, pick up subtle attitudes and underlying beliefs, observe patients' own reactions to their disclosures, and construct a composite picture of the patient's experience as witnessed by the clinician. This process then tends to further convey understanding on the part of clinicians as well as their ability to be helpful.

Thoughtful Self-Reflection

A final purpose of silence is the provision for thoughtful self-reflection on the part of the provider. The opportunity to observe oneself in therapeutic encounters is not something that is familiar to clinicians. The provider generally stays focused on the patient. But when the provider is distracted, the need to eliminate distractions and properly refocus on the patient is important. When providers observe themselves in the context of their encounters with patients, they will learn that a great deal is happening between them and their patients, some of which they will not immediately understand. This includes becoming aware of attitudes, judgments, and feelings. The following data can be retrieved by simply reflecting on one's own thoughts and feelings in the silent periods of a therapeutic interview.

- How am I feeling about what the patient is saying? What am I not saying?
- How am I reacting to the manner in which the patient is communicating?
- How is the context of this interview affecting me and what I do and do not say?
- What am I trying to achieve? How well is it working?
- What do I want to communicate above all else to help this patient?

Just as silence gives patients the opportunity to think through a point or to consider introducing a topic, providers are given the same opportunity to collect and reassemble their thoughts. In actuality, silent periods provide both providers and patients important time-outs that serve the therapeutic aims of the interview.

ANALYSIS OF SILENCE IN PATIENTS' RESPONSES

Sometimes patients are silent, but this silence does not seem to serve the patient therapeutically. The answer as to why the patient is silent is usually a very complex one. It may communicate anger, fear, depression, disinterest, withdrawal, or absence of emotion (Liegner, 1971). Silence can be a response to cultural differences. Davidhizar and Giger (1994) suggest that a number of problems may arise when silence occurs in an interpersonal situation. Among these problems is the different meanings that silence may have from culture to culture. Sometimes patients refuse to talk, and while these cases are not as common as lapses into silence, they are extremely important to understand. There are three reasons patients may refuse to talk: (1) defensiveness against perceived threats, (2) provocation—to get the provider to seek them out, or (3) underlying hostility and resistance.

Defensive Silences

The defensive use of silence demonstrates patients' beliefs that if they are silent and withhold thoughts and feelings, they will not be hurt. Patients who harbor such ideas have usually had repeated exposures to being insulted or shamed when they expressed themselves. Their families may have simply shunned expressions of different thoughts or ideas, or significant mental and physical abuse could have occurred when the patient spoke up or spoke out. In any case, the patient developed a patterned response to withdraw and/or to remain silent in situations they perceived to be threatening. Over time, they may have become unaware of this defensive reaction. Therefore, it is possible that patients will not respond to such queries as: "Why are you quiet?"

A second dynamic behind patients' refusal to speak might be their desire to be sought out. This silence may be conveyed as provocation (e.g., treat me as special). In essence, the provider is being tested. These behaviors are manipulative and tend to cause anger, hostility, and resentment in providers. And, while the original intent of the patient was to secure a helping relationship, the outcome is the opposite—the patient has provoked the provider, who, in turn, prefers to withdraw.

A third and final explanation for silence is harbored feelings of hostility, anger, and resentment. Patients who exhibit silence out of hostility, anger, or resentment communicate these feelings but act as if they did not. These silences are usually cold, rejecting, punishing kinds of silence. Silences of this kind are frequently used in social relationships (e.g., to communicate anger when one's partner is late or has forgotten an important occasion such as an anniversary). They are generally regarded as passive-aggressive. In fact, some individuals will use the ambiguity surrounding silence as a punishment (i.e., "You think you know why I am quiet, but I know you don't know for sure. . . . You will have to suffer with uncertainty until I decide to tell you why I won't speak to you.").

Many providers assume that patients will not exhibit these patterns in their interviews with providers. There are many reasons why patients may communicate their hostility through silence:

1. Providers are generally regarded as authority figures. Patients might have early programming that causes them to be passive-aggressive in the context of dominant-submissive relationships.
2. Patients may fear reprisal if they communicate their anger directly. They may fear being neglected or receiving inferior care.
3. Whatever irritation or upset they experience may be perceived as insignificant in the context of the larger picture. That is, patients may recognize their distress and deliberately minimize it because there are so many other issues of equal or greater importance to them. Nonetheless, the result is the same. The patient contains her feelings and lapses

into silence. Still angry, she extends her silence to communicate passivity which results in a barrier to participatory care planning.

Intervening with Defensive Silences

It is important to understand that the negative use of silence by patients is not easily discussed. In fact, one's first take should always be understanding silence at face value and extending to patients the opportunity to respond at their own rate. However, when silence proves to inhibit disclosures that are necessary, patients need to be helped to open up and get past their destructive use of silence.

There are important steps in dealing with negative, defensive silence in patients. Initially, the provider needs to demonstrate acceptance of the patient's silence. Providers need to listen beyond the silence, reflecting and attending to the patient. This behavior will demonstrate acceptance. Second, providers need to note the context of the silence and if there is a trend. Does the patient lapse into silence about certain topics? Approach these topics with respect. If patients lapse into silences, they are generally more sensitive about these topics. If patients' silences are interrupted, they may become more defensive and be increasingly anxious. The provider runs the risk of permanently cutting short the patients' disclosures.

When asking for verbal replies, it is advisable to begin with neutral themes or superficial material with which the patient feels more comfortable. Providers also need to consider silences as symptomatic of something else. A gentle lead—"I'm trying to understand what's on your mind . . . but, I'm having difficulty knowing exactly what's bothering you," or "I am interested in helping you through this . . . "—is helpful. Exploring the meaning behind patient silences is important. But this cannot be done directly (e.g., "Why are you silent?"). This is done most effectively with a simple suggestion that their silence is a sign that something else is bothering them and that if they share it, they may be able to cope more effectively with it. Patients will frequently experience discomfort if they do not talk, yet discomfort if they do. Exploring resolution of this conflict will enable the patient to feel the provider's support.

NEGATIVE EFFECTS OF USING SILENCE

Silence is not always a helpful technique in patient–provider interactions. It is often difficult to apply in a manner that will achieve maximum benefit and minimize the chance of sending the wrong message (e.g., aloofness, uncaring, coldness) or otherwise being counterproductive. These effects stem from the fact that silence can extend beyond the point of usefulness, thoughts tend to drift, and the focus of the interview can be lost (Collins, 1977). When this occurs, the silence becomes uncomfortable and may provoke anxiety in both the provider and the patient.

Mixed messages about the provider's tolerance of silence can also defeat the therapeutic effects of silence. The ambiguous message, "I accept your need to be quiet but at the same time don't like the stillness in the room," gives two conflicting messages. This situation also results in difficulty in self-disclosure.

The amount of silence depends on the tolerance of both provider and patient and might vary from time to time.

Providers might be needing to fill every lapse in conversation with verbiage. Usually this is attributed to personal embarrassment, self-consciousness, or anxiety. When providers have difficulty dealing with silence, they might inadvertently punish the patient while remaining mostly silent themselves. Punishment can be delivered by insincere or sarcastic responses or simple gestures that suggest, in subtle ways, "If you have nothing to say (ask, talk about) then I won't waste my time with you." A potential therapeutic encounter becomes unproductive when the provider's needs take precedence over those of the patient.

The opposite situation, in which the provider feels more comfortable with silence and the patient's natural mode is to be talkative, can elicit similar outcomes. Essentially the patient will experience little direction from the provider. The patient's need for a response and feedback is thwarted, again because the provider's needs take precedence. Usually when patients do not receive the feedback they need, they will begin to repeat themselves in a second or even third attempt to get a response. They might feel confused and that they are being punished. With patients who are distrustful, silence of any length can evoke anxiety. Also, too much silence from the provider tends to put pressure on the patient to speak when he or she does not feel well or is unable to speak. Generally, an interaction filled with too many pauses or silent periods will result in feelings that the purpose of the conversation is unclear and unfocused.

The tendency to respond in kind can also present problems in the therapeutic interview. In this case, the provider's silence can even become "a game" where the patient offers little, waits to hear from the provider, or simply plays "who can hold out the longest." Communication becomes a game, and the therapeutic benefits of silence are lost.

While effective silence is useful to collect thoughts and determine what should be conveyed next confused, uncomfortable, or resistive silences are seen as unconstructive and should be remedied with corrective measures. An example of confused silence is displayed in this interaction between a provider (counselor) and a patient.

Provider: "Do you think your wife truly supports your decision (to return to school to get a degree)?"
Patient: (Says nothing for approximately six seconds.)
Provider: "You look confused. Did you understand my question?"
Patient: "I don't know what decision you're talking about."

Had the provider not picked up on the fact that the patient had not answered or that the patient looked confused, clarification may not have occurred. One instance of confused interaction can take a toll on the provider's relationship with the patient as patients might interpret too long a silence as disinterest or uncaring. Corrective measures help emphasize the fact that the interview is purposeful and that providers are sincere in their attempts to understand patients.

In summary then, silences can elicit therapeutic gains; however, they can also be detrimental in the course of patient–provider encounters. It is important to distinguish and evaluate their impact so that any corrective measures can be taken before long-range negative effects occur.

CONCLUSION

Virtually all interpersonal relationships depend on verbal communication. In truth, in contemporary Western society, conversation is highly prized. We are often judged by how often and to what degree we engage in conversation. Being socially acceptable is, in part, related to our ability to relate verbally to others. The verbal form of communication is believed to be preferable, at least for some groups. This is not the case for individuals from other cultural groups, where silence is regarded as wisdom.

While the absence of verbal communication implies silence, silence does not imply an absence of communication. It may sound paradoxical, but silence is a form of communicating where meanings are shared nonverbally.

Therapeutic silence occurs when providers deliberately use silence to facilitate patient exploration of problems. The provider conveys understanding or at least a desire to understand the experience of the patient. Silence in itself tends to encourage patients to verbalize if it is an interested, expectant silence.

The major barrier of providers' therapeutic use of silence is their assumption that nothing significant is occurring in these periods. They may judge that their time is being wasted, become bored, and let their attention wander. If providers are able to observe themselves and their patients in these periods of silence, they will learn that a great deal happens in these moments. Listening beyond the surface of the spoken word is facilitated by silent interludes.

Either party can modify the amount and length of silence in an interaction. The giving of silence will eventually result in the giving of silence in return. Silence responses can contribute to the experience of being "known" by the provider, because silence responses are also part of the response referred to as empathy. Short interresponse times may lead patients to feel understood. Sudden changes toward very long silence periods, however, may cause distraction and complicate the process of effective communication. If the provider uses too long a period of silence, the patient may become distracted. Silence and the length of silences thus have to be thoughtfully brought into the interaction to avoid confusing the patient.

Repeated crowding in an interaction can also cause a chain reaction when crowding is reciprocated. The chain reaction where crowding begets crowding, silence begets silence, is referred to as "response matching" and is described further in Chapter 9. Providers can slow down crowded communication by intentionally giving a series of medium-length-silence responses.

Overall, it behooves the provider to be aware of both the positive and negative effects of silences in interviews. Effective interviewing requires skillful application of pauses and silences, where thoughtful observation of the patient directs the pace and depth of the interaction. Otherwise, providers should be asking "Is this an appropriate use of silence, and is it achieving something that will benefit my assessment and the acceptance of participatory care planning?"

The essence of being present with the patient is often thought of as a prime feature of silence. As Pettigrew (1990) explains, the providers' presence can lessen negative effects of suffering as one "comes alongside" and enters that suffering by listening and becoming available. The therapeutic use of silence is frequently overlooked or not thought to be a technique or intervention. In this chapter, substantial discussion was provided to describe its importance.

CHAPTER 9

The Impact and Limitations of Self-Disclosure

One of the most meaningful interactions (with physicians) I had was when the physician cried and said, "I don't know what else I can do."
And what is as important as knowledge? asked the mind.
Caring and seeing with the heart, answered the soul.
—Anonymous

CHAPTER OBJECTIVES

- Define self-disclosure as a therapeutic response mode.
- Describe how self-disclosure may be different by intent and level.
- Describe several therapeutic effects of self-disclosure.
- Identify several types of provider nontherapeutic self-disclosures.
- Describe how to manage requests for self-disclosure from patients and when it is appropriate to do so.

In any human interaction, one is always disclosing aspects of oneself to some degree. In this sense, self-disclosure is unavoidable. Nonetheless, deliberate self-disclosure to facilitate therapeutic aims is a somewhat foreign idea in the history of professional health care. This is due, in part, to the fact that personal self-disclosure was viewed early on as a violation of patient–provider boundaries. In the field of psychotherapy, Freud emphasized the idea of appearing like a blank slate, mirroring back to the patient what the patient is revealing. There was no room for disclosures of a personal kind (e.g., marital status, number of children). However, from the 1960s forward, there was a shift toward a more humanistic approach that viewed provider self-disclosure as being of therapeutic value. In recent years, patients have been empowered to know much more about the training and expertise and even success rates so that self-disclosure has become a responsibility.

Patients are more entitled to know information about their providers that they did not know previously. Still, perceptions of the advisability of provider self-disclosure remain mixed. Although self-disclosure was once judged largely as inappropriate, some level of self-disclosure is now viewed as acceptable and, in some cases, an important adjunct to therapeutic relationship building.

While self-disclosures by providers can facilitate therapeutic aims, they can also be problematic. The issue is one of anticipating the potential impact and judiciously using self-disclosures. The amount and timing of self-disclosures become particularly critical in judging their appropriateness in the therapeutic relationship.

The purpose of this chapter is to present self-disclosures as aids to therapeutic communication with patients. However, before addressing the deliberate use of self-disclosure in the patient–provider relationship, it is important to describe the nature of self-disclosure, present arguments for and against this response mode, and identify types of nontherapeutic as well as therapeutic disclosures.

DEFINITIONS OF SELF-DISCLOSURE

Self-disclosure is defined as instances of openly sharing personal information about oneself, including experiences, attitudes, and feelings (Evans, Hern, Uhlemann, & Ivey, 1989). In essence, provider self-disclosure entails any self-revelation of a personal nature. Such disclosure has been classified among mental health groups as unavoidable, accidental, or purposeful (Psychopathology Committee of the Group for the Advancement of Psychiatry, 2001).

In general terms, all statements beginning with the pronoun "I" could be categorized as self-disclosures. "I" statements, however, are also used to introduce other intentions: advising, interpreting, and expressing opinion. In these situations, the primary impact of the message is some other purpose. Consider, for example, this statement: "I think you should try another solution." This statement begins with "I." It also discloses what the sender is thinking. Still, the major intent is not to share personal data about oneself but to influence the receiver's behavior. This is an example of *advisement*.

Because "I" statements also introduce advisement, interpretation, and the expression of opinion, it is not enough to say that all "I" statements are primarily self-disclosing techniques. A distinction needs to be made between statements made with self-reference and those that are clearly self-disclosures. Self-reference statements refer to "I" or "me" but disclose little personal data about the sender.

Self-disclosure, then, is when an individual reveals nonobvious aspects of the self (e.g., thoughts, feelings, attitudes, or experiences) through a distinct and meaningful self-reference. While "I feel upset with my care in the hospital" is a self-disclosure, "I think you need to close the curtain" is not.

Conceptualizing Self-Disclosure

Self-disclosures may be delivered in very intimate circumstances or be made to many people. Self-disclosures (e.g., "I like you") made in the context of a one-to-one relationship are very different from public disclosures. Public disclosures (e.g., "I'm a registered Democrat" or "I have a BA degree in Biology") made to many persons at the same time are usually more superficial. Although they also reveal the nonobvious, they present much less threat of exposure than do one-on-one self-disclosures.

Self-disclosures can also be conceptualized in terms of the content of the disclosure. Content in disclosures may vary. In social situations, this content may be personal attitudes or the type of work one does. Other disclosures, say, about one's personality, religious beliefs, and perceived body image, are likely to be offered in more intimate situations or when a certain level of trust has been established and a desire for a relationship has been expressed.

Finally, self-disclosures can be categorized as here-and-now, present-experience disclosures or historical disclosures that refer to the past. Consider, for example, the remark, "You make me anxious." This statement refers to the sender's immediate experience. Statements such as "That reminds me of how I felt before my surgery" refer to past feelings. This distinction is important in judging a patient's level of trust. Usually statements made about here-and-now experiences are more threatening than those made about past experiences. When patients feel free to disclose a concern, fear, or impression about their current relationships with providers, it is usually indicative of moderate to high levels of trust.

Intent and Level of Self-Disclosures

There is still another way of classifying self-disclosures that addresses the intent and level of intimacy of the statements. The following types of disclosures will be described in this section: (1) meta-disclosures, (2) irresponsible or accidental disclosures, (3) disclosures in the service of aggression or manipulation, and (4) competitive or attention-getting disclosures.

The first type of disclosure is a meta-disclosure. Typically, *meta-disclosures* are disclosures about a disclosure. For example, "I lied to you because I wanted you to think I was better than I am" is a meta-disclosure. It reveals something about a previous self-disclosing statement (namely, "I told you a lie"). Meta-disclosures are useful in helping providers refocus on the difficulties of understanding the patient. For example, "I'm having trouble understanding what you are saying about your breathing—let me ask some questions" comments on the character of the communication and creates a potential for clearer communication. These statements are also referred to as *process disclosures* because they focus more on the process of communication rather than the content of the dialogue.

Irresponsible disclosures are made without any real regard for the receiver. In the patient–provider relationship, they are forbidden. If a patient is describing, for example, his difficulty maintaining an erection, statements such as "Getting an erection has never been a problem for me" would be irresponsible. Sometimes such statements are also accidental, meaning that the provider really did not mean to share something, but it "slipped out."

Disclosures in the service of other feelings—aggression and anger—are common in social interactions. They are frequently used to punctuate negative judgments. Consider the following dialogue: "You're always cheating on your diet, so how do you think I can help you if you keep doing this? (angry tone) I have never had as much trouble with other patients." Angry disclosures of this kind express aggression. The underlying intent may not be to inflict shame, disgrace, or distress, although that is generally what happens. Providers' frustrations are unleashed on the patient, not only in unhelpful ways but in ways that are hurtful.

Disclosures can also be made to *persuade* or *manipulate* the patient. Persuasion and manipulation are also used in instances where the patient is felt to be resistant or recalcitrant. "Come on now, you can tell me whether you took your medication. I can find out anyway" is manipulative. This disclosure is used strategically to get the patient to disclose when he does not want to. This type of disclosure not only manipulates (i.e., "I'll find out anyway if you don't tell me"), it projects a level of intimacy that is not there. "You can tell me" suggests a level of trust and intimacy that is not present between the provider and patient.

Competitive or *attention-getting disclosures* are also frequently used in social situations. The primary purpose is to gain special recognition. Statements like "Guess what, I'm so cool I just got asked to be the group's representative" could evoke a competitive counter: "I've been the representative for three years already. They want me to be the chair because they like how I handle the budget." The aim is to take the floor from the first person, making oneself better or more important than another.

In provider–patient dialogue, competitive disclosures can occur even though they are clearly disruptive. Consider the following dialogue.

Patient: "I wonder when I'm going to see my doctor. Is he here yet? I think he forgot me today. He's usually here by now. I don't think I can go a whole day without talking to him."

Provider: "That's nothing. I'm going a whole week without talking to my husband. He is on a business trip, and I can't reach him by phone because of the time difference. If I don't get some help with the kids—the babysitter is sick—I don't know how I'm going to work these two 12-hour shifts coming up." (Competitive self-disclosure)

Clearly, the provider's motive in self-disclosing is not patient centered. The provider is focused more on her own problems than on the concerns of the patient. In this dialogue, there is a reverse priority: "You think you have problems reaching someone important to you, wait until you hear this!" The provider's needs seem to take precedence over those of the patient.

THE THERAPEUTIC EFFECTS OF SELF-DISCLOSURE

Self-disclosure on the part of the patient is, without a doubt, essential and hopefully therapeutic. Without patient disclosures, providers cannot conduct valid assessments. Patient self-disclosures also are healing in that they allow the provider to better understand them—and every patient has a basic need to be attended to and understood.

Although controversial, there can be therapeutic value to the patient from the provider's self-disclosing of personal data. The most significant contributions to our knowledge of the therapeutic value of self-disclosure comes from the early work of Jourard (1971), who expressed the view that self-disclosure begets self-disclosure. That is, open-disclosure statements on the part of the provider generate further disclosure on the part of the patient. Provider self-disclosures, however, must meet certain criteria:

1. They must be true statements.
2. They are subjectively perceived statements about the self.
3. They are intentionally revealed to the patient with a therapeutic aim in mind.

Review this dialogue between the provider and patient:

Patient: "I'm worried about my tests. What if they come back 'bad?'" (Self-disclosure)
Provider: "We won't really know until next week."
Patient: "I have problems enough without . . . you know, I don't think I could get through another surgery after all I've been through." (Self-disclosure)
Provider: "You have been through a lot, and I know it wouldn't be easy."
Patient: (Begins to cry.)
Provider: "You know, when I think back on how you have 'held your own'—gone through these last two years, I feel a deep respect and admiration for you." (Self-disclosure)
Patient: (Smiling and tearful) "I didn't know that."
Provider: "Yes. I care. I'm in this for the duration." (Self-disclosure)
Patient: "Then I'll get the courage from somewhere—can't let you down." (jokingly)

This self-disclosure could be of significant therapeutic value. The physician shares some intimate details about his reflections and feelings about the patient. Although the disclosures began at a superficial level, the level of intimacy increased. The conversation culminated with the provider and patient sharing attitudes about the here-and-now of their relationship. The provider evokes self-disclosure by making personal disclosures. These statements encouraged the patient to express the innermost thoughts and feelings that influence the patient's outlook about forthcoming treatments. The nature of these disclosures suggest that there is a context for mutual trust building in this relationship.

There is a tendency for communication to be expressed in symmetry; that is, responses of one kind are likely to evoke similar responses. This tendency for one person to open up on a subject and the other to follow suit is called response matching. *Response matching* means that if providers self-disclose, they are likely to evoke self-disclosure in the patient. Otherwise, self-disclosure begets self-disclosure. When the patient is reinforced or encouraged to continue to talk about a subject in a meaningful way, then the provider's self-disclosure has facilitated the therapeutic goals of the relationship. Thus, social penetration—increasing depth and breadth in disclosures—increases over time. In this way, provider self-disclosures are productive in that they elicit more data and engage the patient in mutual problem solving. The principle of response matching is the primary justification for using self-disclosure in the provider–patient relationship.

There are other therapeutic effects of self-disclosure. These effects arise from the patient's realization that the provider is human. Four effects will be elaborated upon: (1) the sense of being understood, (2) the enhancement of trust, (3) decreased loneliness, and (4) decreased role distance.

The Sense of Being Understood

As previously stated, the therapeutic value of being understood was first documented in the literature by Jourard (1971), who stressed disclosure as a means of understanding the self and the world as another experiences it. One of the major tensions in the provider–patient relationship is the uncertainty about whether the patient will be understood fully enough to choose the best possible intervention. When the provider self-discloses pertinent personal data, the patient can gain reassurance that the provider:

- Listens carefully.
- Is processing the patient's experience.
- Is empathetic.
- Can understand, at the human level, what this illness or injury and its prognosis means to the patient.

In the best of cases, patients whose providers offer brief but well-timed disclosures are more likely to feel that the provider really understands, whereas those patients whose providers never disclose and assume a neutral position are likely to view the provider as impenetrable and therefore impervious to the worrying and suffering that are important to patients and that affect their quality of life. Consider the impact of a self-disclosure like this: "To avoid forgetting to use the waterpik at night, I just use it in the morning but I make sure the reservoir is full."

The Enhancement of Trust

Building on the previous potential benefit, when the patient feels that the provider more fully understands, the patient is likely to sense that he or she can trust the provider. Trust in the patient–provider relationship has two elements: (1) the patient perceives the provider as knowledgeable and competent, and (2) the patient perceives that the provider has his or her best interests in mind. An example of this kind of self-disclosure might be: "Together we are going to get you better."

Decreased Loneliness

Provider self-disclosure can reduce feelings of loneliness in the patient as it alters the level of intimacy in the relationship. The provider's self-disclosure confirms that the patient is not all alone in the process of coping with and fighting his illness. The provider's self-disclosure clearly communicates presence (i.e., "I am present not only as a provider but at the human level"). To some extent, decreased loneliness occurs as patients realize that they are not so different from other people, in this case, the provider. The provider's disclosure can communicate shared experience, and this works directly to alter the personal isolation that the patient encounters. Interestingly enough, the provider's disclosure may increase the attractiveness of the provider. Clinicians have observed that self-disclosure induces liking. Perceived as a reward, the patient feels singled out in a special way to hear the provider's (usually) unexpressed thoughts and feelings. One such example of this kind of self-disclosure might be: "If I were in your shoes, I would feel stressed too."

Liking and self-disclosure are positively associated. When asked to selectively disclose to several clinicians, the patient will disclose more intimate data to those for whom he has a greater liking. Also, at the end of a period of mutual self-disclosure, patients will indicate a greater liking for those with whom they have exchanged more intimate disclosures. The patient who views the provider as someone with whom intimacy is possible will most often apprise the relationship as desirable and be less likely to avoid and more likely to approach the provider. The provider's sense of appeal is a subtle but important factor in many issues concerned with treatment, including the willingness of the patient to be treated by the provider, patient comfort in disclosing intimate details to the provider, and patient compliance with the treatment program prescribed by the clinician.

Decreased Role Distance

A fourth and final potential therapeutic outcome in the provider's use of self-disclosure is that role distance is decreased when providers disclose. Decreasing role distance is controversial in the sense that violation of boundaries is of concern. However, decreased role distance can have the indirect effect of modifying the patient's dependency on the provider and maximizing the likelihood that mutual, collaborative problem solving will occur.

When providers use self-disclosures for the expressed purpose of their therapeutic outcome (e.g., to build empathy), certain steps will ensure success. First, the provider needs to listen carefully to the verbal and nonverbal aspects of the patient's communication. Second, the provider should, while focusing on the patient, express an empathetic response. Third, the provider might reveal a similar personal experience thereby increasing the impact of the empathetic reflection. And, following the disclosure, the provider needs to evaluate the relevance of both the empathic response and the self-disclosure. By using these steps, the provider is increasing the likelihood that the self-disclosure will serve therapeutic purposes.

TYPES OF NONTHERAPEUTIC SELF-DISCLOSURE

Provider self-disclosure when the provider shares with the patient something of a personal nature (beyond name, specialty, and credentials) continues to generate controversy. In part there is little direct evidence that it is helpful or consistently preferable. In a study by McDaniel and colleagues (2007), 85% of the self-disclosures were not helpful to the patient, and 11% were felt to be disruptive to the patient care. In explaining these results, the investigators stated that there was so little time in the space of the interview that the possibility of the provider disclosure enhancing patient disclosure was also very limited. Provider disclosures were more distracting than helpful. Thus, just as there are therapeutic outcomes with the use of self-disclosures, there is also the potential for these disclosures to produce no effects or nontherapeutic results. Providers need to be fully aware of these potential drawbacks.

Decreasing Understanding

There are at least three key difficulties that can arise. First, the provider may express thoughts and feelings, but these will not be within the patient's current frame of reference. This is a common error. In an attempt to make the patient feel better, the statement actually could make the patient feel worse.

Patient: "I've put on a lot of weight—can't seem to get it off."
Provider: "I've lost 20 pounds this year myself. Couldn't feel better." (Self-disclosure)

The topic is weight gain and the difficulties of losing weight. The physician tells of his success. It is obvious that the provider is not at the same place as the patient with this problem, and this might be disconcerting to the patient. The result is more social distance and decreased feelings of being helped. Evans et al. (1989) affirmed that provider disclosures need to relate to patient disclosures in order to keep the focus on the patient's specific and immediate problem. In this way, distraction from the patient is minimized.

Role Reversal

A second major nontherapeutic consequence is that as the provider uses self-disclosure, the patient and provider switch roles. This is sometimes expressed as a boundary issue. The provider, formerly the helper, becomes the helpee. There are circumstances under which patients would benefit from this role reversal; namely, it gets them off the hook. They are relieved of the need to collaborate on their own treatment program. The following dialogue describes this process as the provider is trying to encourage a resistant patient to follow a low-fat diet.

Provider: "There are reasons that the doctor wants you to keep your diet low in fat."
Patient: "I know—but I like salami, chopped liver, fries—a meal is not a meal without bread and butter."
Provider: "I can understand, Mr. S____, that it is hard for you. I've had to eliminate nearly all fat from my diet, and it is difficult to turn my back on things I like so much." (Self-disclosure)
Patient: "What foods have you turned your back on?"
Provider: "Ice cream (my favorite), butter, cheeses, sausage . . ." (Self-disclosure)
Patient: "It probably wouldn't hurt you to have an occasional piece of cheese or an ice cream cone."
Provider: "If I start cheating, I seem to have no control." (Self-disclosure)
Patient: "Maybe what you can do is check into some of those low-fat ice creams or yogurt—my wife eats a lot of yogurt."

In this scenario, there is role reversal. The patient has distracted the provider from the purpose of exploring his own diet restrictions. He has gotten the provider to talk about her own difficulties instead. He is even beginning to give her advice about her problems of coping with diet restrictions. Role reversal is evidenced by the fact that (1) the focus switched to the provider's problem; (2) the patient assumes a helping role; and (3) the provider replies to the remarks in a complementary fashion, reinforcing the reversal of roles.

There is more than one possibility to explain why this occurred. First, the patient may have felt that the provider's questions were too intrusive and wanted to avoid disclosing. Second, the patient might have wanted to avoid changing his eating patterns and simply wants to stop the provider from putting pressure on him. A third possibility is that the patient does want to comply but is unwilling to work with this provider on the problem.

Also, there are various reasons the provider failed to remain a helper in this encounter. First, the provider may not have anticipated negative consequences of a self-disclosure with this patient. The provider may even have been unaware of the patient's desire to take the focus off himself. Second, the provider may have perceived resistance in the patient but decided that expanding on her own experience would increase the patient's trust. Finally, the provider may have some strong feelings about her own problems with compliance and was unaware of these. The patient's questions may have elicited problems that she needs to discuss with her own physician. The surprise element for the provider—Gee, I thought I accepted my restrictions and the realization that this is not the case—may further distract her in refocusing on the patient's problem. Thus, the provider might not be fully cognizant of the role reversal because she is caught up in thoughts about her own problem.

Role reversal is itself reversible. That is, providers can regain their focus on the patient and maintain their professional roles. Ways of doing this include stopping and turning the focus back on the patient's problem, stating that it seems the patient has difficulty with the topic, and regaining control by summarizing what the patient has said about his problem.

CRITERIA TO JUDGE THE BENEFITS OF SELF-DISCLOSURE

Because provider self-disclosure is both beneficial and problematic, clinicians have developed criteria to evaluate its usefulness. Auvil and Silver (1984), for example, have identified four guidelines for judging the merits of a disclosure:

1. Will the disclosure enhance the patient's cooperation, which is necessary to the therapeutic alliance?
2. Will the disclosure assist the patient in learning about him- or herself, to set short- or long-term goals or deal more effectively with his or her problems?
3. Will the disclosure assist the patient to express formerly withheld feelings and concerns that are important for emotional support?
4. Will the disclosure provide the patient with support or reinforcement for important changes or goals he must act upon?

Finally, one rule of thumb to keep in mind in employing self-disclosures therapeutically is that self-disclosure needs to be tied to a goal or aim. If the provider does not have a patient-centered objective for using a personal self-disclosure, then it probably should not be used. If providers are not patient-centered in their use of disclosures, they are probably acting on other motives, including getting their own needs met. Meeting your own needs rather than the patient's is, in most cases, nontherapeutic for the patient. In McDaniel and colleagues' study (2007), 70% of the patients (following provider disclosure) actually returned to their own concerns. They responded to the contents of the provider self-disclosure.

DEFLECTING REQUESTS FOR SELF-DISCLOSURE

There are times when providers are asked by patients to disclose personal data about themselves. Sometimes providers feel that they must self-disclose to be courteous to the patient. Patient requests for self-disclosure are frequently felt to be uncomfortable because they distract from the task at hand. The following discussion addresses ways to avoid self-disclosing when it is not appropriate or when the provider is uncertain of the therapeutic value of doing so. In some cases, the patient's lack of clarity about the intent of the interview will cause a shift in focus to the provider.

Take, for example, this dialogue between a medical student and patient.

Provider: "Mr. J____, I'm here to gather some information about the symptoms you're feeling right now."
Patient: "Who are you?"
Provider: "I'm a medical student. I work with Dr. S____."
Patient: "How long have you been in school?"
Provider: (Feeling somewhat uncomfortable) "Several years."
Patient: "Am I your first patient?"
Provider: "No, I've seen many patients."

This patient might be asking for personal data from the medical student because he is unsure about the purpose of the student and not sure that the student knows what he is doing. The patient is "sizing-up" the student and asks several questions to establish whether the student is competent enough to assume any part of his care.

Self-disclosures on the part of the provider can be uncomfortable. When such disclosures are requested by the patient, they are not readily linked to a patient-centered objective—although it appears that by responding to the request the provider is meeting the patient's need. The need for the information is obscure, and the provider does not know exactly how the information will be put to use. Additionally, there is the threat that what the provider discloses may cause the patient to dismiss or reject the provider. While the provider may not actually be rejected by this patient, the mere threat or anticipation that rejection could occur can make the provider more self-conscious and hesitant. All self-disclosures have the impact of exposing vulnerabilities. And no one, patients and providers alike, is comfortable with feeling vulnerable.

There are cases in which requests for self-disclosures need to be deflected. These cases are determined on the basis of certain criteria that will help the provider know how to respond.

Absence of Patient-Centered Rationale

Does the provider's self-disclosure have a patient-centered rationale? Sometimes complying with the request to self-disclose will benefit the patient directly or indirectly. Benefits that occur directly as a result of provider self-disclosure include those identified earlier: the patient derives a sense of being understood, trust in the provider is enhanced, the patient experiences a decrease in feelings of loneliness, and role distance (between provider and patient) is reduced. Indirect patient-centered benefits include (1) balancing the dialogue, (2) giving the patient an opportunity to relax—a break from the intensity of the interview, and (3) communicating the humanity of the provider so the patient will feel more comfortable in disclosing around a selected topic.

If an invited self-disclosure does not seem to address one or more of these direct or indirect benefits, then chances are the request for self-disclosure needs to be deflected.

Highly Personal Information Requests

In addition to lack of patient-centered purpose, there is still another instance in which the provider will deflect a request for self-disclosure. When a request is too personal and causes provider discomfort, the request should be denied. Examples of these requests vary, but can typically include questions about the provider's age, religion, marital status, if they are dating, where they live, and how much money they make. Sometimes these requests are even more personal and include questions about sexual partner preferences, health status, and other personal life events experienced by the provider and/or the provider's significant others. The questions may be innocuous or intrusive. "Are you married?" seems innocuous. "Do you and your wife fight a lot? Who wins—you or her?" are more intrusive and involve information that the provider would not share with a stranger even if this is a patient situation.

Although the provider may choose to answer and answer honestly, there are other options. If the provider feels uncomfortable with a request, then a statement to the effect, "I'm not really comfortable answering those kinds of questions" is appropriate. It is not required that the provider give an explanation, but explanations such as "I don't discuss my personal life with my patients" helps clarify the provider's response. With these remarks, the provider is setting limits (relationship boundaries) on the discourse. Frequently, the patient means nothing behind the question and may have resorted to social chitchat because nothing else seemed to be important. Nonetheless, the provider still may be uncomfortable and needs to set limits on self-disclosing.

Guidelines in Deflecting Requests for Self-Disclosure

Auvil and Silver (1984) identify five further ways to circumvent a situation where providers' self-disclosure, at the patient's request, may be problematic: (1) expressing benign curiosity, (2) redirecting or refocusing the patient, (3) interpreting the patient's request, (4) clarifying the meaning behind the request, and (5) offering feedback along with limit-setting.

Provided one can be sincere about it, the easiest and most nonthreatening response is benign curiosity. The patient requests personal data and the provider responds with, "I'm wondering why you are asking me this." This reply calls for further information about the patient and gives clarity to the relationship (e.g., "I asked you that because I didn't think you understood about my holding things back from my wife.").

Redirecting or refocusing the patient is a technique to bring the patient back to the original topic that preceded the patient's request. This is done in a manner that indicates that the provider may not have heard the patient's request. It does not negate the fact that the patient did make a request; it simply reestablishes priorities in the therapeutic encounter. The following example illustrates how this is achieved in a relatively benign way.

Provider: "So tell me how this feels when I press here."
Patient: "It hurts but not as bad as it did yesterday."
Provider: "How about here?"
Patient: "Nothing—has anyone ever told you that you have pretty eyes?"
Provider: "What about here, feel anything when I press harder?" (Deflected request for self-disclosure)
Patient: "Yeah, that hurts."

The provider deflects the patient's request by responding as if she did not hear him. This was not done critically or angrily; the provider simply redirects the patient to follow her line of inquiry.

Interpreting why the patient is asking for personal data requires a great deal more knowledge and skill. It is appropriate but less frequently used, especially by inexperienced clinicians, because it calls for judgments that the provider may not be able to make.

Consider the following exchange:

Patient: "Are you married? Do you have kids?"
Provider: "Knowing something more about me as a person makes you a little more comfortable with me, doesn't it?" (Deflected request for self-disclosure and interpretation of the patient's intention)

This type of response requires patients to examine the context of the relationship and their inability or unwillingness to engage in a dialogue about themselves. If patients are not capable of such insight, the interpretation usually loses its impact even though it may successfully deflect the patient's request.

Clarifying the patient's request is a less-presumptuous strategy. For example, "You asked me if I were married, had kids—I wonder what concerns or uncertainties you might have about me." The provider expresses acceptance and positive regard for the patient's desire to know but seeks clarity about why the information is important.

Finally, responding with feedback deflects patients' requests for self-disclosure. Some patients might come across offensively. For example: "What do you like, Doc—blondes, brunettes; big ones, small ones, huh?" Sometimes patients need concrete feedback about their manner. The provider needs to feel that it is appropriate to instruct patients about the effect of their behavior not only on the provider but also on others. For example, "I'm not going to reply to that (patient's name), I don't think many people would."

CONCLUSION

In the most general sense, all communication discloses something about the speaker. Even nonverbal gestures disclose something personal. Still, when statements are made that reveal the nonobvious—a thought, feeling, attitude, or experience—and a distinct self-reference is made, the communication is more deliberately or accidentally self-disclosing. The use of self-disclosure can facilitate open communication that is critical in the establishment of a therapeutic alliance with the patient. When used effectively, self-disclosure can convey empathy, promoting a deeper closeness between provider and patient.

However, the use of self-disclosure is controversial. It may not have this therapeutic effect, there may not be time to use this approach, and the technique could cause negative outcomes. There are various reasons for self-disclosure to be problematic. Essentially, disclosures that miss the target can alienate the patient because the expression would fall outside the patient's frame of reference. Interrupting the flow of the patient's own disclosures can also occur. And as McDaniel and colleagues (2007) found, the probability that the focus will get back to the patient's concerns seems to be lower than we think in the average workday in primary care practice.

There are some very therapeutic outcomes that can occur with self-disclosure that are not a product of other response modes. Trust and the feeling of being understood can be achieved with other response modes to some extent; however, feeling less lonely and decreased role distancing are outcomes relatively unique to this therapeutic response mode.

Self-disclosure is difficult, and it may not be the provider's first choice in encouraging the patient to tell more. Self-disclosure by the provider takes courage and exposes one's vulnerability. Providers are not immune to the fear of rejection or disapproval that comes from disclosure. For these reasons, deliberate use of self-disclosure is a therapeutic response mode that needs to be thought out and practiced. If there is no patient-centered purpose for this self-disclosure, then the provider is not in a therapeutic position to significantly help the patient using this approach.

Although self-disclosure is used in social relationships, its application to therapeutic relationships with patients is still another matter. Provider self-disclosure is a skill that needs to be thoughtfully executed and evaluated. In those who believe disclosure is a pathway to their patients' trust, disclosure may elicit very positive alliances. One of our most important tasks is to understand how much personal information is comfortable for us to share.

CHAPTER 10

The Proper Placement of Advisement

We live in a society where most of our responses are shaped, in some way, by the (expressed) opinions of at least one other person (or group).
—*Gwen van Servellen*

CHAPTER OBJECTIVES

- Define advisement as a therapeutic response mode.
- Describe several misuses of advisement and opinion giving.
- List several helpful principles in using advisement with patients.
- Describe some problematic patient responses to advisement.
- List guidelines that enhance acceptance of advice.

Advice columns (e.g., "Ann Landers" and "Dear Abby") and, to some extent, national syndicated television shows (e.g., Geraldo, Oprah Winfrey, Montel Williams, and, of course, Dr. Phil) serve a common function in our society. They perform the task of helping their audiences choose the better course of action. Sometimes their advice is direct, stating the best way to solve a problem, and comes from them and only them. An alternative approach used is putting the audience into situational dilemmas and creating a form of "groupthink" (i.e., the audience is encouraged to solve the problem together). A form of *audience opinionaire,* sometimes supplemented with invited experts' judgments, is conducted. Audiences learn from this "quick advice" even if it is not totally relevant to their life circumstances. Both the advice columns and the television shows address two aspects of the problem:

1. How one should think when confronted with the situation.
2. What conclusions one should come to at the end of the process of thinking about the problem or dilemma.

In short, what we have in these public media events is mass instruction in problem solving. Along the way, we may even learn something new about such dilemmas as whom you should invite to your wedding, how to deal with a boyfriend/girlfriend who is cheating on you, how to deal with troubled friendships with parents or children, how to cope with overbearing parents, and what to do when a roommate does not pay the rent. The popularity of such media suggest that we are "hungry" for advice.

In our society, people both seek advice and express it. They also like to challenge advice, particularly if the directive is not clearly something that must be followed. Generally, advisement situations generate a great deal of discussion because, by disclosing opinions, one invites open dialogue about what one should do and how it should be done.

In this chapter, the differences between opinion giving and advisement are described. The misuse of both advisement and opinion giving are discussed as they interfere with mutual problem solving in the patient–provider relationship. Finally, principles behind the therapeutic use of advisement are identified and specific guidelines presented. An indirect, open style of advice-giving makes the patient less resistant and suspicious of the provider. It also increases the chances for patients' thoughtful exploration of their own dilemmas.

Advice-giving in the provider–patient relationship has made significant shifts. Formally, the major role of the provider was to give advice and evaluate the extent to which the patient followed the advice. The shift in health counseling toward motivational interviewing infers that simple advice given is inadequate in, for example, motivating patients to change unhealthy behaviors. Another reason for providers to be hesitant to give advice is a function of how the healthcare system works today. Most often, patients are seeing a number of providers and specialists to manage their care over time. Would we hesitate to give advice based on our uncertainty about what other providers and specialists told the patient? Otherwise, we do not want to work at cross-purposes. Is advice-giving so frustrating with some patients (due to their acceptance—or nonacceptance—of it) that we do a poorer job at it? Then there is the issue of accountability when our advice is inferior to the standards of care.

In sum, is the giving of advice, at least in the traditional sense, seen less often—for a number of reasons? Some of those reasons include perceptions that patients are not motivated by simple advice, concern that our advice will differ from the advice of specialists the patient is seeing, frustration due to the patient's lack of acceptance of the advice, and fear of the potential of reprimand if the advice is faulty. What about current healthcare system factors (e.g., the varying length of time we have to see the patient) that drive the extent to which we feel comfortable in our assessment of the patient's motivation and readiness to change?

DEFINITIONS OF ADVISEMENT

Advisement is one of the least studied therapeutic response modes. This is surprising when one considers the ubiquity of advice-giving in our society and the probability the healthcare provider will use advice-giving some time in the course of their relationship with every patient. In broad terms, *advisement* is the act of disclosing what one thinks or feels about another's experience, namely, what you think they should or should not feel, think, or do. It is unilateral in that most of the data and assessment of facts come from the provider and go to the patient.

In specific terms, advisement is the provider's use of suggestions, directives, instructions, or commands. Its aim is to effect change in the patient's behavior, attitude, and/or emotional response. Advice is given at all stages of the health–illness continuum: prevention, treatment, and evaluation of care.

Intensity of Advisement

Advisement can be characterized by the level of intensity. Low-intensity advisement is the process of giving information, opinions, and recommendations, but the patient has maximum control over the ultimate course of action. This form of advisement is very nondirective. For example, telling the patient that if he continues to smoke his health will suffer illustrates that low-intensity advisement sense is not prescriptive. This should not be confused with patients' rights, where patients are ultimately able to reject treatment. High-intensity advisement, on the other hand, is a powerful suggestion, frequently worded as a command. Patients essentially abdicate some control over their behavior. Left to them they will continue to smoke. Providers might state it as a prescription: "I want you to stop smoking gradually so that you reduce smoking to one pack a day. I will see you back here in two weeks and we will see if you are ready to move on from there." Providers get more directive in their advice-giving with patients who have already developed a health problem associated with the condition in this case, smoking. This latter type of advisement is taken up again in Chapter 12 where the judicious use of commands, directives, and orders are discussed.

Advisement differs from the act of giving information and expressing opinions. Essentially, giving information and expressing opinions are preferable because they more likely result in mutual problem solving. In a study of general practitioners discussions with patients about stopping smoking (Coleman, Cheater, & Murphy, 2004), more than three-quarters of these physicians used approaches that would elicit collaboration than approaches that would be confrontational. Advisement, especially high-intensity advisement, can be more forceful and may not be given in a way that is respectful of the patient's thoughts and preferences. Expressing opinions and offering information, on the other hand, tend to communicate respect for patients' views and engage patients in the decision-making process.

Patient Responses to Advisement

Patients' responses to advice often depend on whether the advice was sought. Bertakis, Roter, and Putnam (1991) found that patients were less satisfied in healthcare encounters when providers (physicians) dominated the interview by excessive talking, such as giving too much advice, or when the emotional tone was provider (physician) dominated. Usually, when patients ask for advice, they are open to hearing and modifying the information to fit their individual circumstances. Accepting advice may also be a function of cultural orientation. In some cultures, individualism is stressed and individual rights are valued above all else. Individuals with this orientation may be less inclined to accept advice than are those individuals whose culture stresses conformity.

Advisement, and to a lesser extent, opinion giving, can be misused. Essentially, when providers are telling patients what they should think, how they should feel, or how they should behave, they are implying that they (the providers) know what is best. This position tends to prevent patients from struggling with and thinking through their own problems. Providers do not use advice solely to assist patients. Advisement can be used for ulterior motives such as to avoid uncomfortable patient–provider situations. Some patient decisions are very difficult, and sometimes providers use advisement to avoid uncomfortable silence and to avoid focusing on difficult or painful thoughts and feelings that the patient's situation evokes.

Perhaps the most common misuse of advisement is to solve a problem quickly. In this case, the provider may be given too much credit for the resolution of the problem. Using advice in this way tends to discount the idiosyncratic explanations as to why some suggestions just do not work. It is as much the provider's task to assess why something may not work as it is to offer medically sound advice.

Providers' responses to patients' needs for and reactions to advice are critical. Patients seek provider advice. Patients who openly ask for advice, but are denied, may feel cheated and unhappy with the provider or the service. Sometimes they are given advice but they do not understand this advice and the provider has little time to elaborate. Reactions (e.g., "He said I should . . . but, I don't know why he said that . . . and it happened so fast I didn't think to ask him") can occur on a somewhat frequent basis. Patients and providers alike may be uncertain about the course of action. The ambiguity that exists can be uncomfortable and disconcerting. Although a clear answer may not be forthcoming, some reassurance by the provider that an answer (viewed by the patient as a solution) is at hand is helpful.

A provider's reaction to a patient's accepting or rejecting the advice given is a reflection of the provider's personal need for professional pride and sometimes control. Providers should examine their own needs for affirmation and control so that they are better equipped to manage patients that refuse their advice.

THE MISUSE OF ADVISEMENT AND OPINION-GIVING

Studies seem to suggest that advisement, while common in provider–patient relationships, is frequently problematic. Within the Rogerian client-centered framework, advice is discouraged for four reasons:

1. It is comparatively poor in generating rapport and unconditional positive regard.
2. It can produce more guarded responses in patients who are resisting the advice.
3. It may encourage dependency and diminish learning, which is contrary to developing a collaborative relationship.
4. It tends to increase resistance in the patient, particularly if the advice is given in an authoritative way.

Taking Control from the Patient

Consider the following dialogue between a provider and a young adult patient who is being seen in the clinic for an injury to her arm.

Provider: "So how did you hurt your arm?"

Patient: "I fell while I was snowboarding. It didn't hurt too much at first, but about an hour later, it started to swell and throb."

Provider: (Silence.) "Well, my children are not allowed to snowboard for that very reason. I have three rules: no snowboarding, no skateboarding, and no rollerblading. The same goes for you." (Advisement—indirect)

Patient: (Silence.) "Oh . . . well, I've been snowboarding for 3 years and snowskiing for 10 years, and this is the first time I've gotten hurt."

Provider: "Well, you have just been very lucky, young lady!"

The physician in this scenario approached the patient parentally, suggesting that she was a "bad" girl and "look what happened." His advice—follow my rules—was posed indirectly through a self-disclosure. The effect on the patient was problematic because she judged the self-disclosure irrelevant but also got the point that she should obey him. The patient already felt bad, and the physician's comments might have made her feel worse. His parental tone was annoying to the patient evidenced by her later statement, "I have my own parents, and I don't need his opinion." Further, the physician's comment, "You've been very lucky!" was taken as indirect advice (i.e., "No more snowboarding, young lady!"). Resistance was evoked, though not verbalized. No doubt, the patient felt that her snowboarding was none of this doctor's business. "I came to have my arm X-rayed and set, that's all!"

This patient's experience caused her to request a change in doctors before her next visit for follow-up care. The patient saw absolutely no benefit in continuing with this physician because she did not feel supported, did not learn anything new, could not express her feelings freely without feeling judged, and felt no desire to cooperate. Had the physician listened to his patient, kept his advice "low key," and tried to make the patient feel better, the outcome might have been much different.

By giving direct advice, even disguised, providers can take away from patients the responsibility that is rightfully theirs. This typically puts patients in a state of dependence on the judgment and guidance of the provider. By giving the patient information about the incidence of such injuries—offering low-intensity advice—the provider is supplying patients with data and support for formulating their own decisions and actions.

Altering Negative Effects of Advisement

Consider how the previous dialogue could be altered to achieve a therapeutic aim. Assume that the physician is not only a very competent provider but deeply cares about the health and well-being of his patients. What could he have done? First, he could have explained that he has treated many of these injuries and that this was like the others he has treated. He could also ask his patient to describe how it happened, expressing interest in the trauma aspect of the accident. Actively listening to the patient describe how the event was a shock and what put her at risk would make two points: (1) even though we are pretty certain that we will not be injured, it does happen; (2) reliving the movements she did or did not take that culminated in the injury would have provided her with information about how to prevent future injuries. Data such as, "There is 1 chance out of 25 for this injury to occur" would encourage his patient to consider the odds that it will happen again. The overall purpose of advisement is to alter behavior. Subtle and indirect advice can be more effective than straight-on directives. Phrased as it was in the previous dialogue as a self-disclosure, the advice is indirect but not very subtle.

Unlike advisement, expressing opinions establishes equal opportunity and mutual respect between the patient and the provider. Expressing opinions is assertively interactional. That is, provider opinions are offered as additional information for the patient's decision-making process. Consider, for example, the feelings that these statements evoke: "It's my opinion . . ." and "Based on what I've read (heard, seen), I would say that this course of action is better." Expressing opinions is not making the decision for the patient, it is simply giving the patient the benefit of the provider's knowledge. In contrast, giving advice is a unilateral process of solving problems or making decisions for another (Hanes & Joseph, 1986).

PRINCIPLES BEHIND THE THERAPEUTIC USE OF ADVISEMENT

In some ways, presenting patients with information about their condition is the provider's duty, and neglecting to do so would be very poor practice. The balance that must be achieved is to provide information and opinions without negating the patients' rights to express their own opinions and to ask for further data to come to what they believe is the best course of action.

Less Direct Advice

The first basic principle in using advisement is that for many patients, the less direct the advice, the less likely it is that resistance will occur. To hold to this principle, providers must have an open style—a willingness to have their advice rejected. Advice that must be followed is not advice but rather a command or directive, and when the advice must be adhered to, providers must clearly say so.

Many patients are sensitive to advice, even though they have come to providers for help or a consultation. At its worst, advice communicates that the patient is incapable of self-direction, which can be humiliating and belittling. Many people have received advice that was not helpful or received directives in an unhelpful manner. Just the words, "You should . . ." may be the first and only thing the patient hears before tuning out and turning off. Some individuals have been subjected to critical parental figures and are not able to set their reactions aside when providers begin to advise with parental inflections. Such individuals may also be unable to accept advice from anyone because authority figures have not proven themselves to be trustworthy.

A useful way to present advice to persons who are suspicious of advice-giving is to present the advice in ways that do not resemble advice. Suggesting an "alternative" or "a possibility" lessens the emphatic context of the idea. Presenting ideas as hypothetical is also a way to soften the harshness of advice. The following phrases, juxtaposed on an idea, can soften the impact of direct advice:

- "Do you think this idea will help in your situation?"
- "What do you think about these recommendations?"

- "How do you think this suggestion will fit your lifestyle?"
- "Can you adapt any of these ideas to your situation?"

Providing a Rationale

Another method for giving advice indirectly is to credit it to experience, another source, or another authority. This is called providing a rationale. For example, providers may preface their statements with "Patients who followed this treatment for two years experienced better results," or "According to research on the effects of the long-term use of sleeping medication . . ." Provide ways for patients to rationalize their decisions. In these cases, the provider can appear to be unbiased while at the same time appear to identify with the patient's dilemma. Together they come to a joint decision, although in actuality, it was the provider who swayed the patient to select a specific course of action.

Decrease Confusion

Other response modes used with advice-giving create confusion. One example illustrated in the dialogue between the physician and his patient who suffered a snowboarding injury was self-disclosure used with advice-giving. Was it effective? Most likely not. Nothing was added to the dialogue by the physician's adding personal information about his family. Should the patient comment about the advice he gave to his family or the implicit advice he was giving her? Still another example is when questions are used with advice-giving. Imagine this same patient being asked: "Don't you think that if you continue to snowboard you will suffer an even more serious injury?" This leading question clearly is not one to be answered simply yes or no. The implication is that any patient in his or her right mind would understand this fact (i.e., "What's wrong with you that you don't see this?"). Advisement can inhibit the exploration of a problem by leading the patient to a defensive counterresponse.

Recognize Problematic Patient Responses

Inhibition of further exploration can take many forms. In earlier scenarios between provider and patient, the advice given was ignored and the patient responded, at least initially, with silence. Some typical patient responses to advisement include (1) placating, (2) changing the subject, (3) ignoring the advice, (4) reacting with silence, and (5) passively agreeing with the advice. If the provider is studying the reactions of patients to his or her advice-giving, these problems might be recognized.

Placating is a response that is frequently given by patients. The classic exchange, "You should . . ." and "Yes, I will . . ." establishes that the patient has heard the advice and intends to take it. But is this really the case, or was this the reply because the patient did not want to explore the idea and really had little intention of taking the advice? The response is used to cause the provider to "back-off."

Patients might also change the subject or transition to the next topic as if the advice is "a done deal." The underlying message is, "Let's go on to something else."

Consider the following comments of a patient who is receiving prenatal care from a nurse practitioner in a community clinic.

Provider: "You have been taking care of yourself, right?"
Patient: "Yes."
Provider: "I hope so. You need to control using alcohol and eat well, because if you don't it can cause great harm to your baby." (Advisement)
Patient: (Silence. Feeling somewhat guilty and humiliated.) "When do I have to come back again?" (Change of subject)

The patient probably did not have enough time to seriously answer the question asked of her. Additionally, the advice was levied as a "warning," potentially making the patient feel guilty and ashamed. The patient never really got a chance to explain how well she was caring for herself because the nurse practitioner answered the questions herself. Had the nurse's nonverbal behavior displayed interest and if the questions were open and accepting, the patient might have insisted on some time to really talk about it. The patient may have concluded "There was no talking to her—might as well change the subject"; by transitioning to the next subject or changing the topic, the patient avoids a discussion of her concerns and the advice she was given.

Ignoring the provider's advice with open defiance is yet another potential patient response. Sometimes patients can argue just as convincingly against advice as the provider can argue to support the advice. This can result in "a battle of wits" over who is more right than the other. The provider offers the advice, then is puzzled, maybe even angered, by the fact that the patient does not follow it. The natural counter is, "Why do you even ask my advice if you're not going to take it?!" The provider expresses frustration and might or might not pursue the topic further.

Silence and unelaborated passive agreement are still other responses patients may give to direct advice. Silence occurs when the provider suggests a course of action (i.e., "You should . . .") and gets no answer. Unelaborated passive agreement occurs in circumstances where the provider suggests a course of action, i.e. ("You should . . .") and gets a curt response ("Uh huh").

Guidelines That Enhance Patient Acceptance of Advice

Whether expressing opinions or giving advice, there are specific guidelines that are more likely to ensure acceptance. An important practice is to ask the patient (or patient's family) if they want to hear your ideas or points of view with statements such as, "I have cared for other patients with this illness and have read a great deal on the subject. I could provide a summary if you would like to hear it." If the patient's nonverbal response is avoidance or if the patient argues with your views, it is best to drop the discussion and reestablish trust and harmony before continuing. Remember, you have not changed your mind; you will just wait for another opportunity to discuss the problem.

Advice That Is Tentative

Advice that is tentative is more likely to be accepted. If the provider avoids being dogmatic and makes allowances for the uniqueness of the individual patient, the advice will be more palatable. Questions such as, "What do you think about the suggestions I've given you?" also discourage the provider from being too presumptuous about the patient's readiness to accept the advice. It is always good practice to adapt your advice to both the situation and the patient. If the patient is an individual who rarely appreciates advice, it may be better to cushion the advice with a story, a self-disclosure, or a link with another source or all of these approaches. Additionally, it is important to stay close to the patient's own language, cultural viewpoint, or age-related jargon (e.g., by using the patient's words as you initially talk about the patient's problems). This not only enables providers to further individualize their advice, it decreases the distance that may be felt between the provider and the patient. In the case of young adults or adolescents, it is particularly useful to frame advice in terms that are important to them, because this group is particularly sensitive to criticism and feelings of being put down by adults. After all, if the patient's dilemma was simple, then the solution could be straightforward. By helping patients save face, the provider minimizes threats to the patient's self-esteem and increases the likelihood that the patient will accept the advice or opinions that are offered.

Assessing Patient Readiness

Considerable attention has been directed to processes of change that recognize several necessary steps. A description of the Transtheoretical Model of Change is presented in Chapter 22. According to this model, the stages of change are precontemplation, contemplation, preparation, action, and maintenance. Before offering advice or information or rendering opinions, the provider will need to assess the readiness of the patient. Carkhuff and Rordan (1987) describe a model for determining patient readiness. Essentially, the patient may be at any one of the following five sequential stages: uncertainty and confusion, awareness, understanding, constructive action, or learning.

At stage 1 (uncertainty and confusion), the patient has not yet realized the problem or the magnitude of its effects. Facts and feelings about the situation may be diffuse but still upsetting. Shocked, in denial, or otherwise overwhelmed, the patient is not ready to explore either the problem or the potential solutions. Attempting to give the patient advice at this stage would be useless.

However, in stage 2, awareness, patients are more prone to identify a problem and examine the effects that the problem has on their lives. Advice-giving at this stage might also be futile. The patient is still attempting to sort through the various thoughts and feelings that have been evoked by the problem. It is appropriate to discuss how the problem came about and what the potential consequences are. While the need for intervention can be discussed, the provider will need to refrain from discussing specific solutions.

In stage 3, the patient is increasingly developing a realization and an understanding of the problem. At this point, patients are ready to receive information about solutions. This may be communicated in a variety of forms—as information (written form) or as professional opinions.

In stage 4, the patient is ready for selecting a course of action. This stage is met with constructive intervention and can be supplemented by evaluating the actions taken. In this way, patients' knowledge increases significantly in depth as well as in breadth.

Including your rationale behind the particular piece of advice establishes a guide for patients to judge the wisdom of the advice. Again, it turns the final decision back to the patient. Sometimes, in stage 5, patients will learn more from the provider's discussion of the rationale than they could ever learn with simple statements of advice.

When all is said and done, however, providers must be ready to be wrong about their advice. Also, their opinions may not always agree with the patient's feelings at the time. Premature closure of a topic with the offer of advice can be just as problematic.

CONCLUSION

In offering advice or opinions, providers must be aware that depending on how it is delivered, advice-giving might diminish a patient's responsibility for decision making. This responsibility is rightfully theirs, and keeping patients in a state of dependence on the judgment and guidance of providers minimizes patients' abilities to formulate their own course of action. Sometimes the process of advice-giving does not afford patients the opportunities to sort through their own thoughts and arrive at their own decisions.

Providers may find it difficult to let patients make their own choices. They may be especially inclined to put their expertise to work while infantilizing the patient. Remembering that each patient requires a unique solution to his or her problems enables the provider to forestall the enthusiasm for a "quick fix."

With regard to very tough decisions and courses of action, providers must remember that the lack of advice is just as bad as poorly communicated advice. Uncertainty and indecision are uncomfortable for patients, and patients will not be able to tolerate this uncertainty for long. In the primary care setting, they have come to you for a consultation; they want to know more about their condition or health and are asking for advice or expert opinion. We cannot afford to be caught up in the reasons to avoid advice-giving. Rather, we must understand this response mode, practice giving advice, and study our own approach with patients. Accompanying patients (and patients' families) in the journey to arrive at the best possible course of action requires that providers not be timid about their professional opinions and not be threatened by conditions that deter them from sharing their professional knowledge. There is generally a great deal of diversity in patients' acceptance and understanding of providers' advice. Our challenge is to create a patient-centered collaborative relationship to explore, together, what is best, and this will include giving advice.

CHAPTER 11

Reflections and Interpretations

On the nature of interpretations: An idea under the idea, or a feeling beneath the feeling, can be assisted to emerge, and the process becomes more than an intellectual exercise; it produces an actual shift.
—E. F. Hammer

CHAPTER OBJECTIVES

- Define reflections as a therapeutic response mode.
- Describe how reflections can be therapeutically applied in provider communications with patients.
- Describe ways in which reflections differ by content, intensity, and length.
- Define interpretations.
- Differentiate reflections from interpretations.
- Discuss how reflections and interpretations differ from other therapeutic response modes.
- List several guidelines in using reflections.
- Identify the inappropriate ways in which interpretations are used in social contexts as well as their appropriate use in therapeutic encounters.
- List several guidelines in the therapeutic use of interpretations.

Reflection and interpretation are techniques that have the potential to strengthen the patient–provider relationship and assist patients in making significant changes. Like all other modalities, there are both therapeutic and nontherapeutic uses of these techniques. The practice of these modalities requires in-depth knowledge of self and the development of our own self-reflection skills. With abilities to reflect on self (thought, feelings, and behaviors), the chances of staying within the range of therapeutic exchanges is greater. Certain response modes are known to make a difference in the kind and quality of patient response. For example, reflections or mirroring back to patients what they say or might feel is likely to elicit further disclosure on the part of the patient. This same reaction might or might not be forthcoming with the use of interpretations. By comparing the different effects of reflection and interpretation, we can illustrate the principle that provider responses make a substantial contribution in shaping the patient's self-disclosure and attitudes about the helping process.

This chapter describes each response mode—reflection and interpretation—in detail. Comparisons are drawn between these therapeutic responses. The strengths and limitations of each are also identified, and guidelines for their use are provided.

DEFINITIONS OF REFLECTION

The technique of *reflection* was first endorsed in the work of Sigmund Freud. Essentially, Freud believed that if the therapist presented a human mirror to the patient, there would be growth and healing through increased awareness. From Chapter 9 on self-disclosure, you may remember that this modality can be used to evoke further elaboration from the patient because it presents humanness. However, reflection in a sense is the opposite of self-disclosure. With reflection, the provider withholds his or her personal thoughts, feelings, and experiences. With self-disclosure on the part of the provider, varying amounts of personal information about the provider are shared with the patient.

What is the character of reflection? Reflection can simply be a restatement or paraphrasing of what the patient has communicated; in the classical sense, though, reflection is more than this (Bernstein & Bernstein, 1985). Hill and Gormally (1977) stated that while reflection includes repeating the patient's statement, it should also contain references to stated or implied feelings. The reason for this reflection in psychotherapy is that suppressed feelings need to be connected with current expressions.

Reflections can stem from patients' current or previous statements, nonverbal behavior, reference to the context of the interaction, and even the provider's knowledge of the patient's total situation. Reflections may be phrased tentatively or as affirmative statements. Quite frequently they are stated as observations (e.g., "As you are talking about your surgery, I hear some uncertainty in your voice").

Reflection, then, is a response by providers that redirects the patients' ideas, feelings, and/or content of their message. While reflections may include paraphrases and restatements, they usually display more depth. *Paraphrasing* what the patient said is simply choosing parts of the verbal message and stating these ideas again, usually without extrapolating a primary idea. *Restatement*, unlike paraphrasing, involves reiterating almost word for word what the patient has said. In cases of paraphrasing and restatement, no reference is made to the patients' underlying meaning or attitudes or the nonverbal aspects that give clues to patients' in-depth thoughts and feelings.

Consider the following example. The patient is describing a concern about the anesthesia that will be used in surgery.

Patient: "I still don't know. What if I get real sick from it? They don't really know if they'll be able to use a general anesthesia."

Provider: "They don't know if they'll be able to use a general." (Restatement)

Patient: "That's what they said."

Provider: "So, let me see; you don't know yourself what they'll use or whether they will use a general?" (Paraphrasing)

Patient: "Yeah—it makes me nervous. My mother never could have a general."

Provider: "So as I'm listening to you—I sense that this is very much on your mind—what anesthesia they'll use—and I hear that you are afraid you'll get sick if they do give you a general anesthesia." (Reflection)

Patient: "Yeah—maybe I worry too much, but I do want to know ahead of time. I don't want a general because I'm afraid of having the same problems like my Mom did. Maybe I won't, but it still scares me."

Provider: "Yes, I understand why you are worried."

This series of statements by the provider illustrates the use of restatement, paraphrasing, and finally, reflection. Notice that the reflective remark makes reference to a stated or implied feeling—fear—while both the restatement and paraphrasing did not. Also notice that the reflective response elicited a discussion of depth, while the paraphrasing and restatement allowed the patient to stay with the theme on a superficial level.

Reflections, then, are not only statements by the provider that summarize what the patient has said, they explore what the provider thinks are the patient's feelings about his situation. The provider may reflect the early, middle, or the later parts of what the patient has said, or some part of all phases of the patient's disclosure. Reflection tends to focus the patient at a more in-depth level and at the same time discloses the providers' empathy. Reflection, then, is a demonstration on the part of the provider that he or she understands the patient. Restatement, while similar to reflection, deals more exclusively with the content and words that the patient uses. Reflection deals more with the feeling dimension of what the patient has said.

While it would seem that reflection is an easy response mode to implement, this is not the case. Reflection is a specialized response unfamiliar in the context of everyday conversation. Could you imagine yourself at a party and someone says to you: "I'm feeling kind of sick." And, you answer back: "I can hear you say you're feeling sick, you must feel disappointed that you have to leave the party." Social situations usually elicit response-matching; the detached, objective expressions of reflection are unfamiliar in the context of the give-and-take of social discourse. In fact, for this reason, providers may feel somewhat artificial and clumsy when they first use it. Successful use of reflection is usually more difficult to master than, for example, the therapeutic use of questions and silence because it is a less familiar response.

THERAPEUTIC USES OF REFLECTION

While reflection is an unfamiliar response in social conversations, its use in therapeutic discourse has a substantial history, particularly in psychotherapy. As previously noted in the work of Freud, the term *reflection of feelings* became a well-known aspect of a counselor's approach to people in distress.

Additionally, over the past 25 years, since the advent of Rogerian client-centered therapy (Rogers, 1951), reflection has slowly infiltrated the American, European, and Asian professional cultures. Reflective techniques are now used by a wide variety of providers, who must demonstrate understanding of their client's feelings and experience. Reflection is understood to heighten empathy. The reflective response is excellent in capturing the emotional meaning of the discloser's expressed message and is often used to show the patient that the provider is not only listening but also understands his or her feelings. The desired impact then is to give the patient the experience of being known.

This is achieved by slowing down the interaction, thus giving the patient more time to think out and clarify what was said (Beck, Rawlins, & Williams, 1988). Instead of describing a thought and moving on to the next subject, reflection replays the theme, sometimes doubling the time given to exploring the thought (Goodman & Esterly, 1988).

Reducing Isolation and Loneliness

In the context of dealing with an injury or illness, the patient sometimes has acute feelings of being alone with his problem. Reflective statements, when communicated empathetically, can give patients the experience of being with others that are interested and concerned. As Rogers (1951) so aptly explained, accurate reflections serve as a companion as the client (patient) explores (sometimes) frightening feelings. It is assumed that with sustained experiences of being known by providers, patients feel safety, courage, and company.

Reducing the experience of isolation and loneliness is something that providers can do with skillfully placed reflections. The following dialogue is between a student nurse and a patient diagnosed with leukemia. Chemotherapy has caused the patient's white-blood-cell count to drop, which necessitates the patient's transfer to protective isolation.

Provider: "O.K., Mrs. R____, it is time to move to the other room. Are you ready?"

Patient: "Yes, I am." (Not smiling, looks worried.)

Provider: "You seem quiet right now." (Reflection) "Are you feeling OK?"

Patient: "It is just that Mrs. K____ (her roommate) thinks that I am moving to another room because I don't want to be around her. I've tried to explain, but she doesn't understand."

Provider: "Would you like me to get an interpreter to explain it to her? One of the nurses speaks Korean."

Patient: "Yes, I would appreciate that so much!" (Smiling, then quiet and looking worried again while fighting back tears.)

Provider: "It seems like you are unhappy about something else." (Reflection)

Patient: "I just don't want to go to isolation again. It is so quiet in a room by yourself. Well, at least I can play my music louder." (Smiling, half-heartedly, then looking away.)

Provider: "It seems to me that you are afraid of being lonely in isolation." (Reflection)

Patient: "Yes, I was so lonely last time. The day just drags on and on."

Provider: "Going to isolation must make you feel even more alone since your family is so far away." (Reflection)

Patient: "Yes. Until now, it has been OK that my husband and kids couldn't visit me because I could go in and out of my room as I pleased."

Provider: "You sound very sad." (Reflection)

Patient: "Yes, that is exactly it." (She begins to cry.)

The student nurse stayed with this patient for a few minutes talking about ways in which she could feel less isolated. Subsequently, the patient called her husband.

In this interaction, the student listened empathetically to the patient, observing that the half-hearted smiles could be cues to some distress. Not knowing exactly what was bothering the patient, the nurse used reflection to help both herself and the patient identify the problem and explore the patient's feelings. The patient's self-disclosure seemed to decrease her sense of isolation and feelings of loneliness.

Promoting Positive Self-Worth

As summarized by Bradley and Edinberg (1990), reflection is employed therapeutically to achieve several outcomes. Reflections can impart powerful covert messages of positive self-worth. They obtain feeling responses from the patient. They deepen the patient's feeling state, thus making feelings and attitudes more accessible. Reflections also encourage communication to continue beyond the point where it might have been stopped. Because reflections highlight feelings as well as content, they increase patients' awareness of feelings through a greater sensitivity to what and how thoughts are communicated. Bernstein and Bernstein (1985) suggest that by re-presenting the patient's message, reflections provide patients with new insight. Thus, reflections mirror back to the patient important thoughts and feelings that are made more apparent because of the added attention they receive.

Reflection has become such an integral part of the helping process that the issue is not whether they are useful, but rather, how best to teach reflection. A reflection used mechanically in the absence of empathy, however, loses its impact.

KINDS OF REFLECTIONS

As with most other response modes, reflections differ qualitatively from one another.

Ways Reflections Differ—Content

One way in which reflections differ is in the selected content that the provider chooses to paraphrase. From the whole range of material stated by the patient, the provider will select and paraphrase what the patient has communicated, which may include not only words but nonverbal clues. Because providers will condense what the patient has said, exactly what providers use in their reflections may vary. In some instances, they may focus on the feeling aspects of the patient's communication. In other cases, they may paraphrase the words that the patient used with only minimal reference to feelings.

Ways Reflections Differ—Intensity

Another way in which reflections differ is by level of intensity or depth. Reflections can be graded as light, medium, or heavy, according to their intensity and the insight expected from the provider. Heavy reflections come with high demands, and like interpretations, might be resisted. Generally, the difficulty is that the provider is reflecting that which is obvious to them but may be outside the patient's awareness. Providers might, for example, label the distress that they hear in the patient's tone of voice and refer to rather strong labels (e.g., anger or rage). These labels may be too threatening to the patient, especially if these are feelings that have never been acceptable. The patient's predictable response in this situation is to quickly deny or challenge the validity of the reflection. Other patient reactions may include blocking exploration, ignoring the provider's statements, or attempting to clarify the provider's observations (e.g., "Why? Do I really sound angry?"). The response of the provider can then be changed to use less-threatening labels (e.g., "upset" instead of "angry" and "uncertain" instead of "anxious"). Backing off allows patients to relax, lower their resistance, and explore more comfortably the feeling dimension behind their statements.

Medium-level reflections are less offensive than are heavy reflections. Still, the patient may not understand why the provider's summary includes the labels that are used. Patients will not openly resist medium-level statements and will generally allow the provider to help them see the connection between their verbalization and the provider's impressions. With a little explanation or a passage of time, the patient will usually become open to the connections that are presented.

Consider, for example, the following dialogue.

Patient: "If you want to know the truth, I'd rather you take it (tumor) out right here. It's got to be done. Take this thing out."

Provider: "You want me to take it out here—now? We'll do it. Finding the lump must have been a real shock to you." (Reflection)

Patient: "Good." (Falls into silence expecting the procedure to be carried out, makes no reference to feeling shocked.)

At a return visit to the surgeon's office, the patient offers:

Patient: "This was the shock of my life—I couldn't believe it when I found it. I just wanted to get it out of my body."

Provider: "Yes. . . ." (empathizing with patient) "You caught it pretty early."

The reflection accomplished two things: It acknowledged the patient's request, and it identified the more covert experience of the patient (shock and disbelief about having discovered the tumor).

The reflection re-presents the patient's experience without much addition or subtraction from the verbal and nonverbal aspects of the communication. Feelings were addressed without adding too much new data. The provider was able to demonstrate empathy. While the patient did not initially address the shock that she felt, this aspect of the diagnosis was something the patient addressed after surgery. All in all, the patient was reassured by the provider that what was said made sense and was understood at a deeper level.

Light reflections are rarely resisted by the patient. Essentially, they are comments that the patient may have made him- or herself, usually just before the provider's statement. They frequently come across as "mind-reading" comments. Essentially, the provider puts things together for the patient, sometimes just before the patient is about to reflect these same thoughts. An example might be: "It hurts like crazy" (Patient) and "The pain is hard to deal with" (surgeon). The key to light reflections is that they rarely interrupt the flow of the interaction, and the patient almost always responds in ways that validate the content of the reflection. The patient might reply, "Yeah" or "That's right," and then go right on with remarks that further explore these ideas.

Short and Long Reflections

In addition to the specific content of a reflection and the level of intensity, reflections also differ in how much is re-presented to the patient. Shorter reflections (e.g., a few words) are generally considered better than those that express several thoughts simultaneously. If the provider has been listening carefully, summarizing the patient's communication in a few words is not difficult. The problem arises when the provider fails to respond and allows the patient to roam aimlessly from thought to thought and topic to topic. At this point, providers have probably lost the essence of the discussion and will need to prioritize, using their own frame of reference. To the extent that this frame of reference does not re-present the patient's, the intervention will fail to stimulate awareness and communicate empathy. Capturing the patient's remarks in a few words also presents less demand on the patient. As a receiver, many thoughts and ideas are confusing, need sorting, and are sometimes difficult to decode, so short reflections tend to preserve the steady flow of patient problem solving.

As noted earlier, the therapeutic purposes of reflection are many. They help patients examine their plight, feelings, and attitudes toward their health problems. They invite the patient to explore, in a gentle nondirective manner, their experience. Communicated with warmth and openness, they provide empathy. Sometimes reflections act to reinforce or reward selective patient responses. In other words, as the provider selects from the patient's statements, the attention paid tends to reinforce that which is restated and increases the potential for exploration in this area. Reflection has also been noted to promote relaxation, which may come from the patient's realization that he or she has been heard. Uncertainty about being heard and understood can be lessened through reflective statements. Finally, reflections can be used to clarify the patient's experience so that the provider has a better idea of what is important to the patient.

REFLECTIONS AND INTERPRETATIONS

Reflections Differ from Interpretations

To fully understand reflections, it is important to differentiate them from interpretations. Generally, the differences between these responses are not always clear and distinguishable.

When the patient communicates something to the provider, the provider can use either a reflection or an interpretation to better understand the patient's communication. If the provider fits the message into some language that fairly accurately portrays what the patient said, the provider is using a reflection. If the provider, however, associates what the patient has said with some theory or data about the patient's past experience of life events, then the provider is using an interpretation. That is, if providers give patients their understanding of patient remarks using the patient's point of view, they are more likely using reflective therapeutic responses. If, however, providers attempt to understand patients' remarks through a theory or through the providers' experience, they are more likely using interpretative therapeutic responses. The intent of the reflection is to give the experience of being understood from their point of view or frame of reference. The intention of the interpretation is to convey an understanding of the patient greater than the patient's own understanding of him or herself.

In very simple terms, reflections are simply to let the person disclosing know that he or she has been heard. Reflections are given frequently throughout a single interaction with a patient. In contrast, interpretations are offered much less frequently and only after a great deal of data have been gathered (e.g., at the end of an interview and well into the relationship).

For example, the provider might say, "When first I saw you, you were having difficulty even considering your diagnosis. Now you're saying, 'Why did this have to happen to me? now?' I know this is all very upsetting. This distress will pass—what you're going through is the whole adaptation to serious illness process. At some time in the future your distress will lessen and you'll come to some level of acceptance" (interpretation). This interpretative response accomplishes two goals. First, it links the patient's past and present experience in some meaningful way (that disbelief and current distress are related to one another and both are part of the patient's lived experience of the illness). Second, this reflection reports on a theory of adaptation to illness, where responses occur in predictable sequences. Reflections, however, are not intended to link past and present or give patients a window to a theoretical explanation of their experience.

While reflections do not provide the extra data and insight that interpretations do, they may still provide new information. Reflections allow patients to concentrate, a second time, on material they have shared. This process is likely to generate new thoughts and even new insights in the patient. Reflection promotes exploration that generally is not available to patients if they were considering their circumstances alone, in isolation from a helping person. Reflections also provide new data because it is impossible to re-present material exactly as it was presented. And, even minor or subtle changes can stimulate new thoughts on the part of the patient.

Definitions of Interpretation

A good interpretation, or one placed at the right moment, can significantly increase both patients' faith in the provider and patients' insights into their own experiences. Essentially, the purpose is to facilitate patients to see beyond the surface of their thoughts, feelings, and behavior. *Interpretations* are the explicit statements of providers that give meaning to a segment of patients' feelings or behavior. There are essentially two types of interpretation: one links past and present events, and the other links theoretical significance with patients' experience.

In either case, these interpretations are speculations at best. The linking of past and present events (e.g., about a childhood situation and a current event) assumes that there is some cause-and-effect relationship that justifies the association between these two points in time. Both past and current experience need to have been discussed in the patient–provider relationship at some point in time, but not necessarily at the same visit. Assumptions about a likely connection are highly speculative and not easily verified. Such interpretations are made on shaky grounds because at least one-half of the speculation is completely out of the patient's awareness.

The second type of interpretation, introjecting a theoretical premise, requires both a reformulation of the statements of the patient and the application of a concept or principle. For example, a young mother who is describing a problem with her infant would be assisted by understanding the theoretical explanation for the reasons behind her infant's behavior and her response. This particular theory of growth and development may not be familiar to the young mother. For the theoretical interpretation to really be of value, though, the provider must assess what this mother already knows about stages of infant development and mother–child early interaction.

The major way in which interpretations depart from either restatements or reflections is in the depth of understanding these responses evoke. Interpretations take patients further along the continuum of understanding than do either restatements or reflections. Interpretations actually offer explanations; reflections simply mirror back words and implied feelings. Whereas reflection can be applied early in the helping relationship, interpretations require the collection and analysis of a good deal of data about the patient. Interpretations are offered much later in the relationship. In fact, if interpretations are given too early, it appears that the provider is jumping to conclusions, stereotyping the patient, or simply projecting personal bias. Interpretations are more successful when they are preceded by one or more restatements.

Reflections and Interpretations Differ from Other Response Modes

Therapeutic response modes—the use of silence, questions, and self-disclosure—differ from each other in terms of the direction in which they lead the patient and in the amount of work that the patient will be required to do. That is, the person who does most of the talking, thinking, and feeling may be different depending on the response mode used, and the stage of the relationship. When providers are interested in helping patients explore their problems, reflections are recommended. Providers who are exploring patients' problems from the provider vantage point will use more questions and fewer reflections. Directive statements (e.g., interpretations and closed-ended questions) tend to be followed by talking about symptoms and problems and by less reference to the meanings or feelings behind those symptoms or problems. It is believed that reflections generate less resistance from patients than do direct questions and interpretations because they are less offensive, creating defensiveness to some degree.

Reflections do not attempt to understand patients better than patients understand themselves. Unlike interpretations, reflections do not add much to what is revealed by the patient nor do they fit the experience into some theory or explanation of cause and effect. Reflections are also less likely than advisement to communicate provider values. Less directive than questions, reflections tend to let the patient chart the direction that learning and insight will take.

GUIDELINES IN THE USE OF REFLECTION

If there is one single principle that applies to using therapeutic response modes, it is that of moderation. Moving too quickly and too rigorously in employing these modes is not advisable. Likewise, delving too deeply into the patient's experience is ill advised. Ill-spaced, ill-timed reflection and interpretation can undermine the provider's attempts to obtain data and establish a collaborative helping relationship. How to phrase reflections and how and when to use interpretations are important issues.

Goals for Using Reflection

When the provider uses reflections, the goal is to convey empathy and, at the same time, promote problem exploration. To achieve this balance, several guides are useful. One way to approach reflection is to shift attention from the content of the patient's message to the feelings the patient must have, then silently reflect on how the feeling is associated with the content. The provider can then reflect back the essential thoughts and feelings that have come to mind. Rogers (1951) points out that the provider's tone of voice is critical. Reflections without empathy appear as declarations that have a somewhat judgmental tone. Reflections need to be kept light. These are reflections that simply let patients know the provider has heard and is following their line of thinking. The provider needs to avoid interrupting in order to offer a reflection; pauses can occur that allow some space between the last remarks of the patient and the reflection of the provider. In choosing a paraphrase, the provider should stay within the patient's frame of reference, inserting little, if any, new material and using the patient's own words. Keep the reflections centered on the here and now of what is communicated.

Forming a Reflection

Providers are not always confident about their reflective remarks. Beginners frequently worry about sounding phony. However, skill at forming appropriate reflections can be present in new providers if they have had the necessary training. It is true that providers who concentrate too much on a few key words will miss the patient's message altogether. Inflection at the end of a speculation communicates the provider's uncertainty about the importance of what has been said and/or the understanding that the provider has of the patients' remarks. Reflections that are worded as statements (e.g., as observations) communicate confidence and generally encourage patients to focus on their own experience rather than on the provider's struggle to come up with appropriate terms. Dutiful reflections—offering a reflection because a provider feels it is time to or because a provider feels he or she should—are rarely effective. The provider who uses this type of reflection often lacks the empathetic character needed to make the patient feel the presence of a sensitive provider.

Countering the Awkward Aspects of Making Reflections

Reflections are not always easy to make. There are several common difficulties in learning to give effective reflections. Self-consciousness, awkwardness, inability to capture the patient's words in vivid remarks, and confusion about what aspect of a long message should be reflected are difficulties the provider may experience.

These difficulties can be managed by a number of actions that enhance reflections. Long interresponse times before reflecting allow the provider to sort and examine carefully the patient's remarks. Silently reflecting on what the patient has said, using the imagination to tap into the patient's experience, is also useful. Repeating key words or using metaphors may capture the patient's experience, as will introjecting a disclosure before a reflection when the message is confused.

The most common beginner's problem is a tendency to add too much or to omit important content when re-presenting the patient's experience. Sometimes this results in serious distortion or exaggeration. If the provider is a beginner, it is important not to sound too mechanical. If this happens, reflections are presented stiffly and sound strained. Voicing reflections under one's breath is helpful. It is also important to recognize that one may need to use 50 to 100 reflections before feeling authentic when using this response mode.

Usually, in the beginning, the provider feels like an echo. There does not seem to be time to think through what one is going to paraphrase. Silence response modes or pauses, however, can stimulate creative associations and evoke metaphors. Statements like, "You feel you're on slippery ice" (fear) or "You must feel like you're in a corner and can't get out" (helplessness) are vivid images that help capture the essence of the patient's story.

When the patient talks too quickly or too long without giving the provider an opportunity to introject a comment, reflection is difficult. Sometimes the patient has presented confusing or even contradictory messages, and precise interpretations are not always possible. Reflecting the most useful parts of a complex disclosure is a skill that develops over time. One strategy is to reflect silently, assess the most important aspect of the message, and reflect it back verbally to the patient. If the patient communicates contradictory or confusing material, it is advisable to reflect the contradiction. For example, "I've heard you express good and bad things about this change; on the one hand . . . but . . ." If the confusion is complicated, the provider may offer, "It's hard to really know how you're feeling about this change." Remember, the patient may not be confused at all; it may be that the provider's ability to track and comprehend all that the patient has said is limited. In this case, it is better to disclose one's inability to comprehend the patient's feelings.

Avoiding Overuse of Reflections

Reflections can be used too frequently or indiscriminately. When this occurs, the provider may appear disinterested. Collins (1977) suggests that "parroting" can appear as mimicry and can make reflection and other nondirective techniques seem ludicrous. Consider the following dialogue between a person in pain and a medical student.

Patient: "I have pain in my shoulder."
Provider: (Scanning patient chart) "You have pain?" (Restatement)
Patient: "Yes, right here—my left side—it hurts a lot."
Provider: "Your left side is really painful—it concerns you?" (still thumbing through chart) (Reflection)
Patient: "I told you twice—my side hurts. Aren't you going to look?"

Understandably, the patient is getting agitated with the provider. This overuse of the reflective technique actually worsens the inattention that the patient experiences. Notice that one therapeutic benefit of reflection is establishing empathic understanding, yet this use of restatement and reflection, which is ill-spaced, actually communicates the opposite.

INTERPRETATIONS USED IN SOCIAL AND THERAPEUTIC CONTEXTS

Interpretations go beyond patients' surface messages and into the less-obvious meanings and motivations behind remarks. Because they deal with less obvious material, they are subject to error.

In Social Contexts

In social situations or social relationships, interpretations are received negatively. There is no justifiable reason to support interpretations in these interactions. Frequently, they make the receiver feel vulnerable and the sender feel superior. All providers who are trained in interpreting patients' remarks need to be extremely careful to avoid slipping into this mode outside the therapeutic relationship. In truth, the provider may get into very complicated situations and come across as arrogant.

Consider, for example, the provider who meets an eligible dating partner, and after learning something about the young lady, offers this explanation about her hesitancy in accepting a date. "From what you've told me, you've been burned badly. Many girls I know carry around excess baggage. You probably struggle with problems of intimacy coming from your early childhood years." These interpretative remarks are interesting and might even be accurate. However, the balance in this social relationship has shifted. The young woman is left to believe that she has major problems—some she did not even know about. Her reaction may be to hesitate further—why would she consider getting to know someone who makes such giant leaps with just a little knowledge of her? She may feel badly about the labels that have been thrust on her.

Because interpretations violate the norms of social relationships, they are not comfortably employed in therapeutic relationships. And the way interpretation is misused in social relations can color provider attitudes in using interpretations in helping situations. In addition, providers may hesitate to use therapeutic interpretations because they are concerned about the response matching tendency in the patient. An example might be: "You need to know what to do with . . ." (provider); "It's clear to me that you need to know what to do with . . ." (patient). That is, provider interpretations may be matched with the patient's interpretation of the provider. In reality, this type of "turnabout is fair play" rarely occurs, although providers do worry about the possibility.

Therapeutic Uses of Interpretation

Interpretations, however, are response modes that can provide comfort to the patient. Interpretations can be experienced both as providing new information and providing new order to old information. A sound interpretation by the provider can increase the faith and confidence of the patient in the provider. Thus, interpretation has the potential to decrease patient anxiety and increase feelings of security if it reflects the patient's self-experience.

Consider the following dialogue between provider and patient. The patient is in much distress over the physician's refusal to discharge him early from the hospital. The nurse caring for this patient has observed his course in the hospital and has read his chart describing his past history and multiple hospitalizations related to his chronic illness.

Provider: "It seems you're upset you can't go home earlier—I understand that."

Patient: "Yes, they said that I would. . . . I can't take this much longer."

Provider: "I think you're also reacting to the long struggle you've had with repeated hospitalizations."

Patient: "It seems this is going on and on and nobody can help me like they should."

Provider: "You may be more angry with your illness than with any of us."

Provider: "We are safe targets for this frustration. It happens a lot with our patients . . ."

Note here how the past is drawn into the present and how the nurse suggests that the healthcare team, not his illness, is the target for his stored-up frustration and futility. The patient learns that his reactions are not random and disconnected but form a continuity that reveals a problem over time and, in this case, is related to his acceptance of and adaptation to his chronic illness.

In this way, interpretations can translate a set of apparently unrelated or surface-related events into a coherent whole. This process in turn creates a more meaningful understanding for patients and deepens their awareness of what is happening to them. Said differently, the need for receiving interpretations is a need for creating new meaning from a series of events that evoke helplessness. Even minor interpretations can be perceived as helpful by someone who is struggling to make sense of frustrating or unmanageable situations.

The use of interpretative remarks in helping relationships has not always been judged helpful or advisable. In fact, there are some psychotherapeutic schools of thought that view interpretations as irrelevant and dangerous. Cognitive behavioral therapists, for example, generally regard theoretical interpretations as, at best, chancy and interpretations linking past and present as unimportant to the process of supporting growth in the patient. What is important is what is manifested here and now. The reasons that the past relates to the present are not critical to achieving behavioral changes. Some clinicians view provider interpretations as mere projections of the provider's own conflicts or dilemmas. If interpretation is putting on the patient what is truly only relevant to oneself, then providers could be making gross errors in their assessment and treatment of patients.

A more moderate view suggests that interpretations can be therapeutic, and because no single therapeutic response will do in all situations, it is better to have more options. Thus, interpretations are suitable options if utilized properly. Most providers caution that interpretations should be offered only when the patient has established a connection and is about to expand his or her insight in a particular area. Research indicates that interpretations that are much more removed from the patient's awareness are more likely to be resisted. Thus denial, blocking, and inattention on the part of the patient are important clues that the patient's readiness to hear and deal with the implications of the interpretation is not what it needs to be. The patient should be able to listen to, ponder, and ultimately understand the interpretation if it is to be successful. The patient's readiness to receive an interpretation is felt by some to be more important than the accuracy of the interpretation.

It is possible to plot reflection and interpretation on the same continuum with the expectation that as the provider moves from simple reflections to restating material not immediately within the patient's awareness, the depth of interpretive responses increases. That is, reflection begins with a restatement of remarks. When comments are made to link previously unrelated statements, the provider is moving into the realm of making interpretations.

GUIDELINES FOR THE THERAPEUTIC USE OF INTERPRETATIONS

Patient exploration of situations, dilemmas, or problems must be preserved. Principles for the effective use of interpretative remarks stem from this idea. The basic outcome—to enhance patients' sense of control over the situation and to allow them to grow in knowledge—directs the choice and placement of interpretations.

Placing Interpretations after Reflections

Interpretations placed after reflections tend to make problem exploration go smoothly. Also, interpretations that start out simple and build on increased perceptions of the situation are likely to be less obtrusive.

Validating Interpretations

Interpretations need to be evaluated and validated. Validation can include comments such as, "Can you see the connection I described?" or "How does this idea fit with your thinking about this situation?" Delivering a few interpretative remarks with adequate evaluative follow-up generally permits more self-exploration than does direct unsubstantiated interpretations. Interpretation, though, can lead to the abandonment of self-exploration with the result of silence, denial, or blocking. Usually, interpretations made tentatively are less likely to cause patient anxiety and therefore preserve the flow of patient self-disclosure. While an interpretation may be true, there may be several others that are also true. The provider's interpretation may be true but not salient. For this reason, evaluative comments are needed to help both provider and patient put interpretative remarks in perspective.

A common problem when making interpretations is the juxtaposing of one theory with every instance. Using one principle to explain all behaviors within and across groups of individuals is a faulty application of interpretations. No theory exists that adequately and accurately explains a single behavior across individuals. Interpretations using theory, then, are always tentative.

To summarize, effective interpretations can be made by even the beginning practitioner. However, adequate observations of the patient and a theoretical basis on which to draw one's conclusions is essential. The delivery of an interpretation will meet with more success if it is communicated as a tentative suggestion, inviting the patient to collaborate in validating the idea. Sometimes self-disclosure (e.g., "I'm wondering how your frustration about your discharge is related to the total experience of your illness") presents the interpretation in a mild, nonobtrusive fashion. Or, a question in the service of interpretation can be delivered more palatably (e.g., "Do you see a connection between your frustration with discharge and the experience of your illness as a whole?").

Using Interpretations Sparingly

Interpretations need to be used sparingly. Because accurate interpretations require thoughtful reflection by the provider, the ability to deliver several interpretations in a single discourse is not the point. In fact, patients who are encouraged to stay on this intellectual plane may miss the feelings associated with several interpretations offered at the same time.

CONCLUSION

Reflections and interpretations are two additional therapeutic response modes. While they are similar to some degree, they are also very different. Interpretations move the patient to a deeper level of exploration of experiences because they mirror the patient's behaviors and feelings that may not be within the patient's immediate awareness. Because of this, they are also more open to error if the provider misses some of the critical information about the patient. If reflections are tied closely to the patient's current experience, and providers correctly paraphrase words and feelings that are reflected in the patient's story, there is less chance for error. When empathically expressed, reflections disclose that the provider is present, listening, and respectful of the patient's need to direct the focus.

Patients receive reflective remarks as a request to elaborate (Lussier & Richard, 2007). Reflections acknowledge the patient's right to have opinions, to make decisions, and to think for oneself. With reflections, patients are doing most of the thinking and feeling. According to Levine (2001), reflective listening is the most valuable skill for giving the patient the assurance that the concerns expressed are truly being heard. Interpretations can elicit deeper understanding and even reduce anxiety in patients by explaining why they feel confused or out of control. The major drawback of interpretations over reflections is that the latter can be more provider-driven and therefore, less patient-centered. In the case of interpretations, providers are doing most of the thinking.

Guidelines in using both response modes include forming reflections and interpretations so that they can be understood, phrasing them accurately, using them sparingly, and presenting them in ways that are least offensive to the patient. Timing is important, particularly with interpretations, so that the revelation is accepted or, at the very least, provides useful material for discussion. Interpretations should never be presented as accusations or moral judgments but rather as supportive remarks offered as tentative explanations. Finally, whereas reflections can be made early in the provider–patient relationship, interpretations are best reserved for a period when provider–patient rapport has been secured over time. If not, the patient is likely to react negatively, and there are likely to be missed readings of patients thoughts and concerns.

While reflections express the patient's experience from the patient's frame of reference, interpretations tend to express the patient's experience from the provider's frame of reference. While experience in patient–provider communications would generally help, specific training in these modalities is essential. Deficiencies in knowing how to employ these modalities are not confined to the new provider.

CHAPTER 12

The Judicious Use of Confrontations, Orders, and Commands

Confrontation without a solid relationship created through the communication of empathy, respect, warmth, and genuineness rarely is helpful.
—G. M. Gazda, W. C. Childers, and R. P. Walters

CHAPTER OBJECTIVES

- Define confrontation.
- Differentiate between levels of confrontation.
- Compare the use of motivational interviewing versus confrontation and describe how each are different in intensity.
- Differentiate between factual and experiential confrontation.
- Describe how one would regulate the intensity of confrontations.
- Differentiate commands and orders from confrontations.
- Identify ways of assessing compliance to commands, orders, and directives.
- Describe appropriate ways of summarizing directives to patients.

Up to this point, the therapeutic response modes that have been presented are largely facilitative, where providers do not judge or overreact to patients' healthcare decisions. Rather, providers try to facilitate an atmosphere in which patients feel comfortable and will share their concerns and worries about their disease and treatment. Essentially, the idea is to show empathy, confirming the value and worth of the patient and establishing trust. Additionally, the use of questions, advisement, reflections, and interpretations can be rather gentle techniques to prompt patients to engage in collaborative problem solving. These approaches respect the patient's readiness to change. The question is, is it more appropriate in selected instances to express judgment and urgency? Providers must draw on their expertise and experience, and sometimes this requires being more forceful in their approach. The contribution of these types of modalities (confrontation, orders, and commands) is that they ensure feedback that is clear and concise and expresses the seriousness of moving ahead quickly to preserve the patient's life and welfare.

In this chapter, the judicious use of confrontation, orders, and commands is discussed. It is through the use of supportive communications—empathy and unconditional acceptance—that providers establish their therapeutic connection with the patient. Confrontations, orders, and commands involve being judgmental and evaluative. These responses are usually employed to ensure action—to cause a response so necessary that the avoidance of action has serious consequences. These response modes are not, however, useful in long-term behavioral change situations. In fact, confrontation, for example, is considered counterproductive in cases in which the patient needs to reverse a pattern of behavior (e.g., alcohol or drug use). In these instances, the closest example of something like confrontation is the approach to "present contrast," where the provider confronts patients with the difference between what they say they are doing or want to do and what they are actually doing by giving pointed feedback. The purpose of this technique is to build awareness in patients, which should reinforce motivation to change.

Historically, the use of confrontations, orders, and commands involved the sequential escalation of provider power. Power and authority rested in providers, with minimal recognition that the patient was an active participant in his or her own care. Sometimes providers decide that they need these more direct approaches to clearly state the seriousness of the situation and get the response they are looking for in the short run. Confrontations are more indirect, orders clearly state one or more recommendations, and commands demand a specific response (avoidance of which would involve critical consequences). Quite often these responses are used together. That is, orders or commands are often given in an encounter where confrontation has occurred.

Despite the fact that our orientation to behavior change discourages the use of confrontation, there are times when this modality is appropriate. Without confrontation, we rely on patients' changing through stages, based on their own unique readiness. Still, confrontations, orders, and commands can have an important role in health care. For example, one form of physician order is the medication prescription. If this is needed to get the patient better, to prevent the patient from transmitting the disease to others, and may result in threats to morbidity and mortality, are we going to operate on the patient's own motivation and readiness to take the medication? Are these instances in which it is important to exercise authority and strongly insist that the patient follow orders? Not all patients are willing or able to participate collaboratively in their care. But, clearly they need this care. So, while we limit "ordering" the patient, we will not eliminate orders from our repertoire.

CONFRONTATIONS: DEFINITIONS, LEVELS, AND TYPES

Definitions of Confrontation

Confrontation is the deliberate use of statements or questions to point out to another individual certain discrepancies. As previously indicated, using the behavioral change theories, presenting discrepancies, is one such technique. These discrepancies may be (1) differences between what persons say and what they do, (2) differences across several elements of communication or statements made over time, and (3) differences between what individuals should do and what they are actually doing.

The value of confrontation is that it offers alternative views about what is really going on. Assuming that patients are truly interested in the provider's point of view, feedback about discrepant behavior can be informative and can actually contribute to patient insight. When this feedback comes from a healthcare provider, it is generally presumed that the observations are valid and have some bearing on the patient's well-being. In some cases, the providers' observations may be more complete than the patient's. Confrontations that increase patients' knowledge or self-awareness stem from providers' extensive experience and high level of expertise. The point is not to withhold this expertise but to challenge it in a way that the patient can use this important feedback.

Levels of Confrontation

Confrontations may be more or less intense. And, like interpretations, they may be more or less threatening. Low-level confrontations are less intense and consequently arouse low levels of emotional response. Consider this dialogue between patient and provider; the provider is speaking to the patient about the necessity of a low-fat diet:

> **Provider:** "OK, Janice, now I know you like fast foods, but, if I catch you at a fast-food restaurant I'm going to get upset." (Smiling)

This confrontation delivers a message—despite an urge for fast foods, the patient must avoid them. This confrontation is low level because it is offered in a friendly manner. It is also delivered in a jovial, somewhat ambiguous fashion. Is the doctor really that serious or not? It might arouse negative feelings in the patient, but it does not really pose a threat. While the patient might make use of this feedback, the informality may dilute the chance to use this as a teaching moment. Therefore, this confrontation and feedback seems to be too weak.

Confrontations that are moderately intense but are not so direct as to damage collaboration are middle-level confrontations. Consider the following dialogue between the patient just described and her provider.

> **Provider:** "Janice, I know you like fast foods, but, if you continue to overindulge, you will gain more weight and your ability to control your diabetes will get harder and harder. I have had lots of patients in your situation and have seen this happen time and time again. Did you read the information the nurse gave you?"

There is nothing ambiguous about this confrontation. This confrontation is more intense, and the need to comply is clearly articulated. The physician, without a doubt, wants to warn about the seriousness of the situation and uses emphasis. The physician wants to "arm" the patient with important information and expects that the patient will hear it loud and clear.

There are also instances in which confrontations might be too strong. Typically, these high-level confrontations arouse intense feelings and can be perceived as very threatening. They are highly unlikely to encourage change and more likely to upset patients. Consider this third adaptation of the same patient–provider encounter.

> **Provider:** "Janice, I know you enjoy fast foods, but you've got to cut them out of your diet. I can't continue to treat you if you self-indulge like this."

This confrontation reproves the patient. It may make the patient feel inadequate, "bad," and ashamed. It does not elicit constructive problem solving nor does it empower the patient to correct her unhealthy eating patterns. The purpose of the confrontation is lost in the idea that the provider may decide to release the patient. As such, the threat is actually the loss of a provider, not the loss of health. This confrontation is very threatening and is likely to arouse very strong negative emotions.

Gazda, Childers, and Walters (1982, p. 143) addressed the problems with strong confrontations. They stated that if confrontations are too strong, five undesirable outcomes may occur; patients might:

1. Respond defensively, with explanations and rationale, building a wall against the provider's influence.
2. Be driven away.
3. Become angry and go on the attack.
4. Pretend to accept the advice but actually ignore it.
5. Feel helpless and become inappropriately dependent on the provider.

Any one of these undesired responses reduces the probability that further communication between provider and patient will be constructive.

If the confrontation is too weak, however, the outcomes can be equally undesirable. There are three undesirable outcomes as a result of confrontations that are too weak; patients might:

1. Lose respect for the provider. Otherwise, the patient may assume that the provider does not really believe in what they are talking about or that they lack the courage to be forceful about their judgments.
2. Neither notice nor pay attention to the providers' statements.
3. Receive the confrontation as reinforcing. The impression given to the patient is that the discrepant behavior is really OK (i.e., "You shouldn't eat fast foods—but, it's OK if you do").

In the example of the provider who confronts the patient about unhealthy eating patterns, we note that the first example (low intensity) resulted in the patient's feeling confused about the convictions of the provider. The high-intensity confrontation, however, runs the risk of causing a defensive response that ranges from high levels of dependency to withdrawal from the provider.

In summary, the intensity of any confrontation needs to be strong enough to elicit positive actions but not so strong that it immobilizes the patient. To achieve this aim, it is important to regulate the intensity of the confrontation. In accordance with patients' reactions, confrontations can begin as gentle statements with feedback and progress in intensity if patients demonstrate confusion or fail to grasp the seriousness of the situation.

Types of Confrontation: Experiential or Factual

Confrontations can also be described as either experiential or factual. That is, providers can speak from their firsthand experience of patients' behavior, or they can present data of a factual nature that will provide the patient with information and feedback. For example, if providers state that the patient is trying to avoid fast foods but is not able to, the confrontation is experiential. Otherwise, the provider learned this about the patient through firsthand experience with the patient. Two observations communicate discrepancy: the patient's attempt to avoid fast foods and apparent inability to be successful. If the provider, however, states, "Janice, if you continue to eat fast foods the way you are, your blood sugar levels will fluctuate significantly," then the provider presents clinical judgments that are substantiated by factual data about the disease and its management.

Confrontations, as has been explained, present discrepancies. They may be more or less intense and more or less threatening. They may reflect the provider's direct observations of the patient and/or draw from the provider's expertise and knowledge in the field, or both. For any confrontation to play a positive role in change it should be coupled with trust and empathy. High levels of trust and empathetic responsiveness in the patient–provider relationship are prerequisite to effective confrontations.

Easing into Confrontations and Regulating Intensity

The procedures of easing into confrontations and regulating intensity have been described in the literature in some detail. The following six steps seem to follow logically and ensure that confrontations occur when the patient–provider relationship itself is substantially strong enough to permit the provider to confront the patient. In this case the provider has:

1. Established a relationship built on trust and caring.
2. Used empathy, positive regard, respect, warmth, active listening, and genuineness in building this relationship.
3. Laid a foundation for the purpose for addressing the patient's unique concerns and problems.
4. Avoided appearing overly judgmental and critical in instances in which there was no emergent threat to the patient.
5. Identified any discrepancies that were obvious and planned an approach to communicate them.
6. Defined the provider's role and level of commitment to the partnership.

Returning then to our scenario between the physician and the patient who is overindulging in fast foods, and therefore placing her health at risk, the following process exemplifies how to prepare the patient to receive the confrontation.

The physician first empathizes with the patient about how difficult it is to resist fast foods and even supports the patient in having made some attempts in this direction. To communicate further respect and appreciation, the physician may ask the patient how she sees the problem and what solutions she would propose. Before zeroing in on this patient's difficulty, the physician speaks generally about other patients' difficulties and/or what she has learned through her professional experience and research of this problem. At this point, expressions of tolerance, if not previously expressed, may be given: "I know, it's tough," or "The most difficult thing is to resist those 'Golden Arches.' " Finally, the physician states clearly and succinctly, "Eating fast foods is going to prevent you from staying well. You're going to need to change this pattern—I don't expect you to do it without help. But we are definitely going to get very serious about this."

In most cases, this process is sufficient to both gain the patient's attention and increase his or her interest in making changes. If the provider determines that what is really called for is a great deal more forcefulness, there are five specific ways in which this confrontation could be strengthened:

1. The more personal the reference is, the more direct the confrontation. By making it clear that it is the patient's behavior, and nothing else, that is the issue, the confrontation becomes decidedly more direct.
2. The more concrete the examples are, the more difficult it is to challenge the accuracy of a confrontation. For example, the physician could remind the patient that she is becoming more noncompliant than she was six months ago.
3. The more recent the events are, the more powerful the examples. Behaviors that occurred in the past are less threatening, even if they reflected poor judgment on the patient's part. The physician could remark, "In the last month you've shown me you cannot go a week without going off your diet."
4. The more behaviors, not just words, are dealt with, the more pressure can be applied because behaviors are not easily dismissed or invalidated. Thus, the physician's reference to specific examples of going off her diet cannot be argued.
5. The more using what the patient has said or done earlier to contradict what she is saying or doing now, the more a confrontation is strengthened. The physician may comment, "The last time you were in this office you said you would stay on your diet, yet you tell me you didn't."

Considering that providers can either strengthen or weaken confrontations, and that they can even do both within a single encounter, it is important to consider general instances in which confrontations are appropriately intense.

Most patients will respond to simple first-level confrontations; however, there are instances that require more direct approaches. When patients are asked to make changes, these changes are not always easy to implement. Some changes involve altering rather deep-seated patterns, and patients are not easily convinced that the change is worth it. In this instance the provider will have to decide whether there is time to use one or more motivational interviewing approaches.

In the following dialogue, the nurse practitioner is trying to persuade an elderly patient to adhere to a low-fat diet. The patient is recovering from hepatitis that was incurred as a result of a blood transfusion at the time he was hospitalized for hip surgery. The patient was hospitalized but has been discharged and is receiving follow-up care and instruction because his liver damage was significant and recovery has been slow.

Provider: "Mr. O____, I've looked at your test results, it looks like you're going to have to stay on your low-fat diet for a while more."

Patient: "But, I love chopped liver, poor-boy sandwiches, pizza . . ."

Provider: "I know it's hard being on a restricted diet—have you ever been on a restricted diet before?"
Patient: "A low-salt diet . . ."
Provider: "And did you stick to it?"
Patient: "Mostly . . . yes. I had a stroke."
Provider: "So you stuck with it because you were afraid something bad would happen to you?"
Patient: "Uh huh."
Provider: "Do you know why you are being kept on a restricted diet?"
Patient: "No—not really, no."
Provider: "The liver and gall bladder are involved in digesting fat. Your liver was traumatized because of your hepatitis. It cannot work as well as it should. So, we need you to keep fat out of your diet so we can give your liver a chance to heal. Right now, your liver needs a rest."
Patient: "But I've been on it (the diet) a long time—how long will it last?"
Provider: "The liver needs time to heal—especially when you are older."
Patient: "But I love corned beef and cabbage, a beer before dinner, and . . ."
Provider: "I know, but, for now, you really need to stick with your diet. I'll get you a copy of the revised food list. Later we can be a little more lenient; but for now the thing you need to do is stick to it."
Patient: "So, you think I'm better off, huh, if I give this another try?"
Provider: "Yes, I can't really release you from the restrictions until your tests are better."
Patient: "Sure I can't have just a little chopped liver?"
Provider: "No, I'm afraid not. It's not going to be this bad forever. Try to think ahead to when your liver is healthy. Going back over the information I gave you, what would happen if you ate lots of fatty foods?"

In this scenario, the patient expressed how difficult it was to abide by the dietary restrictions. Chances are, he was cheating on his diet but not enough to feel the effects. At first, low-level confrontation strategies were used. Then the nurse practitioner intensified his confrontation in several ways. He presented factual information that had specific meaning to the patient, was raising discrepancies and provides an example of confronting with expert knowledge. By not giving in but repeating and more emphatically stating the need to remain on the diet, he gave the patient very clear messages. Also, by applying authoritative leverage by suggesting to the patient that he was under orders, he gave the patient very clear information that, for his own welfare, under no circumstances was this order to be changed, at least not at this time. Finally, by asking the patient to look at the discrepancy between what he wanted to do and what would happen if he did, discrepancies are raised again.

Healthcare providers are particularly committed to promoting and maintaining health. If they observe that patients are doing things that run counter to these values, they are likely to become more concerned and even express judgment. Patients who resist necessary health-promotion or disease-management recommendations generally require skilled confrontational approaches as in the use of confrontations by presenting discrepancies as was used in this case near the end of the dialogue.

ORDERS AND COMMANDS AS EXPLICIT DIRECTIVES

Confrontations are frequently associated with two additional therapeutic response modes—orders and commands. Orders do not refer exclusively to written orders that are typically found in the patient's chart. Rather, what is meant by *orders* (and commands) is the provider's action to elicit change by insistence. When a patient must adhere to a course of action and this course of action is related to an emergent life-and-death situation, providers need to issue an order if it is within their authority to do so. Orders and commands are used to increase the probability that a certain action will occur immediately. They are delivered with authority and require immediate response. In many respects, giving orders or commands is simply directing patients about what the provider wants them to do under serious circumstances.

There is yet another important element—the demand aspect of the directive—that separates commands from simple directives. In the scenario between the nurse practitioner and the hepatitis patient, the provider gave directives (e.g., "For now, you really need to stick with your diet," and "I can't really release you from the restrictions until your tests are better"). These directives were clear and firm. They were, in fact, statements of the medical order; stating that the patient must stick to his diet expressed a demand quality. Phrased differently, it would have been a directive but not a command. For example, the nurse practitioner's statement, "I've looked at your test results, and it looks like you're going to have to stay on your low-fat diet for a while more," comes across as a directive but the tone is less insistent. While it is clearly a directive, it is not expressed as a strong command.

Differentiating Orders and Commands from Confrontation and Advice

Orders and commands in health care differ from confrontations and advice-giving. Also, orders differ from commands—both need to be followed—but *commands* denote the critical and immediate necessity for the action or change.

It is the provider's responsibility to see that every order is understood. Thus, in our scenario, the nurse practitioner spent time giving the patient information about liver damage and the healing process, as well as feedback about his specific condition—his liver-function tests did not warrant the relaxing of restrictions. To avoid confusing the issue, the nurse practitioner was clear and succinct in his presentation of facts and imperatives. This is a requirement of issuing orders: procedures or steps to be taken need to be worded simply. When orders are very complicated, requiring many steps, and/or when the patient's memory and concentration are impaired, orders need to be followed with written instructions.

Pharmacists and nutritionists are particularly aware of the need to specify orders in writing. Usually there are so many important details that these orders need to be written. Consider what would seem to be a very simple instruction about a patient's medication.

- "The doctor wants you to take these medications two times a day."
- "Take two capsules of this medicine and one pill each time."
- "Take these medications after your meals—in the morning after breakfast, at night after dinner."
- "This medication should be taken within an hour after eating."
- "Continue taking these medications until they are gone—7 days for this medication, 14 days for the second medication."
- "While you are on this medication, you should drink ample amounts of water—eight glasses a day."
- "Also, you should avoid alcohol while taking these medications."
- "If you have excessive nausea or drowsiness while taking these medications within the first day or so, you should call and speak to your physician."

It is obvious that this information is more than good advice. Embedded in these instructions are orders.

As with advisement, an order is always more acceptable to a patient when the provider has established a relationship and uses the language and knowledge of the patient. This is an important principle with all patients but particularly so with patients who have low literacy levels. Providers need to accompany orders with ample explanation and time for the patient to respond and ask questions. When possible, orders need to be linked with the patient's own goals—for example, to be able to eat certain foods again.

In the scenario between the nurse practitioner and the patient, the nurse practitioner was not certain that the patient knew enough about his condition or treatment to understand the medical order. And, the patient responded as if he were confused or puzzled. It was important for the nurse practitioner to notice the patient's verbal and nonverbal responses, because both gave clues about the patient's readiness to hear, accept, and implement changes. While head nodding or the patient's reiteration of the directive are good signs, blank stares, confused expressions, and repeated questioning about the necessity of the order are not. Such signs suggest that the patient will have difficulty following the orders. The provider must ascertain both the patient's intentions to comply and the reasons he may be reluctant. In some cases, orders can be revised to incorporate the specific preferences of patients. However, in most cases, orders are to be followed precisely as they are given. And, even though the provider may want to relax the order, as in the scenario between the nurse practitioner and patient, orders generally can not be altered.

Responsibility for Assessing Adherence

Once an order is issued, members of the healthcare team must evaluate the patient's level of adherence. Nonadherence to treatment plans, especially medication regimens, is a common problem, particularly among patients with asymptomatic chronic illnesses such as diabetes and hypertension. However, these patients are not the focus in this discussion. The patients important to this discussion are those facing urgent health issues. When a patient is found to be nonadherent under these circumstances, what the provider does is critical. Still, some principles applying to chronic conditions that are not immediately life threatening do have applicability here. In each instance, the provider's response is important in further modifying the patient's behavior.

In our scenario, the nurse practitioner did not assess the patient's level of adherence but assumed it was less than what it should be. It is also possible that the nurse practitioner did not want to arouse the patient's defensiveness by suggesting that he was lax in following the medical regimen. Assessing nonadherence, however, is extremely important for several reasons. When nonadherence or incomplete adherence occurs, the medications do not reach therapeutic levels for them to work the way they should. The original order may need to be changed or extended. Special adherence education and support might be required. Frequently, the patient's responses to one aspect of his treatment will raise issues of his adherence to other aspects of his treatment. The reasons for poor adherence are multiple, including fears, suspicions, lack of knowledge, cultural beliefs, past experiences with healthcare providers, trust in the provider and the treatment, treatment side effects, and demands of the particular medication regimen. Providers are encouraged to review sections of this text that address health literacy and patient adherence to treatment.

Generally, it is advisable to accept some part of the blame for patient's nonadherence if it is appropriate. In truth, patients are only one aspect of nonadherence process. Additionally, to induce shame or guilt in the patient is likely to be counterproductive. For example, in the earlier scenario, the nurse practitioner replied that he would get the patient a copy of the revised diet outline, recognizing that if he had discussed this with the patient, the patient might be more knowledgeable and receptive. This does not mean that the provider totally ignores the patient's role in nonadherence but conveys the collaborative nature of the two working together to achieve the treatment goals. Although the seriousness and immediacy of the problem should be made the focus of the discussion, there is still opportunity to explore and problem solve with the patient how he could be more adherent (see Exhibit 12–1).

Commands Differ from Orders and Directives

Sometimes commands fit into the category of needing to be delivered immediately. These directives, like orders, are phrased as necessities, but the seriousness of the context is usually more apparent. Directives that command not only convey that a behavior is mandatory, they imply immediacy.

"Take this medication now" is a command. The behavior is mandatory and the immediacy of the action is clear. While some providers may be uncomfortable with commands, the skill of issuing both orders and commands is a necessary addition to their less-directive response modes.

In issuing orders or commands, which should be communicated clearly and simply, it is extremely important that the patient not only understand the action he or she is to take but also that these orders or commands are not mistaken for advice or extraneous information. Unlike advice, orders and commands must be followed. Because there is much at stake in noncompliance, verbal orders are best complemented by written instructions. In cases of orders and commands, the inference that the patient has a choice to not comply or to

Exhibit 12–1 Assessing and Exploring Patient Nonadherence

- "What do you remember about (specific action or change directive)?" (open-ended question to explore)
- "How are you doing with (specific action or behavior change)?" (open-ended question)
- "There are probably things that keep you from (specific action or behavior change)." "What are yours?" (normalizes and encourages exploration of barriers)
- "Looking back at it, what do you think helped you do it or kept you from doing it?" (open-ended question, still exploring barriers and facilitators)
- "What did you think you should do instead?" (open-ended question, encouraging problem solving)
- "What happened when you did it?" "What happened when you didn't, or did it only partially?" (open-ended questions, exploring evaluation of attempts to change)
- "Given the same situation again, what would you do?" (open-ended question, problem solving)

---

comply only partially must be avoided. Also, the patient must understand that noncompliance or partial compliance cannot be dismissed or excused.

If, for example, the patient will die if he or she does not follow a directive, the expected action must be clear and the importance must also be clear. Should the provider wait several months when this fate is immediate? No, the patient's health and welfare requires an immediate warning phrased as an imperative. Orders and commands must always be received as critical advice. Discussing difficulties that the patient may have to endure (such as social losses due to changes in behavior) fail in comparison to the necessity of immediate changes. Order can, but should not, be perceived as a choice not to comply. In the earlier scenario, the patient wanted to negotiate a relaxation of the diet restrictions—"sure I can't have just a little chopped liver?" The responsibility lies with healthcare provider to reaffirm the seriousness of these directives.

Summarizing Directives for Patients

Closing discussions with patients when confrontations, orders, and commands have been used is sometimes complicated. Essentially, the provider must assess not only what has and has not been understood but also how it has been understood. Usually, to assess the patient's response, the provider will summarize the important points of the discussion, including any directives given. Some providers will prompt the patient with a gentle command using the "teach-back" approach (e.g., "Tell me what you heard and what you plan to do") to assemble all the essential facts of the discussion. Asking patients to assemble the points they remember is a good way to assess the level of shared meaning that exists between provider and patient as well as any misconceptions patients may have about what the provider said. If directives have been successfully used, the patient will be armed with feedback, including awareness of adverse consequences that direct him or her toward healthy choices.

As in any interview or consultation encounter with a patient, patients need to be told that the session is ending. This awareness can prompt patients to ask questions or clarify points that were not clear to them. They should understand that if they are unsure about a directive or are feeling that they could not comply, they have limited time to address their concerns and need to know how they can clarify issues or what the provider said once they leave the office visit or hospital. It is very important for the patient to understand how to get further information because the likelihood is that other things will occur to them as they leave or when they talk to friends and family members. In all cases, it is important to summarize the exchange in a positive manner.

Providers need to focus on the shared understanding, consensus, and plans that have come from the discussion with the patient. Additionally, providers may take particular notice of gains or progress made in previous attempts to adhere to medical directives thereby raising self-confidence and self-efficacy in the patient that he or she can manage his or her critical health problem.

CONCLUSION

Assisting patients to cope with illness and manage disease requires more direct strategies as well as more supportive approaches such as empathy, trust, respect, and warmth. While many times providers will opt for behavioral change theories that respect the patient's stage of readiness and strive to avoid confrontation (Elder, Ayala, & Harris, 1999), there are specific instances in which it is appropriate to make more deliberate and assertive efforts to convince patients to change or take on a new behavioral approach to their problems and do this quickly. Providers are acting on their best clinical judgment and evidence-based practice. Most providers would agree that the seriousness of the situation dictates, in part, what strategy they will use. If their patient is in immediate threat for death or disability, they would more likely think more active and assertive strategies are appropriate if not essential to the health and welfare of their patients.

It is widely understood that the action potential of confrontations, orders, and commands are best delivered when providers have earned the right to use these techniques. Confrontation can be more or less harsh, but they are important, action-oriented therapeutic responses. Confrontations deal openly with patients' displayed discrepant behaviors or with discrepancies between what patients should do and what they are actually doing. The most threatening type of confrontation is the one that deals with the present and is accusatory. Patients usually respond defensively to these high-level confrontations, so it is important to assess the need and wisdom of using confrontations of this type. In actuality, a provider has many options in any given encounter—beginning with a mild, low-level confrontation and proceeding with more direct, intense confrontations.

Although orders and commands are frequently used along with confrontation, they are actually separate strategies to promote change. Both orders and commands are directives; however, commands are usually issued more forcefully and require immediate response. Situations requiring rapid response are best treated with commands.

Confrontations, orders, and commands are frequently preferred over advice and opinions. Advice can lack strength and influence, while confrontations, orders, and commands, even mildly phrased, do not. Patients who are at risk for ignoring advice and instruction require strongly stated imperatives. For example, if the patient is going to die in a year if he continues to do what he is doing, you are going to confront him with this fact. It is your duty to share this factual information. Will you wait for his readiness to change before explaining this to him? Not likely. You will do it immediately.

While confrontations, orders, and commands increase self-awareness and help promote change, their distinct contribution is that they stress the seriousness of the situation, punctuating the necessity to listen and comply with providers' directives. Just as we cannot rely completely on this approach, neither can we abdicate our responsibility to use these responses in appropriate contexts. Because these modalities are frequently used in a context of punctuation with affective involvement by the provider, it is necessary that providers be aware of their own emotional responses. Additionally, as noted by Weiner and Cole (2004) in discussing clinician communication in training for advance care planning with dying patients, emotional self-awareness needs to be accompanied by emotional self-regulation capacities.

PART III

Communications to Ensure Comprehensive and Continuous Patient-Centered Care under Challenging Circumstances

Most people would agree that communication can be difficult. Under the best of circumstances, we can get poor results. Individuals can fail to send messages in ways that they can be understood. What is said is not always perceived and processed in the manner that we intended. By definition, human communication can be problematic.

What if we upped the ante, so to speak, and tried to communicate in already difficult interpersonal circumstances. Would we need to quadruple our skills and knowledge? Most likely—because to communicate effectively in these instances we have to know a considerable amount about the specific so-called difficulty. In health care, we are confronted time and time again with challenging circumstances—circumstances that are intense and emotion laden, circumstances with a high risk for not turning out well, circumstances in which patients successfully resist our good judgment and good care.

In this section of the text, specific attention is drawn to communicating with patients and others under challenging circumstances. We communicate with patients and families who have barriers due to low literacy. Some circumstances include communicating under conditions of conflict and crisis. It also means that we communicate with patients who display significantly negative or resistive behavioral patterns. What is difficult for one provider may be elementary to another, so the situations chosen for discussion in this section of the text may or may not be challenging to most providers but at least for the beginning clinician, they should be. Barriers to communication in these situations have been amply described in the literature.

In Chapter 13, Communicating with Patients of Low Literacy, the challenges of communicating effectively with those who by virtue of education, language, ethnicity, culture, and previous experience or lack of experience may have difficulty in understanding U.S. health care and navigating the health-care system is addressed in detail. Specific steps in assessing level of health literacy and recommendations for shaping communications to meet the needs of these communities are described.

In Chapter 14, Communicating with Patients with Chronic and/or Life-Threatening Illness, the concepts and principles of communicating with patients take on particular specificity. Knowing what patients may be experiencing at a certain phase is important in establishing how to respond therapeutically. Knowing how the threat of patient noncompliance factors into disease management is yet another dimension of communicating with these patients.

In Chapter 15, Communicating with Patients in Crisis, the deficits in communication that individuals in crisis typically exhibit are detailed. Patients' subsequent reactions to the stimulus and crisis events are discussed. Finally, guidelines for communicating effectively with individuals in crisis are presented.

Providers who are engaged in the management of chronic disease and life-threatening illness must know a great deal about patients' actual and potential responses to illness. Managing care includes managing responses to illness (and treatment). We are to be both healers of disease and healers of maladaptive coping responses. Communicating with patients who display emotion, specifically when the display is negative, can be moderately to extremely difficult for most providers. In the final chapter of this section, Communicating Effectively with Patients Displaying Significant Negative or Resistive Coping Responses (Chapter 16), the emotional situation is really the challenge. The specific behavioral response is the challenge. If we asked a thousand healthcare providers which specific patient behaviors caused them problems or created substantially negative effects, we might develop a significant level of consensus. The difficult patient behaviors discussed in the chapter have also been addressed elsewhere in the literature. The accusatory, complaining, demanding, aggressive, and self-pitying presentations usually arouse emotions in providers. These emotions are soon followed by defensive and/or aggressive reactions—reactions that unfortunately aggravate a preexisting bad situation. Understanding these patient behaviors, their underlying causes, and what providers can do to avoid interpersonal traps are essential to communicating effectively with patients.

In summary, Part III of this text addresses communication skills at a somewhat higher, advanced level. This is not to say that the basic generic skills presented in Part II are not useful. Rather, generic skills must be added too. Experiences with actual patients in the context of health and illness provide depth and wisdom for our communicating effectively as health professionals.

CHAPTER 13

Communicating with Patients of Low Literacy

Speak properly, and in as few words as you can, but always plainly; for the end of the speech is not . . . to be understood.
—William Penn

Broadly speaking, the short words are the best, and the old words best of all.
—Sir Winston Churchill

Think like a wise man but communicate in the language of the people.
—William Butler Yeats

CHAPTER OBJECTIVES

- ☛ Discuss the problem of low literacy in the United States.
- ☛ Differentiate between literacy and functional health literacy.
- ☛ Discuss the relationship of education and functional health literacy.
- ☛ Identify at least four barriers to health literacy.
- ☛ Discuss the potential relationship of low health literacy and poor health outcomes.
- ☛ Identify populations at risk for low health literacy.
- ☛ Describe ways to assess health literacy in patient populations.
- ☛ Describe ways the provider can assess and enhance health literacy among patients.
- ☛ Identify the importance of using "plain language" in speaking to patients.
- ☛ Describe how to deal with shame related to low literacy in interactions with patients.
- ☛ Describe specific ways systems of care might deter or promote health literacy.

Knowing the degree to which patients or patients' families understand what you communicated and its significance is the single most important challenge of communicating with persons with low literacy. On the flip side is the question of to what degree you understand them. How often would you admit: "I really can't be sure"? Although seldom noted, the reality that neither you nor your patient understood completely what was communicated is rather high. Provider's mode of communicating with low literacy patients is critical in determining desired treatment outcomes. Low literacy has been associated with poor knowledge of disease, poor adherence to treatment regimen, problems in self-management, and even clinical outcomes. Descriptive as well as randomized controlled studies have reported the link between low literacy and these outcomes. This chapter addresses the concepts and strategies for communicating with persons of low health literacy and strategies to assess literacy levels and plan accordingly. Strategies in this chapter include using the smallest amount of information at a visit, reinforcing information with visual handouts, repetition, using the words of the patient, and using stories.

THE PROBLEM OF LITERACY IN THE UNITED STATES

Illiteracy poses a major barrier to educating patients about their illness and its treatment. Young (2004) goes as far to say that it is a *national epidemic*. Glassby (2002) refers to the problem of health illiteracy as *the hidden handicap*. To understand the problem of health literacy, providers need to have a working knowledge of the problem of low literacy or the ability to read and write and calculate basic math and the extent to which it affects patients' abilities to understand aspects of their illness and to follow the treatment that is planned for them.

Beginning knowledge of the prevalence of literacy deficits suggests that it is far more pervasive than expected. Recent research has shown that the U.S. population suffers high rates of low literacy. The now classic study instrumental in identifying literacy problems, 1992 National Adult Literacy Survey (NALS), revealed that 1 out of 5 people in the United States are functionally illiterate (Kirsch, Jungeblut, Jenkins, & Kolstad, 1993). Furthermore another 27% were estimated to be marginally literate. Taken as a whole, slightly more than half the U.S. population may have difficulty communicating with healthcare providers or understanding the important meaning and instruction of providers in their conversations with their patients. These patients and their families present a special challenge in that they may not easily understand materials and instructions presented even at the sixth-grade level. Frequently, they feel ashamed to reveal their illiteracy and may not try to engage in dialogue with the provider to risk revelation that they are not understanding what is being said (Parikl, Parker, Nurss, Baker, & Williams, 1996). Not surprisingly, there is a circular situation with neither patient nor provider comprehending what is needed.

FUNCTIONAL HEALTH LITERACY

According to the Ad Hoc Committee on Health Literacy for the Council of Scientific Affairs, American Medical Association (AMA, 1999), the results of the National Adult Literacy Survey raise serious concerns about patients' abilities to function adequately in a healthcare setting. Whereas *literacy* speaks generally to the ability to read and write, *functional health literacy* refers more specifically to the skills and knowledge necessary to understand illness and treatment and the ability to navigate the healthcare system. These skills include understanding how to read and interpret medication prescriptions, appointment slips, and referrals and understanding the concept of follow-up of illness through additional medical appointments. Health professionals value functional health literacy in their patients for several reasons.

1. Health literacy can empower patients to form an active alliance with their providers enhanced chiefly by the patient's ability to understand basic medical terminology and procedures.

2. Informed patients are more likely to initiate and sustain self-management behaviors that will result in health-promoting behaviors and improved health outcomes.
3. Patients who do not understand health providers' instructions are less likely to receive quality medical care (AMA, 1999). This is particularly a problem with the elderly who bear the greatest burden of disease but are known to have low levels of health literacy (Safeer & Keenan, 2005).

A primary underlying purpose of providers' communications includes improving patients' health literacy. Maximizing patient encounters to improve patient health literacy is complicated by a variety of personal, patient–provider, and system factors that are not always under the provider's control. Nonetheless, the goal is to advance the patient's understanding of illness and treatment through singular or sequential contacts with the patient and family.

According to the Institute of Medicine's health literacy report (2004c), although there is no direct evidence of the impact of health literacy on health outcomes, there is sufficient evidence to support its importance:

> The report states that studies have shown that people with low health literacy understand health information less well, get less preventive health care—such as screenings for cancer—and use expensive health services such as emergency department care more frequently.

In a report by the Agency for Healthcare Research and Quality (2004), it was concluded that low literacy is not only associated with poor understanding of medical advice but with adverse patient outcomes and even negative effects on health. Taken as a whole, low health literacy can lead to substandard care. It was noted that patients with low literacy had poorer health outcomes (intermediate disease markers, measures of morbidity, and general health status) but also poorer use of health services.

The research is marred by a number of methodological issues (reliance on cross-sectional designs, inconsistency in type of health literacy measure used, and problems with generalization due to small and selective sample sizes). Further, most studies measured short-term knowledge gain and immediate health outcomes without building in measurement of long-term effects. An issue of importance is whether these relationships would hold up over time and what exactly is the nature of this relationship. For example, it has been shown that literacy also correlates with economic and insurance status, which are linked with use of health care and preventive health services. The impact of health literacy on health service use could be confounded by many other related factors.

Nonetheless, the literature supports a positive and significant relationship between level of health literacy and patient outcomes in a wide array of patients with chronic conditions: HIV (Kalichmann & Rompa, 2000; Miller, Brownlee, McCoy, & Pignone, 2007; Miller, Liu, et al., 2003), hypertension (Williams, Baker, Parker, et al., 1998); diabetes (Williams, Baker, Parker, et al., 1998; Schillinger et al., 2002; Rothman, Malone, Bryant, et al., 2004); asthma (Williams, Baker, Honig, et al., 1998), and open heart surgery postoperative care (Conlin & Schumann, 2002). Others have studied the risk of hospital admission associated with health literacy (Baker, Parker, Williams, & Clark, 1998), the use of preventive health services, and use of health services in general (Baker, Parker, Williams, Clark, & Nurss, 1997; Baker, Gazmararian, Williams, et al., 2004; Miller et al., 2007), as well as the associated costs of hospitalization with low literacy patients (Marwick, 1997).

The U.S. Department of Health and Human Services, in its report *Healthy People 2010*, included improved health literacy as an objective (11-2), stressing the need for equity in health care. In this document, health literacy is defined as: "The degree to which individuals have the capacity to obtain, process, and understand basic health information and services needed to make appropriate health decisions."

According to this document, health literacy includes the ability to understand: (1) instructions on prescription drug bottles, (2) appointment slips, (3) medical education brochures, and (4) medical directions and consent forms, plus (5) the ability to navigate complex healthcare systems. Health literacy is not simply the ability to read materials. "It requires a complex group of reading, listening, analytical, and decision-making skills, and the ability to apply these skills to health situations."

Health literacy includes both verbal and written comprehension and numeracy skills. Understanding cholesterol levels, calculating how many medications to take and when, and reading labels all require math skills, and, while most of it is simple math, still the probability that any one patient with low literacy skills may not understand what to do is significant enough to address. In addition to basic literacy skills, health literacy includes background information about how the body works, what infection and injury mean, how the body recovers with medical intervention, and the relationship of lifestyle patterns and illness (e.g., nutrition and obesity).

Unlike basic literacy skills, health literacy is not necessarily related to years of education. A person who has attained a graduate degree may not function well in a healthcare setting nor understand the importance of preventive care. A person who is well educated but was educated more than 20 years ago may no longer have an accurate understanding of many chronic illnesses. Other reasons accounting for poor health literacy include the individual's previous exposure to chronic illness and healthcare environments. Likewise, someone who has not graduated from high school may be particularly knowledgeable about how to navigate the system and the meaning of chronic illness due to their own history of a chronic disease or the treatment of a close family member. Due to the complex nature of healthcare forms and regulations, not even a person with excellent literacy may interpret his or her lab tests with ease, and not even a physician could help a patient complete insurance forms or use the best insurance coverage plan. All things considered, it is important to conduct an individualized assessment of the patient's knowledge and ability to function in the healthcare setting.

BARRIERS TO HEALTH LITERACY

It is difficult to propose an approach to solving the health literacy problem without first identifying the factors and barriers to health literacy. The state of the science in studying health literacy is preliminary, with many studies focusing on the assessment of literacy and others on the connection of literacy with health-seeking behaviors, with a minor concentration on the factors that influence health literacy. This is, in part, due to the absence of a conceptual framework from which to view the problem in a broader context. The following discussion places health literacy in a context affected by multiple barriers, some of which are mutable (within the provider's control) and others which are not.

Barriers to achieving health literacy are multiple and occur at many levels: individual-level barriers (demographic, health status, complexity of illness/treatment, illness experience and healthcare system exposure), patient–provider relationship barriers, and system-related barriers (number, length, and quality of encounters, patient-centered care delivery). Figure 13–1 is a diagram of these factors and illustrates how they may interact with each other to affect level of healthcare literacy.

Individual-Level Barriers

There are certain populations that, as a whole, are vulnerable to low levels of health literacy. Age, culture, language, education, and income all play an independent and collective role in affecting individuals' level of health literacy. The following populations are at particular risk for poor health literacy: youth, the elderly, those with low socioeconomic status with no health insurance, minority and marginal or vulnerable populations, the medically or cognitively impaired, and the medically underserved.

Vulnerable populations are those that, by virtue of their position in life, are at risk for health problems but also for problems in self-management of their

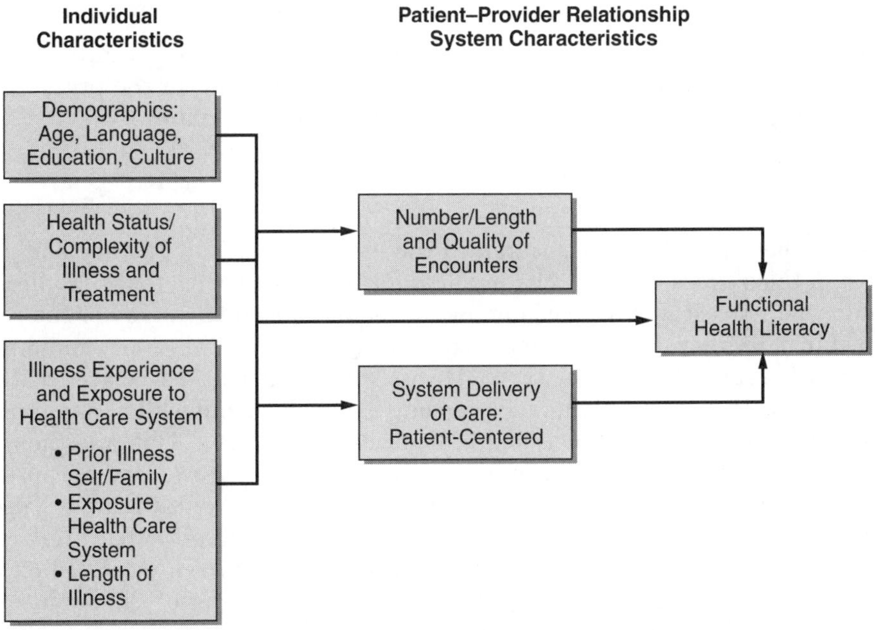

Figure 13–1 Multiple Interacting Factors Affecting Functional Health Literacy.

disease. Typically they are populations that exhibit more than one risk simultaneously. They may be elderly, poor, from minority groups, and immigrant. They may have limited comprehension of English and little to no formal education. Sarkar, Fisher, and Schillinger (2006), in a study of the relationship of self-efficacy and diabetes self-management across race/ethnicity and health literacy, reported that self-efficacy was associated with self-management behaviors in four of the five self-management behaviors but not medication adherence. These investigators concluded that further study of the determinants of and barriers to self-management were warranted. It was suggested that self-management skills and knowledge be expanded to include ethnically diverse populations across the span of health literacy.

Vulnerable populations have been shown to be at risk for disparities in health care and health. The AHRQ *National Health Disparities Report* lists a number of reported facts that substantiate that vulnerable populations are at higher risk for healthcare disparities:

- Minorities are more likely to be diagnosed with late-stage breast cancer and colorectal cancer compared with whites.
- Patients of lower socioeconomic position are less likely to receive recommended diabetic services and more likely to be hospitalized for diabetes and its complications.
- When hospitalized for acute myocardial infarction, Hispanics are less likely to receive optimal care.
- Many racial and ethnic minorities and persons of lower socioeconomic position are more likely to die from HIV. Minorities also account for a disproportionate share of new AIDS cases.
- The use of physical restraints in nursing homes is higher among Hispanics and Asian/Pacific Islanders compared with non-Hispanic whites.
- Blacks and poorer patients have higher rates of avoidable hospital admissions (i.e., hospitalizations for health conditions that, in the presence of comprehensive primary care, rarely require hospitalization).

At Risk Populations

A number of studies have examined the association of low literacy and age. Most of the studies examine the problem for the elderly with fewer studies on youth and adolescents. In a comprehensive and noteworthy study of the relationship of literacy and mortality in the elderly (Sudore et al., 2006) found that limited literacy (using the REALM) was independently associated with a nearly twofold increase in mortality among 2,500 black and white, community-dwelling elders without functional difficulties or dementia. This was the case even after adjusting for a number of confounding factors (demographics, socioeconomic status, co-morbidities, self-rated health, health-related behaviors, access to health care, and psychosocial status). While limited literacy is prevalent in the elderly, no prospective study to date was conducted to link literacy with mortality in this population. Noting the aging of the population and the prevalence of chronic disease in the elderly raises the question of how literacy plays a role in both co-morbidity and mortality. It is possible that low literacy is implicated in health screening and continued use of appropriate health care. Because of the impact of low health literacy on hospital visits, healthcare expenditures, and poor health outcomes, much attention has been placed on adults and the elderly. For youth, the issues are different, but the problem of use of health services and following preventive practices may be similar to that of adults and the elderly. The relationship of low health literacy and adolescents' willingness to follow disease prevention messages and health promotion practices has been studied. Brown, Teufel, and Birch (2007) reported that in addition to age, difficulty understanding health information and belief that kids can do little to affect their future health decreased their interest in and desire to follow what they were taught about health. The investigators concluded that more attention should be placed on increasing student interest in health issues and feelings that they could control health outcomes.

To illustrate this further, low literacy has been associated with use of preventive healthcare services (Miller & Degenholtz, 2003) and the nature of outpatient encounters (Roter, 2000). Culture and ethnicity have also been studied for their influence on health literacy. Language and education affect health literacy in that not all literature is comprehensible, and this might affect patients' growing repertoire of information about disease and treatment.

Given multiple problems in these areas increases the risk that their healthcare literacy will be very low. These individuals may have difficulty finding or accessing health providers, completing healthcare forms, making decisions when offered alternatives, describing their history of healthcare problems and the course of treatment, understanding the role of preventive health care, understanding the relationship of risky behaviors and health promotion and disease prevention, self-managing chronic or acute health conditions, understanding directions on health information sheets, and making decisions about their care. Recognizing individuals with these deficits is important early on, and, as suggested, sufficient time and attention needs to be given to bringing these individuals to a place of even basic understanding:

- Patients do not recognize what they do not know: many patients do not know what they don't know. These groups frequently include the elderly, those with impaired judgment, and those with limited exposure to disease and healthcare systems.
- Patients think they know but do not know: many patients harbor misconceptions about disease and treatment. They have no reason to doubt their understanding so rarely ask questions to clarify what they believe.

An example of this kind of misconception would be the following: A 34-year-old Hispanic male with HIV infection and Hepatitis C expresses the opinion that he thought that he could not transmit Hepatitis C to someone else *unless his liver touched the liver of this person*. What is lost in the translation here is a knowledge of how disease is transmitted and the effect of the disease on body systems. Another example is the patient who interprets the directions on their medication bottle reading *take twice a day* to mean *take two pills at once*.

In each of these examples, there were apparent barriers to effective communication, including patient low levels of health literacy, language problems, and misunderstanding of disease (how disease and treatment work).

- Shame associated with poor literacy: there have been a number of reports that patients may be ashamed of their inability to understand written or verbal messages. Feelings of shame may prohibit them from asking important questions to clarify what they do not know (Parikl et al., 1996).

This type of patient may be unresponsive to questions by the provider, may appear relatively silent and withdrawn, and may wait to be asked questions. In this case, use of open-ended questions is the preferred format. They may also answer "I don't know" and avoid eye contact rather than engage in discourse about the topic.

The identification of the barriers just listed focuses almost exclusively on what the patient brings to the encounter. In addition to these factors, several other facets affect patients' health literacy and ability to communicate effectively. Patient–provider encounter, health and treatment complexity, and system issues affect patient–provider communications and the degree to which individuals are more or less health literate.

Provider–Patient Encounters/Relationship Barriers

It has been previously suggested that the provider–patient encounter may affect health literacy favorably or unfavorably. Provider training has been studied for its ability to favorably affect professionals' abilities to identify and reach patients with low literacy, and this occurs across disciplinary boundaries. Bass, Wilson, Griffith, and Barnett (2002) examined residents' abilities to identify patients with low literacy skills. Olson, Blank, Cardinal, Hopf, and Chalmers (1996) and Youmans and Schillinger (2003) explored the pharmacist's role with the needs of low literacy patients appearing to have problems understanding medications.

A good deal of the health education literature has relied on improving the written word to communicate more effectively with patients and their families. The assumption is that if the materials are sufficiently user-friendly, the problem of low literacy has been addressed. The problem with this assumption is that it does not account for the impact of the relationship between providers and patients. In this case, it is not only the quality of the printed matter but the interpersonal approach to the patient. Several theorists have attempted to describe the essence of the patient–provider relationship that will successfully affect patients in positive ways. Several of the interventions described in Parts x and y (listening, pausing, and judicious use of silence) are included in explanations of what makes for therapeutic communications with persons of low literacy.

It has also been suggested that the patient may or may not understand the provider and, if confused, may not ask for clarification. The presence of an interpreter is not always the answer because what may occur is that the relationship focus shifts from patient and provider to interpreter and provider. Although necessary at times, the use of an interpreter may be problematic because the issue is establishing a therapeutic alliance with the patient. The appropriate use of interpreters has been addressed in several publications.

A considerable amount of attention has been focused on health professionals and the necessity to train providers to both assess for health literacy and respond accordingly. These approaches need to address barriers. Health professionals and patients may differ in age, gender, socioeconomics, educational level, culture, national origin, and sexual orientation, to name a few. These differences are not always celebrated, nor are they taken into account in each and every instance.

System-Level Barriers

System factors that may act as barriers are perhaps the least explored category. They include the mission of the institution, the system of delivery of care, the proportion of providers to patients, time and schedule of care activities. If the mission of the institution is to serve primarily low-income populations at risk for disease and illness who have not perhaps received adequate screening and preventive care, then the philosophy may be to focus on methods to enhance receptive approaches to gain the trust and confidence of the population they serve. However, if the system of care is such that the ratio of providers to patients is inadequate and the time provided for medical visits is limited, then organizationally the attention to improving health literacy may be compromised. Studies of provider–patient ratios and health outcomes, including patient satisfaction with communication received, indicate the importance of a system that *talks the talk and walks the walk*.

Paasche-Orlow, Schillinger, Greene, and Wagner (2006), in a careful account of the system-level barriers, suggest that changes need to occur at the level of organization and delivery of healthcare system to improve the overall quality of U.S. health care and produce a more health-literate society. They advocate that *comprehension* should be a standard in clinical care to the extent that it is a basic universal precaution. To effectively do this, providers will need system-level supports, including time, education about assessing and addressing health literacy deficits, and built-in incentives, to encourage this facet of their roles. Above all, these structures and incentives, including reinforcements, should be targeted for vulnerable populations. It is in these populations in particular that a variety of biophysical, economical, environmental, and cultural factors influence the health and health care to those with limited literacy. Summarizing the nature of the link between the system and outcomes for those that have literacy deficits, Paasche-Orlow and colleagues propose three distinctive organizing principles:

1. Promote productive interactions between provider and patient to improve communications, exercising universal precautions to assure comprehension, improving providers' communication capacities, and developing communication technology platforms.
2. Address the organization of health care, making patient-centered care a system property and streamlining, simplifying, and targeting vulnerable populations.
3. Embrace a community-level ecological perspective, using intervention models that acknowledge the multilevel nature of population vulnerability and advocate and develop an independent and trusted public health voice.

COMMUNICATION INTERVENTIONS TO IMPROVE HEALTH LITERACY

Health providers have an important role in assessing, planning for, implementing, and evaluating health literacy and problems directed at enhancing health literacy. It has been estimated that up to 80% of patients forget what their doctor has said as soon as they leave, and nearly 50% of what they do remember is inaccurate. By assessing and addressing health literacy, providers can improve communication with their patients and increase the probability that patients will understand what they say, which may lead to better adherence to treatment and, ultimately, better health outcomes. Healthcare systems can enable providers to play significant roles in addressing literacy issues. Table 13–1 describes the elements of healthcare systems promoting health literacy.

Perhaps the very first thing health providers need to know is how to identify individuals with low levels of health literacy. Because patients with low health literacy often feel shame and a sense of inadequacy, they may hesitate to ask the provider to repeat instructions or explain treatment or other important relevant information (Safeer & Keenan, 2005).

ASSESSING HEALTH LITERACY

Reviewing the literature on physician assessment of health literature, Safeer and Keenan (2005) bring attention to the fact that health providers do poorly in assessing literacy. The usual approach is to identify the patient's potential understanding by obtaining the patient's level of education. Safeer and Keenan also indicated that the grade level of the patient may underestimate the level of illiteracy and, as the age of patients increases, declining cognitive skills, decreased sensory abilities and increased time since formal education placed people at greater risk for poor health literacy.

There are a number of health literacy assessments that have been used for research purposes, including TOFHLA (Test of Functional Health Literacy in Adults; Baker, Parker, et al., 1997), the short-measure S-TOFHLA (Baker, Williams, et al., 1999) in English or Spanish to measure language proficiency, the REALM (Rapid Estimate of Adult Literacy in Medicine; Davis, Michielutte,

Table 13–1 Elements of a System Promoting Health Literacy

Time to construct reading materials using plain language and illustrations.
Opportunity to test and evaluate all written materials and medical instruction information sheets.
Provider–patient time to communicate to exceed 6–10 minutes.
Advocacy for health literacy in the organization and recognition of the value of assessing health literacy.
Providers knowledgeable and skilled in concepts of and assessment of limited literacy.
Opportunity to conduct feedback loop (patient is asked what she or he does and does not understand as well as time for provider to clarify patient's communication).
Development of population-based health literacy best practices.

Askov, Williams, & Weiss, 1998), or more recently, the REALM-R (Bass, Wilson, & Griffith, 2003). The REALM-R is a new eight-item measure to rapidly screen for health literacy problems. The REALM is easy to administer and is quick, whereas the TOFHLA provides a formal overview of patients' abilities to comprehend material but is generally more time-consuming and less practical in the everyday clinic setting. Thus, the short form of the TOFHLA was designed. Another instrument, developed to be used exclusively with Spanish-speaking patients, is called the Short Assessment of Health Literacy for Spanish-speaking Adults (SAHLSA-50; Lee, Bender, Ruiz, & Cho, 2006) and is based on the REALM. This instrument contains 50 items and could be used in the clinical setting to screen Spanish-speaking patients for low literacy. The shorter versions of the S-TOFHLA (in Spanish or English) or REALM-R may be useful in the community clinic setting; however, the provider interviewer approach is key in assessing health literacy. The S-TOFHLA is useful in measuring written comprehension but does not capture language competency. Recently, the BEST (Basic English Skills Test) has been tested for its use as an oral interview that can be used in the emergency department (Downey & Zun, 2007).

Basic medical language is usually graded on a continuum, as in the REALM; there are terms that are easy to understand (at the third-grade level or below), moderately difficult (at a fourth-grade to sixth-grade level), slightly more difficult (seventh and eighth-grade levels), and most difficult to comprehend (high school level). Asking the patient if he or she has heard any of the words in the category *moderate* (fatigue, prescription, depression, nutrition) may give the provider some idea about whether the patient is at the very low end of health literacy or may be healthcare experienced and knowledgeable to the point that he or she is very health literate. As suggested in the REALM, a provider might ask a patient whether he or she has heard the term and secondly, what he or she thinks it means. In this way a provider captures both recognition and comprehension, both of which are needed to understand a patient's disease and its treatment.

There is still another assessment tool that has been developed, and it can be used as a quick screening tool in the primary care setting (Weiss et al., 2005). The Newest Vital Sign (NVS) uses a nutrition label (the ice cream nutrition label) and six questions to ascertain patients' comprehension. It takes approximately three minutes to complete. Fewer than four correct answers indicate a patient may have limited health literacy. The English version has been shown to have good reliability; however, the reliability of the Spanish version was not as good and was explained as a function of so many subgroups of Latino subjects tested. The investigators recommend further testing of the NVS. This tool is available online only at: http://www.annfammed.org/cgi/content/full/3/6/514/DC1 (Weiss et al., 2005, p. 516).

Because little has been done in the assessment of health literacy in adolescents, Chisolm and Buchanan (2007) validated a tool specifically to examine the TOFHLA for the use in adolescents. They found that the reading comprehension component of the TOFHLA was valid for adolescents. While most literacy tools have been used and validated for adults, there is an ever-pressing need to have adolescents make healthcare choices, which requires them to be knowledgeable about health promotion and disease prevention.

One of the most practical and conventional assessment tools is the *teach-back* method, also referred to as the "feedback loop" or "closing the loop" (Schillinger et al., 2003). The idea behind this intervention is that in order to fully understand patients' comprehension of the information given to them, it is important to assess their grasp of the content that was communicated. It is suggested that both consumers and providers use this method to increase the effectiveness of their communications with each other. The patient is asked to restate the information in his or her own words, not simply repeat what the provider said, to better ensure that the information is both understood and remembered. Thus, this strategy is used to assess the comprehension of medical information and aid in the patient's remembering what it is that the provider taught them. When the patient's understanding is inaccurate or incomplete, the provider repeats the process until he or she is confident that the patient understands the information needed to be compliant to the treatment regimen or recommendations for health promotion. Patients can also be asked to act upon the information given as if they were, in real life, performing the action. For example, they would read the prescription bottle and demonstrate the number of pills they would take of this and other medications twice a day. They could also demonstrate their knowledge of how many pills they will take in a single day as well as morning and evening intervals and what secondary conditions are needed (e.g., before meals/after meals, avoiding use of alcohol, and reporting significant side effects).

In the use of the teach-back or closing the loop techniques, it is important to avoid a "test-like" atmosphere. Rather the provider is testing how well the patient was taught. By putting the responsibility on the provider, he or she avoids the feelings of shame and anxiety that may result from the patient feeling like they failed the test and disappointed the provider.

Provider: "So what the instructions mean is that you will need to take this medication in the morning before you have a meal. You are free to eat after one hour from the time you take this pill. But, if you forget to take it before 2:00 in the afternoon you need to wait until the next day."

Provider: "Now, I want to see how well I did in explaining everything you need to know in order to take your medication. What's important about taking this medicine in the morning?"

Patient: "I have to take it before 2."

Provider: "Ok, you got one part. The other important thing to remember is that you need to take it before you eat and wait until one hour before you have something to eat."

Each time we conduct a teach-back we find out how the patient has processed our instructions and what needs enforcement. We used the example of instructing about medication use, this same technique could be used in teaching them about other parts of their treatment or in their understanding of their illness and symptoms.

If the patient is unable to repeat what was told to them, the provider will need to assess what the problem is and how he or she might reframe the teaching. If the provider chooses to repeat the information, it is advisable to restate the material without using the same words. Usually try to simplify because it may be that the first attempt was beyond the patient's comprehension. Another approach is to repeat the material several times in the course of the discussion to assess whether the patient is getting more accustomed to the words used and the principles behind the messages.

This method is also used to determine whether the patient has the technical skills to handle management of their disease whether it be giving themselves insulin injections or simply how they are going to organize their medications in their weekly medication tray.

Baker and colleagues (1996) have identified several cues to indicate that the patient may have difficulties in comprehending the healthcare medical encounter. Table 13–2 lists several indicators that will help enhance providers' skills in assessing patients.

DOCUMENTING HEALTH LITERACY PROBLEMS

The patient's medical record contains a wealth of information about the patient's health condition and the plan of care. What is often missing is information about the patient's comprehension of his or her disease and treatment. A simple approach to documenting patient comprehension is to provide a flow sheet with the essentials of what is required for the patient to adequately self-manage their care. For example, for a diabetic patient on insulin, such a chart might include the complications of not controlling sugar levels, the beginning signs of insulin shock, how to measure one's glucose level, how to inject insulin, and what diet and exercise plan will be recommended.

One section of the flow sheet could indicate that this information was covered, and the second section could indicate the provider's perception of the patient's level of comprehension. Added to this flow sheet may be indications about what information needs to be reinforced or supplemented. The documentation of health literacy problems is critical because of its associated link with patient adherence to treatment regimens.

PRACTICAL APPROACHES TO IMPROVE LITERACY AND ENHANCE COMMUNICATIONS

A multitude of agencies have concern about the health literacy in the United States regardless of where the public falls on the health–illness contin-

Table 13–2 Potential Indicators of Poor Health Literacy

Ambivalence about asking staff for help (tends to avoid being an imposition).
Reserves questions until after leaving the examination room (may ask another staff member in passing).
Asks a question and then withdraws it as if he or she really understands when he or she does not.
Misses appointments and does not call to reschedule (may give no reason).
Nonadherence to treatment plan and medication regimen (may simply reply, "I forgot").
Quiet and unassuming in treatment room.
Comes with adult companions who can offer advice or reword what provider says.
Delays making decisions about treatment options and asks for things to be put in writing.

uum. Disease prevention initiatives cannot be effective if they do not address the probability that communities cannot easily understand messages that are broadcasted or communicated in narrow circles.

Public media are instrumental in communicating disease-prevention and health-promotion information. Viewing these messages will inform providers about works. Notice that messages are brief, and persons who are or are not yet affected by the disease speak (they are persons like the majority that may be at risk). Context of the message is important, and usually the audience can identify with the context.

An example: A young Hispanic couple and young children are pictured in the context of a loving family unit. The words are: "Protect YOUR family!" (from HIV/AIDS). What is known about this population is that the family (*familia*) is a high priority, and the man in the family is strong and powerful. Thus, the concept of *machismo* is intrinsically addressed in the message to take positive action. As is, this message has significant impact on those who read it; although the message is very brief, the context makes it powerful. Few who read this message are likely to forget the content.

The literature on improving health literacy through good communications with patients and their families is extensive. A list of references is provided at the end of this chapter. Table 13–3 provides a composite list of approaches that are recommended and/or have been used in communicating to patients with limited health literacy.

In summary, health literacy needs to be assessed and specific steps need to be taken to enhance the effectiveness of each encounter. Certain populations

Table 13–3 Communication to Improve Patient Health Literacy

Take a moment to develop a *gestalt* of the patient and situation (demographics [age, gender, ethnicity, educational level], culture, cultural similarities and differences, presenting problem and history, previous treatment plan), including first response.

Assess the patient's health literacy (not educational level).

Assess in a manner that avoids suggesting that this is a test and that it is shameful to not know.

Be aware that the patient's level of comprehension may be at even fourth grade or lower.

Use small, brief, and simply worded messages.

Communicate messages at a pace the patient can follow.

Place these messages in some context known to and valued by the patient.

Repeat material at selected intervals, being careful to use similar but not the same words.

When possible, supplement information with visuals: cartoons, videos, pictures.

Choose visuals that the patient can identify (shared fears, values, or goals).

Initially use the patient's words, then carefully move to the known medical terms for the condition or treatment (presuming the patient will never comprehend a medical term may be as humiliating to the patient as shaming him or her for not knowing).

Draw pictures if there are no pictures or diagrams to use.

Tell stories about other hypothetical cases (while protecting the confidentiality of case materials) that would pique the interest of the patient.

Use the teach-back or return demonstration technique to judge how much the patient has understood and retained.

Using the patient's level of understanding, carefully fill in any gaps or correct misconceptions (patients will rarely understand the first exposure).

may have unique presentations based on their exposure both to illness and to treatment. At the very least, providers need to make sure that patients advocate for themselves; on a regular basis at patient–provider contacts ask:

1. What is my problem?
2. What are you going to do?
3. What am I supposed to do?
4. Why is it important for me to do this (take medication, follow a particular diet and exercise program, monitor my blood glucose levels)?

In the context of these questions and answers, the patient should become more familiar with how the body/mind works, how the disease/illness/injury affects the body, how other conditions might result from this primary condition, how long it will be before he or she sees improvement, and what the alternatives are in treating the condition the way the provider suggests. All this should happen in the context that the patient may have very limited accurate and complete information and that in-depth learning will require repetition of facts and ongoing decisions that will be expected of them.

IMPROVING HEALTH LITERACY WITH PATIENTS WITH CHRONIC DISEASE

Patients with a chronic health condition may appear to know a great deal about their health status and medical treatment. Over time, their exposure to the healthcare system, different medication regimens, different providers, and information they have gleaned from printed materials or the Internet have given them some foundation to self-manage their care. What they might not know are the particular patterns of disease self-management that may affect their health behaviors. They may not understand that, as their treatment is prolonged they are likely to tire of the routine and even experiment with altering their care plan. They may also lapse into nonadherence due to the long-term demands of their illness. If they do not have a good alliance with their provider, where there is open communication, and an environment that is shameless, they may not inform the provider about what steps they have personally taken to give themselves "a break."

Among those at particular risk for literacy-associated self-management problems are those with chronic illness, the majority of which are elderly and not only have chronic diseases but also more co-morbid conditions. According to Schillinger and colleagues (2003), the impact of low literacy on health of persons with chronic disease, has brought attention to persons with lower health literacy have more problems managing their care, has greater rates of utilization of health services, and has poorer health outcomes.

Consider an 88-year-old elderly woman living alone in a one-bedroom apartment. She is taking medications for diabetes, high blood pressure, osteoarthritis, depression, and several over-the-counter vitamins and minor pain supplements with the notation "prn." She understands that she must take medications on a regular basis but several times a week finds that she is just not able to read the prescription on the bottle or remember if she already took her medications. She has several prescription aids to help her (e.g., weekly pill box and refrigerator magnets). She knows she has several pills to take and can not read the writing on the pill bottle, so she just takes one, the one she thinks she needs to take. Then an hour after, returns to take a second pill. This time she remembers the doctor told her to take two pills twice a day so she takes four ($2 \times 2 = 4$), thinking she is doing the right thing . . . what her doctor said.

Occasionally, her daughter calls and asks: "Are you taking your medication, Mom?" She is not sure that she is, but she does not want to bother her daughter, so she replies: "Yes . . . I know how important my pills are." The discussion ends there, and because her daughter is an hour away, there is no investigation as to the reality behind the reply.

Although this example seems exaggerated, this event occurs more often than we would think. Unless the patient's overdose does not create a problem, the misunderstanding can go unnoticed for sometime.

IMPORTANCE OF USING "PLAIN LANGUAGE"

Using plain language is only one tool in the briefcase of the provider. For health providers, it is not as simple as it would seem. Health providers are trained and skilled at knowing and using medical terminology in their relationships with other providers. To some degree, this language is abbreviated and is specific to the setting in which health care is provided. Think of all the shorthand versions providers use to communicate with one another. Sometimes medical terminology is abbreviated to allow providers to talk about medical conditions in front of patients and family without their fully understanding what is being said and its significance.

Using plain language requires a paradigm shift, where there is a conscious awareness of the importance of communicating openly and effectively with patients and their caregivers. Plain language is such that the very first time a patient reads or hears a message they can understand what is communicated. Even what providers may regard as plain language may not be plain enough. The U.S. Department of Health and Human Services, in its *Quick Guide to Health Literacy*, lists the various elements of plain language: (1) presenting important points first, (2) organizing complex thoughts and ideas into understandable parts, (3) using simple terminology and language and defining technical terms whenever used, and (4) using the active voice instead of passive voice in making statements to the patient. Active and passive voice are clearly different. The following is an example of the use of active or passive voice using the same message.

Active Voice: "The clinical specialist will contact you by telephone to set up an appointment for you to come back next week."

Passive Voice: "To provide you a new appointment for next week, you will be contacted by telephone by the clinical specialist."

These messages virtually contain the same information, but as they are read, the message in the active voice is easier to follow and to understand and, controlling for all other factors (e.g., stress at the time), is more likely to be retained in the patient's memory. Using plain language is just one step in ensuring your message will be received as you intended. But because groups differ in how and what they understand, not all messages will be received similarly across groups. A case in point is patients whose primary language is not English and whose culture is other than the predominant culture; thus, there is a true need for cultural and linguistic competence in sending and receiving messages.

Consider the following dialogue, carefully identifying the problem areas in the discussion with the patient.

Provider: "Many people have diabetes. You have what is called diabetes type II. Diabetes occurs when the pancreas doesn't produce enough insulin or the body can't effectively use the insulin that the body does produce. Diabetes type II occurs later on in life but many younger people are being diagnosed with this condition now."
(Pause.)

Patient: "Diabetes . . . the 'sugar disease'?"

Provider: "Actually, diabetes can be controlled with proper diet and exercise. However, if your diabetes cannot be controlled, there are medications you will need to take, and you will have to monitor your blood glucose level on a regular basis. This is how we will know whether the medication is working for you at the dose we prescribe. It is very important that we treat this condition because serious consequences can occur if it is not. You may have heard about retinopathy, impotence, kidney diseases, or even heart disease associated with diabetes that has not been effectively treated."
(Pause. No response by the patient.)

Provider: "Do you know what the signs and symptoms of diabetes are?"

Patient: "No . . . what are *signs and symptoms*?"

Provider: "Signs and symptoms are what is going on that are typical with diabetes. Some of them are unusual thirst, frequent urination, weight changes (either gain or lose weight), blurred vision, extreme fatigue, cuts that are slow to heal, tingling in your hands or feet, problems in getting or maintaining an erection. As you can see, diabetes affects many bodily functions. So today I want to give you a list of directions to follow. I want to see if we can control your diabetes with exercise and healthy eating. To get you in to check your blood glucose level, we will have the nurse practitioner set up an appointment for you today."

Analysis of the communication in this clinic visit of a patient being diagnosed with type II diabetes pinpoints many potential problems and needs for change in the dialogue providers have with someone who has health literacy deficits. First of all, the information shared with the patient is accurate and the aspects covered are typical. They include: a description of what the patient's condition is, what this means in terms of the body's functioning, what the provider will do, what the patient may need to do, and why it is important for him to follow the medical regimen. What is problematic, however, is how this information was presented and the level of discourse between the patient and provider. All else considered, although the provider expected to see compliance to the plan, the patient may not have been in a position to be a truly informed decision maker.

In analyzing this interaction, note whether the messages were in "plain language." Remember that plain language would mean something different to different groups. The following words could be misunderstood by many with low literacy:

Pancreas: *Many people do not know what a pancreas is, where it is, or even that it is a part of the human body. It is not something visible and people rarely talk about their pancreas.*

Signs and symptoms: *Average people do not talk in terms of signs and symptoms. They may not understand that things that occur are considered in clusters. They are more likely to understand them as single isolated events.*

Concept that the body produces insulin: *Again, average people may not have heard the word or know what insulin is and where in the body it is located. They may not know that it is the function of the pancreas to make insulin because they did not know about the pancreas either.*

Age and diabetes: *The data about the late onset of diabetes II raise the issue of what is diabetes I and diabetes III. Patients might wonder if they were supposed to know they were going to get diabetes when they were younger. The issue of risk factors for diabetes was indirectly touched upon in a short discussion of diet and exercise. Patients are not likely to understand this issue or why the provider raised the issue.*

Diabetes and control: *Providers cannot be certain that the patient knows what it means to "control" diabetes. Control may mean getting things to slow down; but how does this jive with making the body effectively use insulin.*

Blood glucose level: *The person with low literacy may not know what glucose is and what it is doing in the blood. Monitoring blood glucose means what? Does that mean something is attached to the blood vessel that sends messages to the doctor when the blood gets too much glucose? What does "regular basis" really mean?*

Consequences: *retinopathy, impotence, kidney disease, heart disease: The majority of these concepts may be unfamiliar to the patient, or if familiar, the patient may not understand that these consequences do not all occur or occur at the same time.*

Exercise and healthy living: *Exactly what does this mean? Does it mean joining a gym, eating only fruit and vegetables, cooking without wine and oil? The concept of exercise means something different to people as does the concept of "healthy living," which may include native foods that would be contraindicated in a diabetic diet.*

On first appraisal, the provider is not only accurate but is communicating what generally should be explained about the patient's condition. However, in the analysis of the discourse, several problematic words and concepts appear. What is equally concerning is the manner in which the provider conducted the discussion. Despite pausing, examine the fact that she asked only one question about what the patient understood ("Do you know what the signs and symptoms of diabetes are?"). It should be noted that this opportunity for the patient to share his level of knowledge comes late. And, while the provider tries to explain signs and symptoms, the patient is inundated with new and unfamiliar terms. The patient did not make good use of the pauses, perhaps thinking that any questions he had would be answered later or perhaps reacting to the moment of learning about his disease for the very first time. What occurs over the entire discussion is a cascade of overloading the patient so that he appears overwhelmed and retreats into silence, possibly thinking that the only way to understand this provider is to go home and talk to the friends and family around him. The provider had a final opportunity to complete the feedback loop by having the patient discuss in his own words what the provider said, but she does not take this opportunity to do so. To add to the difficulty of the discourse, the provider, while well intended, slips in a message in the passive voice, which is more difficult to understand than one in the active voice.

For the purposes of learning from this example, consider this same discourse using some of the principles of communicating with those with limited health literacy.

Provider: "You have a condition called diabetes. Have you heard about diabetes before?"

Patient: "I think it is the sugar disease. My father had it and lost a toe."

Provider: "Sometimes people talk about diabetes as 'the sugar disease.' What it really means is a problem with your pancreas (pancreas is a word used to describe an organ in your body that makes insulin which is necessary for everyone and everyone has a pancreas). So when someone has diabetes, their pancreas is not making enough insulin or their body is not using it the way it needs to. Do you understand what I said?"

Patient: "Well . . . I have a pancreas . . . everybody does . . . it's not working, so I have diabetes. But how do you know I have diabetes; you didn't look at my pancreas?"

Provider: "Right, I didn't, but we take blood tests and we can tell if you have too much glucose (blood sugar) . . . also, when you came in you said you were 'tired' and lack energy to do the regular things you usually do, were always thirsty, peed a lot, and had gained weight. Your blood test, together with these things (we call them signs and symptoms) . . . we think you are diabetic."

Patient: "Well, what are you going to do?"

Provider: "You and I will be partners. I need your help, too. We will talk to you about the exercise you do and what you eat and how you cook your food."

Patient: "I don't know . . . my wife does the cooking."

Provider: "So it is going to be important that she also understands what diabetes is, what the plan is, and what can be expected if you follow the plan. We would like to have your wife come in next time we see you. The nurse will schedule a visit for you."

The previous dialogue is exemplar in the use of some principles of communicating with persons with limited health literacy. Notice that the information was cut into sections (breaking complex information into smaller chunks). Notice also that the pace was much slower than in the previous attempt (slow down the pace of information giving). Considering the previous dialogue, this provider tried to use simple language, avoiding technical terms when possible. When technical jargon was used, it was done sparsely, and the provider took care to define terms (use simple language and define technical terms). Finally, the active, not passive, voice was used, simplifying the messages considerably (use the active voice). The differences in communication between the first and second dialogue point to several important issues. The second dialogue occurs in the context that the environment values the importance of health literacy, provides the time to implement health literacy best practices, seeks and trains providers in the concepts and principles of enhancing literacy and consequently encourages patients and their families to be active participants in their care and treatment decision making.

CONCLUSION

In summary, it appears that the problem of health literacy is far more pervasive than initially thought. Health literacy has a direct impact on the quality and quantity of communication between the provider and the patient and community caregivers. Further, health literacy appears to be associated with health outcomes, disease management, and use of health services. The exact mechanism by which health literacy affects health outcomes and disease management is not completely known. However, it has been suggested that health literacy has a direct impact on quality of self-management, which, in turn, affects health outcomes. Sentell and Halpin (2006), in a secondary analysis of the data from the 1992 National Adult Literacy Survey, concluded that literacy inequities may be a significant factor in health disparities having powerful effects on work-impairing conditions as well as long-term illness.

The relationship of education and self-management is also not completely clear. Schillinger, Barton, Karter, Wang, and Adler (2006) suggest that it may be that literacy mediates the relationship of education and self-management; however, more research needs to support this premise. The idea here is that education level does not need to be related to self-management and disease control if it is only associated with health literacy, explaining why some people who are very well educated may not understand self-management tasks while those with little to no schooling might be very health literate. The reason for this is that there are several factors associated with health literacy, including age, exposure to illness and healthcare systems in the past, and the system of care that fosters health literacy. Evaluating patients' level of comprehension and planning a process of effective communication with patients and caregivers who have deficits in health literacy has been suggested as a universal precaution because of the relationship among health literacy, patient self-management, and patient safety. This chapter provided an overview of the concept of health literacy, its relationship to health outcomes, and use of healthcare services; an analysis of barriers to health literacy; and some general concepts, principles, and interventions that are effective in communicating with low literacy populations. The resources listed here are intended to provide additional information in communicating orally and in writing with populations who experience health literacy deficits, with the understanding that health literacy is modifiable and each healthcare professional has a role in improving health literacy in the context of patient population and the particular setting in which he or she is delivering health care, disease management, and health promotion services.

Resources

American College of Physicians: Promoting Health Literacy. *Health Literacy Solutions*. ACP Foundation's Patient-Centered Health Literacy Program. http://foundation.acponline.org/health_lit.htm.
[ANNO]
The ACP Foundation website defines health literacy, addresses solutions, and establishes goals and objectives for change. The overriding goal is to improve the health of the nation by increasing persons' ability to obtain, procure, and understand basic health information needed to make appropriate decisions that affect a person's health.

American College of Physicians Foundation: Promoting Health Literacy. *Health TiPS: What You Can Do*. http://foundation.acponline.org/hl/htips.htm.
[ANNO]
This link describes health sheets (4-in. × 6-in.) that contain information patients need to know to manage their disease, and does so at or below the fifth-grade reading level. These sheets are in English and Spanish and are designed specifically for low health literate populations. They are disease specific: After Your Heart Attack, COPD, Dementia, Diabetes, HIV/AIDS, Hypertension, Opioid Pain Medications, Pain, Peripheral Artery Disease, Restless Legs, Smoking, Healthy Shelter Living, Medicare Part D.

American Medical Association Foundation Health Literacy. http://www.amaassn.org./ama/pub/category.8115.html.
[ANNO]
This site contains information about patient education and links to other resources on health literacy.

Harvard School of Public Health National Center for the Study of Adult Learning and Literacy. http://www.hsph.harvard.edu/healthliteracy.
[ANNO]
This site provides information, tools, educational materials, research reports, and an extensive reading list on health literacy.

National Center for the Study of Adult Learning and Literacy (NCSALL). www.ncsall.net.
[ANNO]
NCSALL is a federally funded research and development center focused solely on adult learning. It is the purpose of NCSALL to improve practice in educational programs that serve adults with limited literacy and English language skills through professional development programs and support for research use.

National Institute for Literacy. http://www.nifl.gov/.
[ANNO]
Literacy information and resources are provided as well as research and funding opportunities. This is a federal agency that provides leadership on literacy issues of national concern and is a repository for current comprehensive literacy research and policy.

Pfizer Clear Health Communication Initiative. www.clearhealthcommunication.org.
[ANNO]
This site presents an overview of the meaning and problem of low health literacy. It also discusses a new assessment of literacy measure, Newest Vital Sign (NVS), to be used in primary care settings. A link to a research report evaluating the measure cited in the *Annals of Family Medicine, 3*(6), 2005 is provided.

Plain Language Action and Information Network. www.plainlanguage.gov.
[ANNO]
A resource that also includes examples of words and phrases that are quite often confusing and could have implications for using them in the healthcare setting (e.g., take "daily," "cool," "awful," "bad"), depending on one's experience with the English language and various subgroups of the population.

Project to Review and Improve Study Materials (PRISM). The Group Health Center for Health Studies (CHS) Readability Toolkit (2006). http://www.improving chroniccare.org/index.php?p=Health_Literacy&s+38.
[ANNO]
The toolkit was developed to help research teams communicate information about studies in plain language.

Quick Guide to Health Literacy: Strategies. Improve the Usability of Health Information. http://www.health.gov/communication/literacy/quickguide/healthinfo.htm.
[ANNO]
This website provides an overview of concepts, ideas for improving health literacy through communication, navigation, knowledge-building, and advocacy. Examples of health literacy best practices are given, and suggestions for advancing health literacy programs at the organizational level are provided. It addresses a series of fact sheets on health literacy, practical strategies for improving health literacy, and resources, including websites and publications on health literacy.

Scientific and Technical Information: Simply Put. www.cdc.gov/communication/resources/simpput.pdf.
[ANNO]
This resource from the Centers for Disease Control and Prevention, provides a guide to help you translate complicated technical and medical jargon into materials that is interesting and holds of attention of patient populations.

M. Wynia and J. Matiasek. *Promising Practices for Patient-Centered Communication with Vulnerable Populations: Examples from Eight Hospitals*. The Commonwealth Fund, August 2006. cmwf@cmwf.org.
[ANNO]
This reference re-post on "promising practices" as observed in eight selected hospitals includes having passionate champions, collecting information on patient needs, engaging communities, developing a diverse and skilled workforce, involving patients, encouraging awareness of cultural diversity, providing effective language assistance services, and addressing low health literacy. Finally, these hospital practices should be tracked over time.

Books and Book Chapters

Baur, C. R. (2005). Using the Internet to move beyond the brochure and improve health literacy. In *Understanding Health Literacy*. Schwartzberg, J. G., Vangeest, J. B., & Wang, C. C. (Eds). Chicago: American Medical Association.

Doak, C., Doak, L., & Root, J. (1996). *Teaching Patients with Low Literacy Skills.* (2nd ed.). Philadelphia: J.B. Lippincott.

Neilson-Bohlman, L., Panzer, A., & Kindig, D. (Eds.). (2004). *Health Literacy: A Prescription to End Confusion*. Washington DC: National Academies Press.

Schwartzberg, J., Vangeest, J., & Wang, C. (Eds.) (2004). *Understanding Health Literacy: Inspirations for Medicine and Public Health.* Chicago: American Medical Association.

Special Issue on Health Literacy. *Journal of General Internal Medicine*. (2006). Published on behalf of the Society of General Internal Medicine. *21*(8), 803–900.

U.S. Department of Health and Human Services. (2000). Health Communication. In: *Healthy People 2010*. (2nd Ed.). Washington, DC: U.S. Government Printing Office.

Weiss, B. (2003). *Health Literacy: A Manual for Clinicians*. Chicago: American Medical Association.

CHAPTER 14

Communicating with Patients with Chronic and/or Life-Threatening Illness

The human potential for resilience in situations of extreme threat is indeed remarkable.
—Judith F. Miller

CHAPTER OBJECTIVES

- Describe responses to dealing with illness and/or injury and the patients' corresponding communications.
- Identify the meaning of illness and/or injury to the client and/or family.
- Define several sequential phases in the adaptation to illness or injury.
- Discuss the specific impact of responses (e.g., powerlessness, helplessness, and hopelessness).
- Discuss providers' corresponding reactions to illness and injury in patients.
- Describe several coping skills that providers may use to fend off the professional stress syndrome.
- Discuss the barriers and facilitators of communication in end-of-life care.

There is something "special" about patients who face death and life-threatening illness and something "different" about those who deal with chronic illness. We make these observations and subsequently categorize patients by disease stage and its potential impact. Yet, can we be sure that these categorizations are correct? All patients are special; all patients are different. Why do we categorize patients? We do so because there are particular things to look for with patients who have certain chronic or life-threatening conditions. There are communications that might be unique. And these conditions, at least theoretically, pose differences in the way patients should be cared for. Our first assumption is that patients with chronic debilitating diseases or terminal illnesses are significantly different from those with an acute disease or mild, albeit persistent, chronic disorder.

Are there differences? And do these differences call for unique approaches? Are there differences between patients with chronic illnesses and those with life-threatening advanced disease? For example, do patients who are experiencing the debilitating effects of arthritis differ from those who are dealing with advanced stages of cancer or AIDS? One is a chronic debilitating illness; the other, a life-threatening one. Still both might be depressed, lack energy, worry about their future, and experience pain and other limitations. Although many issues are common to both, most providers would agree that the differences between these patients raise particular concerns that make the care of each unique.

In this chapter, the similarities in communicating with these two categories of patients are discussed in depth. Issues of coping and adaptation are described along with the psychological responses of helplessness, powerlessness, and hopelessness. Interventions and communications that address these patient psychological responses are discussed; additionally, principles of communicating with terminal patients about their prognosis and end-of-life care are explored. The stages of adaptation to illness and injury affect patients' emotional states and the character of their communications with providers as well as friends and family. It should remembered that they are coping with a number of symptoms as well as their realization and acceptance that they have an important affliction. These symptoms could be fatigue, pain, sleep disturbance, breathing difficulties, gastrointestinal disturbance, sexual dysfunctions, fevers, night sweats, weight gain or loss, exhaustion, and deficits in daily functioning. These ongoing aspects of their illnesses affect their adaptation to their illness and their communications with providers.

Illnesses or debilitating conditions to which these principles apply include any number of illnesses or diseases such as cancer, AIDS, congestive heart failure (CHF), cardiopulmonary disease (COPD), strokes, chronic renal or hepatic disease, arthritis, asthma, diabetes, and any number of psychiatric and neuropsychiatric conditions (e.g., depression, panic disorders, and Parkinson's disease). Some conditions are not life threatening but chronic and debilitating (e.g., arthritis and asthma). Still, they can significantly alter a patient's quality of life and present the patient with another set of losses. Infrequently do they cause death. In contrast, other conditions (e.g., lung cancer and COPD) limit a patient's quality of life and also significantly shorten their lives. Still other diseases have both life-threatening and chronic dimensions. This would be the case with CHF, kidney failure, and certain nonaggressive but life-threatening cancers.

THE PROCESS OF DEALING WITH ILLNESS AND INJURY

Most beginning healthcare professionals do not immediately grasp the importance of understanding how patients respond to illness and injury. Some providers react defensively, claiming they are neither psychiatrists nor psychologists. However, in our roles as healthcare providers, we cannot adequately care for and communicate with patients unless we understand something about how they experience and adapt to their illness and injury. Patients communicate with providers in the context of their response to their illness or injury. Providers at any point in time can be seen as caring or insensitive based on patients' responses to them.

The Meaning of Chronic and Life-Threatening Illness

Patients respond to illness and injury in ways that are similar to coping with any stressful life event. In short, patients may have long histories of adapting to stressful life events, and this history influences how they will respond to their current illness. They have developed their own unique lifestyles and ways of dealing with unwanted, unpleasant, and painful situations, including illnesses and injuries. Many illnesses run courses that are unpredictable and uncontrollable and therefore, are overwhelmingly threatening to life as the patient has known it. Other factors affect patients' experiences of illness; they include their beliefs, knowledge, experience, values, and cultural meanings they attach to illness. The specific coping responses that a patient demonstrates may be common, but how these are displayed and responded to are a function of many unique personal characteristics. Therefore, in the next section describing stages of adaptation, be cognizant of the fact that the presentation of these stages in patients will take unique shapes depending on their individual differences.

Stages of Adaptation to Illness and Injury

While each patient has a unique pattern of response to illness or injury, there seems to be certain responses or series of responses that can be generalized from one patient to the next. The process of adaptation, particularly to traumatic illness or injury events, has been studied extensively. Essentially, specific responses typify each stage of illness and injury on a timeline (Table 14–1).

For example, the awareness or discovery of disease carries with it emotional reactions of denial and disbelief. Emotional reactions to acute illness and/or chronic conditions, wherein repeated exacerbations occur, might manifest as anger and depression intermixed with beginning resolution. And in terminal stages of illness, resolution and acceptance are commonly observed, but the experience of the stage is uniquely tied to the provider's responses and communication skills.

One well-known theorist established a conceptualization of the process of adaptation that has significantly influenced the way patients' emotional reactions are viewed. This theorist was Dr. Elizabeth Kübler-Ross. Addressing the issues surrounding death and dying, she composed a compassionate account based on her interviews with patients. These observations were published in her classic work, *On Death and Dying* (1969). Essentially, Kübler-Ross identified five sequential stages that patients go through once they become aware that they are dying—denial, anger, bargaining, depression, and finally acceptance. Many factors contribute both to how a patient progresses and to the intensity of any one response. Kübler-Ross documented these reactions from a

Table 14–1 Illness Trajectory and the Adaptation to Illness Process

I. Phase or stage of illness:	Discovery	Acute and chronic	Terminal
II. Event timeline:	Diagnosis (with or without symptoms)	Symptomatic, depending on exacerbations and remissions	Significant physical decline
III. Adaptation stage:	Denial and disbelief	Anger, depression, beginning resolution	Ultimate resolution and acceptance

composite of statements made by patients, including their affective reactions to an awareness of their illness.

Other conceptual frameworks are similar to this classic description. Today, there are many frameworks from which to choose. Engel (1960), for example, poses a model of adaptation to chronic illness that specifies stages built on the grieving process. The model includes shock or disbelief, developing awareness, restitution, resolution of the loss, and idealization. Crate (1965) used the concepts of disbelief, developing awareness, reorganization of relationships with others, resolution of the loss, and identity change. Many theories differ only in terms used or in the number of stages or substages that were observed. A recent review of the lived experience of healthy behaviors in people with debilitating illness (Haynes & Watt, 2008) explained that spirituality and focus/adaptation were key in helping patients cope with resolution of the implications of living with their chronic illness.

Providers engaged in disease management (caring for patients with chronic illnesses) have conceptualized the adaptation process for these patients in a similar manner. Identifying the emotional reactions of patients who are facing rehabilitation, the following four categories have been used to describe specific stages: (1) fear and anxiety, (2) anger and hostility, (3) depression, and (4) resolution and acceptance.

Any categorization is largely a question of semantics, and healthcare providers should observe and report their own observations of patients' emotional reactions and the particular sequential arrangement of stages. The most important principles to guide our observations are that (1) patients do have emotional reactions to their illnesses or injuries and (2) these reactions change over time.

Since this early research, a number of studies have addressed the process of adaptation and have suggested further guidelines for understanding patients' responses. First, it has been documented that some patients seem to harbor certain reactions longer than others; this includes the observation that some patients never demonstrate certain reactions (e.g., anger), while other patients remain in one stage (such as denial), throughout their illness. Second, unlike the original notions about sequential stages, the process of evolving emotional reactions appears to be more complex. For example, in the case of many chronic and terminal illnesses, there are a series of events that can potentially trigger additional cycles. The initial diagnosis of a terminal illness may trigger one sequence, but the reappearance of symptoms or the advent of new symptoms can trigger additional cycles. In studies of patients with cancer or HIV, there are a series of events that herald new emotional responses. The initial diagnosis can trigger a strong emotional reaction. During the course of the disease, the appearance of opportunistic infections and symptoms may trigger additional trauma. For HIV patients, a patient's appraisal of an irreversible decline in his or her CD_4 count or percentage can signify his or her inevitable demise—and additional responses of anxiety, anger, and depression.

Fear, Anxiety, Disorganization

Psychosocial adaptation to illness involves many emotional reactions to illness that significantly affect a patient's communication behaviors. Fear and anxiety (mild or intense) are generated by an awareness of illness and injury.

Conceptualizing adaptation to life-threatening disease, Molassiotis (1997) used a stressor-adaptation model to describe the adaptation to illness of cancer patients treated with bone marrow transplant. He explained that stage 1 is divided into two distinct substages and these affect how patients will experience stages 2 and 3. The substages are the primary and secondary appraisals of the disease. He continues to say that the prognosis of the disease (e.g., of a short survival period) will lead to more severe psychosocial maladaptation. Underestimating the prognosis of the disease cannot occur if we are to fully understand the phases to follow.

Logically, it would be presumed that minor illnesses or injuries would evoke mild fear and anxiety and major illnesses or injuries would cause severe anxiety and fear. However, remember that the patient has a unique response and perception of the disease that we might not share. Studies have shown that objective appraisals of illness and injury events do not always parallel patients' subjective evaluations. Therefore, a minor illness may create severe distress and a major illness, mild distress. In this way, minor illnesses may create more distress—and major illnesses, less distress—than they seem to warrant. Patients' expressed fears reflect their appraisal of the severity of their illnesses. They may not verbalize their fears, but they behave fearfully, such as watching every move the physician makes and listening carefully to remarks made to the physician's assistants. Will the physician reveal the real seriousness of the diagnosis to the nurse? Will the nurse display concern that is not readily apparent from the physician's demeanor? Patients monitor providers' communications to determine what they think they do not know.

Patients are frequently unable to put their fears and anxieties into terms that all providers can understand. Anxiety tends to lack definition, while fear is more circumscribed. That which is making the patient anxious is not readily expressed. Fears, on the other hand (e.g., "I'm afraid the doctor is not telling me everything," "I'm afraid my incision will get infected," "I'm afraid my medication will affect my sexual performance," and "I'm afraid of the pain"), have specificity. While no one questions the appropriateness of the patient to experience fear or anxiety, those reactions may be underdiscussed. One reason for this is that because these reactions are considered "normal," it is not necessary to discuss them. This reaction to a patient's experience of fear and anxiety and, similarly, to any additional emotional reactions (e.g., anger and depression) is nontherapeutic. It is a standing recommendation that providers openly discuss a patient's emotional reactions to his or her illness regardless of how appropriate or commonplace these reactions are.

Anger and Hostility

Anger is both a reaction to stress and a statement of protest. When patients recognize their diagnosis as something tangible, the natural response is to object. Questions such as, "Why me?" may be quickly replaced with the denial, "Not me." Patients who are reacting angrily to their diagnosis have registered the underlying meaning (i.e., a shortened life span in the case of a terminal illness or an impaired quality of life with the advent of a chronic, debilitating illness). When stressors are insignificant, the natural reaction is a milder form of anger (e.g., irritation). In the case of either chronic or terminal illness, the reaction is not irritation; the feeling is much stronger. It is inconceivable to think that patients who are diagnosed with a chronic asthmatic condition or cancer would be irritated. Whether chronic or terminal, these conditions are "earth-shaking" or "life shaking." We can understand the impact of these diagnoses if we focus on the primary and secondary implications of these conditions. Depending on several factors (e.g., the patient's outlook, culture, religion, and previous history with stressful life events), these responses may be severe or modulated. Sometimes expressions of anger are present but communicated in ways wherein they go unnoticed, or they are misunderstood. For example, a patient who learned of a cancer diagnosis and recently underwent surgery and experienced dependence and confinement could react by communicating objections to the care she receives. A limited analysis would lead one to conclude that she pulled out her nasal gastric tubing because she did not like being fed this way, the tube was irritating her nasal passages, or she did not understand the necessity of the procedure. While these factors may have something to do with her behavior, this limited explanation is very shortsighted. The insult she experienced as a result of her diagnosis explains, in greater depth, her reactions and communications. Being angry at everything and everybody is a potential reaction and a real experience for many patients. Providers and family members who are targets of this anger should understand the fact that there is seldom anything personal in the patient's response. Patients have limited outlets for their frustration, stress, and misery; it is understandable that the objects of their anger may be the very people the patient needs and relies on the most. Most providers understand that patients are actually communicating frustration surrounding the indignities of their illnesses. And, witnessing this protest may be far better than observing the patient passively acquiesce and become "victim" to their condition. This is why depression, the next reaction or stage, is more difficult to observe and respond to.

Depression

Most patients, sometime during the course of their illness, will experience and report being depressed. According to Sharpe, Sensky, Timberlake, Allard, and Brewin (2001), the diagnosis of any potentially chronic illness has significant ramifications for patients' lives, and it has been observed that many persons, early on in the course of their disease, experience depression. Some may admit to being sufficiently depressed to contemplate and attempt suicide. Depression can be more intense if there is an insufficient outlet for angry feelings, limited support, and intense feelings of powerlessness and hopelessness. Patients who exhibit depression along with hopelessness are prime candidates for suicide attempts and must be watched very carefully. In cases of chronic illness, the routines of treatment allow little flexibility, and a release of anger may be curtailed. In cases of terminal illness, the patient's appraisal of his or her powerlessness over the disease can cause more anger than he or she is capable of releasing appropriately. Thus, intense, suppressed anger is associated with depression. Patients who suppress anger may also hide feelings of depression. They may mask their real feelings with comments that they are "OK," "fine," or "pretty good." They may even smile and attempt to be cheerful. This veil of well-being is thin and will soon become obvious to the astute provider.

Some patients will explore their feelings with providers. They may complain that they lack energy and feel tired; they also may report outbursts of crying or an overwhelming sadness and a sense of isolation from other people. These disclosures are clues about the depth and intensity of depression, and coupled with behavioral responses (e.g., prematurely composing a will), they expose the significance of these reactions and the need to evaluate the patients' capacity to resist depressing thoughts and feelings.

Resolution and Acceptance

The acute, demanding phases of illness do not prevail over time or ebb and flow. As if to give the patient a respite, whatever physical and functional decline is to occur may plateau. The crisis does not remain a crisis. One patient experiences a new opportunistic infection and gets better from it. Another patient becomes more dependent, maybe requires life support, but eventually this event recedes in importance. In both cases, stress lessens, and the patient prepares for the next major health event. For most patients, the end of health-related stress means recovery or rehabilitation. Even if the outcome is less than what was hoped for or expected, or the prognosis remains grim, a sense of relief occurs.

Having a chronic or life-threatening illness causes patients to reflect on their life events and accomplishments. Thoughts of having "too little time" cross the minds of the chronically ill because years of healthy life will be reduced; thoughts of "too little time left" concern a terminally ill patient because the temporary nature of human existence is acutely apparent.

Maintaining a feeling of being in control and sustaining hope despite an uncertain or downward course are extremely important to these patients (Miller, 1983). Averill (1973, p. 23) identified three categories of control that are important for individuals who are experiencing stress. As applied to patients, these categories are (1) behavior control—the patient's reaction to direct environmental demands, (2) cognitive control—the way in which the patient evaluates or interprets events, and (3) decisional control—the ability of the patient to choose courses of action from among reasonable alternatives. Chronically ill patients may find that the intrusions into their lives by the healthcare system threaten their personal privacy and integrity. The ability to control this environmental intrusion and maintain privacy can preserve a patient's sense of dignity. Additionally, communicating to patients what is happening to them and engaging them in decisions about their care and treatment (thereby promoting cognitive and decisional control) gives to patients the regulatory ability that preserves their rights to self-determination regardless of their compromised functional abilities.

As chronic health problems become more severe and limit even further the patient's ability to function, feelings of hopefulness will bolster the patient. Hope enables patients to avoid overwhelming despair. Despair may occur as a result of the roller-coaster effects of the illness, when remissions and flare-ups are multiple, or as a result of the decline that becomes more permanent than transient. Assisting the patient to identify realistic and immediately relevant goals helps that patient cope with feelings of despair. Not only does this augment and confirm the patient's value, it provides a necessary distraction.

Chronic and/or life-threatening illnesses create a number of condition-related stresses, particularly losses. These have been described in research studies and include fear of pain, disfigurement or body-image change, fear of dying, and loss of work and family roles. When accompanied by actual experiences of pain, fatigue, loss of energy and appetite, self-regulatory functioning, and restricted mobility, patients' adaptive capabilities are taxed at very high levels. These occurrences, collectively, present a supreme challenge for both patients and their significant others (see Exhibit 14–1). The resourcefulness of most patients is remarkable. They employ a high level of coping potential in dealing with their disease. Some patients dredge up coping capabilities that they, themselves, did not realize they had. Otherwise fragile individuals may demonstrate a remarkable degree of coping once they are faced with the reality of their health status. If, however, patients cannot cope with the demands of their illnesses or have difficulty accepting the realities of their decline, they may remain anxious, angry, or depressed. Consultation on cases is warranted.

Exhibit 14–1 Losses Associated with Chronic and Life-Threatening Illness

Alteration in health-status losses

- Energy and appetite
- Strength, vitality
- Cognitive capabilities
- Ability to communicate
- Muscle coordination and mobility
- Bowel and bladder control

Loss of body parts, alterations in body image

- Organs
- Hair
- Weight

Alteration in roles

- Loss of occupational role
- Loss of family/marital partner

Alteration in self-esteem, self-concept

- Loss of control
- Loss of identity
- Loss of self-respect
- Loss of independence

Alteration in relationship with others/loss of significant others

- Loss of friends, partners, spousal support
- Isolation from social networks

Alteration in quality of life

- Pain
- Fatigue
- Diminishing finances

Source: Reprinted with permission from Inspiring Hope, in *Coping with Chronic Illness*, J. F. Miller, ed., p. 290, © 1983, FA Davis & Company.

In summary, all patients do not proceed through stages of adaptation to illness in the same manner. The process is not linear: one, two, and then three. The process is circular. Thus, it is always important to understand the limits of applicability in using conceptual frameworks. The advantage of such models is that they provide a point of departure; the major disadvantage is that the model inadequately describes a particular patient's unique experience.

Recurring Responses: Helplessness, Powerlessness, and Hopelessness

Managing the care of patients with chronic and/or life-threatening illnesses requires the provider to be intimately and knowledgeably associated with the patient's response of feeling out of control. Among the most devastating experiences of any chronic or life-threatening condition are recurrent feelings of helplessness, powerlessness, and hopelessness.

Researchers have shown that extended exposure to threat and/or harm produces a state of helplessness. When threats are outside an individual's control, are global (affecting many aspects of the person's life), and are also unpredictable, feelings of helplessness can be intense. *Helplessness*, then, is a condition that is both perceived by and induced in patients who are experiencing illness. Learned helplessness occurs when patients realize that despite all they do, nothing will help their situation. Thus, repeated exposures may reduce an individual's overall coping capability.

What happens when patients encounter helplessness over time? Patients encountering prolonged, sustained helplessness will develop perceptions of powerlessness. *Powerlessness* is the recognition that the patient cannot significantly affect a specific outcome. The patient's sense of power or powerlessness is directly related to his control over his or her illness—both the primary and secondary consequences of his or her illness. A sense of powerlessness has been attributed to individual personality predispositions, and theorists will also argue that this emotional reaction is also situationally defined.

Feelings of sustained helplessness can result not only in feelings of powerlessness, but eventually, hopelessness also. *Hopelessness* is a feeling of despair that causes a patient to give up. In fact, if powerlessness persists, a state of hopelessness will occur. Hopelessness is also associated with depression and suicidality, and although it may be temporary, it may, nonetheless, result in a deteriorated physical and mental status.

That which alleviates helplessness will help to prevent hopelessness. The primary issue in dealing with a patient's hopelessness is to anticipate and prevent it. Once again, the three categories of control—behavioral, cognitive, and decisional—are relevant. Giving patients explanations about their decline as well as control over treatment decisions (when possible) can minimize hopelessness, and reminding patients that there is something or someone to live for can alter the resulting apathy.

PROVIDER RESPONSES TO THE CHRONIC AND TERMINALLY ILL

Certain patient conditions make healthcare providers anxious. Patients whose circumstances are perceived to be fragile certainly create anxiety. To some extent, providers can become overwhelmed with the same feelings of helplessness, powerlessness, and hopelessness that their patients experience.

Provider's Fear and Anxiety

A common retort of providers who choose not to work with these patient groups is: "I could never work with them. Isn't it just too depressing?" Fortunately, there are many who have sufficient emotional self-awareness, who can monitor their own fears and anxieties and thus be free to become deeply committed to the care of these patients. Some providers who initially regard these patients as "depressing" learn to appreciate the rewards and satisfaction that come from caring for them.

There has been a great deal of literature directed at helping providers communicate effectively with the terminally ill or with patients who are facing death. In the professions, the most challenging aspect of caring for patients is managing the feelings about the patient's experience and the feelings of powerlessness that are subsequently evoked. With the terminally ill and their families, the task of managing feelings is especially difficult. For example, the care of cancer patients can create feelings of despair. But, observing how patients adapt to and integrate the basic facts of their illnesses may reveal that these patients are indeed not to be pitied. Patients learn and come to terms with the realities of decline in health and functional status but, in doing so, do not always give up hope. Physically, mentally, socially, and spiritually, they are very much alive. Experienced clinicians frequently remark that they learn much about living from their patients who are dying.

Like caring for acutely or terminally ill patients, caring for chronically ill patients also lacks appeal. Sometimes the routines for caring for the chronically ill appear repetitive and boring. There is rarely any drama associated with chronic illness. With some exceptions, these illnesses are relatively predictable as is their course of treatment. Chronic illness among the elderly frequently precipitates early placement in a nursing home. The burden of repetitive home care activities is trying on families.

Coping and Counseling Skills

Coping efforts serve two main functions. First, they manage or alter the problem that is the source of stress (problem-focused coping), and second, they regulate the stressful emotions that are engendered by the stress (emotion-focused coping). Lazarus and Folkman (1984) explain that individuals who face stressful events or situations use both forms of coping. Patients, then, employ coping mechanisms to deal with the problem (their symptoms of pain and fatigue) and to alter the emotional distress they feel as a result of their symptoms (pain and fatigue). Promoting adaptive behaviors in patients necessitates recognizing not only the symptoms (the problem) but the patient's evaluation of the symptoms that cause distress.

Guides for assessing a patient's coping status are outlined in Exhibits 14–2 and 14–3. Exhibit 14–2 outlines specific interview questions that are useful for gathering information from patients about their coping abilities. Exhibit 14–3 identifies avenues of investigation that will help clinicians come to an

Exhibit 14–2 Disease Management: Assessment of Coping Status—Patient Interview Probes

- "What concerns do you have about your illness?"
- "What do you expect from your treatment?"
- "What helps you to reduce stress?" (Former stress-busting measures might be employed in the current adaptation to illness.)
- "In dealing with your illness right now, what works best? What doesn't seem to work well?"
- "Is there a support system for you? Do you feel it is adequate?" (When people are ill, they call on friends or family to support them; however, this system may not provide the support the patient needs.)
- "What barriers keep you from getting the support you need or want?" (How optimistic are you about getting the care and support you need?)
- "Considering the symptoms you are having right now—how well are you dealing with them?" (Address each symptom one at a time.)
- "Overall, how much does your health limit you? How would you rate the quality of your life?"

overall appraisal of a patient's coping behaviors and his or her risks for maladaptive responses.

Patients who experience chronic and/or life-threatening illness will cope better if they are aware of and understand how their personal ways of dealing with their illnesses are important to their health and how they may prevent

Exhibit 14–3 Provider Guide to Assessing Patients' Coping Capabilities

- What is the patient's current condition? Health status, prognosis?
- What is the patient's current knowledge of his or her illness and awareness of the significance of his or her diagnosis?
- What is the patient's present mood, affect, feelings of control, and level of self-confidence about dealing with his or her illness?
- What are the patient's primary coping responses at this time (denial, anger, etc.)?
- To what extent is denial used, and what level of denial is manifested (first order, denial of facts; second order, denial of implications of facts; third order, denial of illness outcome)?
- What and how adequate is the patient's support network?
- How available are self-help and/or home health care resources to the patient?
- What are the patient's spiritual/religious needs?
- What stressors, secondary to health status, are particularly significant—financial, loss of family/social support, stigma and/or social alienation, loss of independence?

unnecessary hospitalizations. Most patients are not aware of how their illness creates stress and how their lifestyles and beliefs about self, others, and health affect them. This lack of awareness occurs in patients who (1) lack knowledge of the stressful events and chronic strains that contribute to their health problems, (2) believe that looking at how they cope is only necessary when a crisis has occurred, and (3) believe that changing the ways in which they deal with stress and their illness will not be necessary once they feel better. Some patients believe that learning new ways of coping will cost lots of money, and if they change an aspect of their lifestyle, this may cause other problems for them and for other people around them.

The coping efforts of an individual are influenced by many factors (e.g., personal factors and available coping resources). The cognitive mediating process that is important in determining an individual's perception of threat is cognitive appraisal. The patient's perception of and processing of health-related problems will determine any given emotional reaction. If a patient does not see a health-related condition as a problem, a threat is not perceived, and the patient does not call into action any additional resources to handle the problem. To understand why patients who are exposed to the same event react differently, we draw on the principles of cognitive appraisal. Through the cognitive appraisal process, the individual's way of processing information, the patient evaluates the significance of stressful health-related events. In primary appraisal, the patient evaluates the extent to which an event is relevant or irrelevant, benign or threatening. Threatening events are deemed either immediately harmful or capable of harm. Otherwise, the patient evaluates both the immediate and the potential anticipated threat of events. In secondary appraisal, the patient evaluates the magnitude of the problem by assessing the extent to which something can or cannot be done. When the patient's reaction is one of hopelessness, an evaluation that no available options exist has usually occurred and the event is threatening.

Whether patients perceive an event as threatening, the particular coping responses they use are determined by available resources. The resources available to individuals clearly affect coping abilities (Pearlin & Schooler, 1978). There are many constraints that mitigate the use of any available resources once the event has been evaluated as threatening. They include socioeconomic factors that determine access to healthcare resources and sociocultural values and beliefs that define illness and shape a patient's responses to actual or potential illness.

It is important to understand the impact of coping on health, mortality, and morbidity. Research has shown that the effects are significant. Coping, for example, has been shown to influence the duration, frequency, intensity, and patterning of neurochemical stress reaction. Coping can also affect health negatively by increasing the patient's risk for morbidity and mortality. Research on maladaptive coping responses for example, catastrophizing, may adversely affect health outcomes (Drossman et al., 2000) and perception of pain (Geisser et al., 1994). Other examples include patients who cope with stress by resorting to the use of lethal substances such as elicit IV drug use or even tobacco when clearly the life-threatening potential of these actions is known. Thus, engaging in any high-risk behaviors in order to cope with stressful life events exposes the patient to higher risks for morbidity and/or mortality.

Yet another very important way in which coping responses influence morbidity and mortality is the appropriateness of the response in light of the threat. For example, many patients who suspect that they have a health problem delay seeking medical screening or treatment. Medical attention then can be significantly delayed when patients do not evaluate the situation as threatening or use a response that does not directly address the significance of the signs or symptoms that they are experiencing.

Understanding the use of denial to cope with health-related threats is important. In still another classic conceptual framework, Weisman (1972) describes three levels of denial pertaining to the diagnosis of life-threatening illnesses:

First-order denial is simply a denial of facts. Signs of recurrent illness may be explained away as insignificant. New breast changes in a patient with a history of breast cancer may be explained away as too minor to be upset about.

Second-order denial is denial of the implications of the facts. Thus, the patient may acknowledge the facts—breast changes—but deny the significance or meaning of these changes. In denying the significance of these changes, patients minimize the importance of their primary diagnosis. Many patients go through phases in the course of their prolonged illness wherein they "will their illness away." They are tired of being hypervigilant; they do not want the restrictions that their illness imposes. Most patients will be brought back into awareness with minimal confrontation; others may need additional support and counseling. Sometimes patients do not deny their illness altogether but "fractionate" their illness, rendering it significantly less threatening. Fractionating *means that patients have cognitively broken their illness into smaller, manageable parts; while this process can be adaptive, an undesirable result is that symptoms may be evaluated as considerably less important than they really are. Or, the patient may focus on some small part of the illness (e.g., weight loss), thus minimizing the secondary implications of the serious illness (cancer).*

Third-order denial is denial of the ultimate outcome of the illness or prognosis. For persons with life-threatening illness, this is a denial of eventual death. For persons with chronic, debilitating illness that is not life-threatening, it is denial of the ultimate immobility and loss of function that may occur over time. In this case, patients acknowledge the reality of their illness (diagnosis), and even recognize the immediate consequences of their condition (e.g., pain, fatigue, and weight loss). They do not, however, accept their ultimate prognosis. The issue of death is avoided. Patients may believe and talk as if they will experience little functional decline. They may even plan future events as if their state of health will remain the same.

Denial is a powerful coping response in which certain perceptions are not processed in usual ways. Patients and their families use this response to control the anxiety and distress that they experience as a result of their illness and the changes they encounter throughout the course of their illness and treatment. Assisting patients to cope requires providers to intervene effectively with the presenting health problems. This means employing interventions to control symptoms and the disease process.

Intervening with presenting health problems is a partial picture of how providers must interact with patients and their families. As previously indicated, treating patients' reactions to their health problems is imperative to effective disease management and successful self-management support. This means that providers will communicate to patients about the responses they are likely to have, how these responses change over time, and what they can do to manage any distress they experience as a result of their health-related changes. It also means providing resources and instruction to patients such as how they can monitor and manage their symptoms and conditions.

There are certain patient attitudes and beliefs that are indicative of low-level awareness about stress and chronic illness. But, how do we know when patients need instruction about stress and coping? The following list of statements about stress and coping with illness cover basic principles that will assist all patients to cope more effectively with the impact of the illness. Patients should know that:

- Stress can contribute to their inability to cope effectively and their ability to perceive themselves as capable of dealing adequately with their illness.
- Coping effectively with their problems can help them feel more adequate and enhance their self-efficacy in disease management.
- Their attitudes, beliefs, and cultural backgrounds influence how they deal with problems.
- Their responses and coping capabilities are important in their recovery.
- There are more than a few ways in which to cope with their disease and impending consequences.
- When their resources are limited and stress is overwhelming, they are at greater risk for a health-related crisis and rehospitalization.
- Stressful life events (e.g., loss of a loved one) affect their coping abilities, but chronic strain (e.g., dealing with chronic pain) also significantly affects their coping ability.
- Active coping (e.g., through diet, exercise, and stress management techniques) as well as asking for support from providers, friends, and family are effective coping responses.
- Generally, when they repress their feelings, refuse to think about their problems, or dwell on them for long periods of time, they are coping maladaptively.
- Friends and family can either help them cope more effectively or cause them to cope ineffectively.
- Teaching them a systematic problem-solving process can help them cope more effectively with each phase of illness and illness demands.
- It is possible for them to cope effectively with some problems and at the same time, ineffectively with others.
- Feeling hopeless or helpless about their problems needs to be checked or monitored so that they will feel more efficacious in managing their illness and will use adaptive coping strategies.

Approaches to Truth Telling and Patients' Capacities to Receive Information

Providers play a significant role in balancing a patient's awareness of his or her illness and the emotional distress evoked by this awareness. It is generally understood that all patients need to maintain some level of denial in order to remain hopeful. Thus, telling patients about their illness and prognosis is guided by certain professionally shared assumptions. First, patients have the right to make decisions about their health and well-being. Depriving patients of information is denying their rights to informed choices. Second, patients' health and well-being and the condition of their bodies belong to them. Providers discover and determine facts about patients; however, these facts are for the patient, not the provider, to dispose of. While providers may recommend and conclude facts, they are not solely responsible for deciding on courses of action. Remember, the provider–patient relationship is based on mutual respect and trust. If providers, particularly physicians, withhold essential facts from patients, they are violating the ethical basis of the relationship.

In cases of terminal illness, providers face additional responsibilities related to truth telling. Terminally ill patients have certain responsibilities to address before death. Settling personal affairs, making provisions for significant others, and making peace in a spiritual way may be tremendously important to patients. Failing to be truthful and factual with patients denies them the opportunity to bring closure to their lives.

Providing information, then, is an appropriate function and an important obligation. Many providers, however, question the advisability of disclosing information, particularly in relation to prognoses. Providers are concerned about the emotional reactions of their patients and the consequences of adding stress. Some believe that to evade the facts is a better course of action, particularly when the prognosis is poor. Some research, however, has shown that the majority of patients feel they should be fully informed. This research reveals that among those patients who were informed, the majority were glad that they were told. Among those undergoing diagnostic testing, the majority want to be told the truth. This disparity between what providers feel comfortable revealing and what patients want to know is a serious one.

A primary concern behind providers' hesitancy to inform patients about a poor prognosis is the fear that the patients' awareness will result in negative outcomes. Providers anticipate strong negative reactions, including unnecessary dependency, excessive worry, and even clinical anxiety and depression. They are concerned that these reactions will considerably alter the patients' quality of life. In some cases, concerns about patients' suicidal potential influences providers' willingness to be truthful. Although suicide is of concern, particularly in devastating illnesses (e.g., cancer and AIDS), it is also true that the potential for actual suicide is greatly exaggerated. Providers who are sensitive to patients' suicidal expressions sometimes assume that if they broach the subject of strong emotions and suicidal thoughts, they will actually provoke self-destructive responses. Yet while some patients consider suicide, many more do not. Providers must recognize that patients, in all probability, simply want an opportunity to communicate their fears, frustration, grief, and sorrow.

In contrast to perceived negative consequences of informing patients is the evidence that patients who are told not only prefer to know but experience positive change. The initial awareness can create an imbalance, but after the initial upsetting event, patients regain composure. The positive effects of this awareness are also observed in family members. In general, there is less tension and desperation, which can result in improved communications and feelings of serenity that can be shared by the patient and family alike.

Underlying the issue of truth telling is the fact that patients actually know a great deal more than they are told. Many patients deduce the nature of their condition without being presented with factual information. Staff frequently do not realize that patients come to conclusions that they do not disclose to providers. Providers who believe that patients only know what they have told them are underestimating the situation. As mentioned elsewhere in this text, patients gather data from the nonverbal responses of staff and significant others. Silences, efforts at evading topics, false reassurances, and pessimistic attitudes are frequently picked up and processed by patients. Patients are also able to read their own bodies and establish for themselves that they are weaker, less alert, and irreversibly dependent on others. Patients may remain silent about what they know, because they assume that the silence of providers and significant others means that they do not want to talk about the inevitable. This phenomena of each party not disclosing to the other is called *mutual denial*. It can appear that patients have joined a conspiracy of silence to protect those involved from feeling uncomfortable. Because patients generally know more than what they are told, providers run the serious risk of losing patients' trust and confidence by withholding any aspect of their condition. Providers must be aware of their own reactions to patients' conditions and give careful consideration to how these feelings affect their communications with patients.

Guidelines for initiating dialogue with patients regarding their diagnosis and prognosis are outlined in many professional textbooks. Because providers' responsibilities differ with respect to their professional discipline, specific guidelines should be sought from these professional textbook sources. There are, however, some general guidelines that should be followed. First, all patients should be informed about any harmful or potentially life-threatening aspects of their current condition. Second, any negative outcomes of potential treatment regimens, including surgical intervention, should be communicated clearly and stated early. In all cases, the patient should be encouraged to ask questions about the level of threat and the probability that treatment options will yield negative or positive outcomes.

When providers approach issues of negative prognosis or terminal status, the actual discussion should be thoughtfully planned in advance. These conversations should not be initiated without providing patients the opportunities to clarify and react to the information. Abrupt announcements or short-lived explanations are nontherapeutic. Some providers will ease into a conversation by first asking questions (e.g., "Well, I suppose you've been wondering just what's going on") or by leading with a disclosure (e.g., "This news is difficult for me to tell you," or "I wish I could give you better news"). By easing into the subject, providers can assess the patient's tolerance and capability to pursue the subject. Because the provider has offered an opening, the possibility of a frank and open discussion is provided. Patients who feel sufficiently secure will reveal the extent to which they have assimilated the implications of the facts. In addition to offering the opportunity to discuss the facts, providers must recognize that once the subject is raised, there may be a continuing dialogue where many concerns will surface and will need to be handled patiently and repeatedly. Different concerns arise as different people and various members of the healthcare team are brought into the discussion.

The uncertainty surrounding a terminal status is difficult for most patients and significant others to deal with. Patients and significant others frequently ask for exact estimates of survival time. Usually, providers render an estimate very cautiously because predicted survival does not always match actual survival time. Sometimes providers will err toward optimistic estimates. Such estimates, however, are not always helpful; although they may sustain hope, this hope is unrealistic. For those families who need to coordinate the many aspects of dealing with the loved one's actual demise (e.g., gathering family members from long distances), overoptimistic predictions are a disservice to the patient and the family.

Concerns about Communicating with Patients and Family around End-of-Life Care

There is considerable concern about whether communication is adequate around end-of-life care. These concerns have been presented in a number of professional journals, all raising the issue: how can communications be improved?

An editorial in the *American Journal of Respiratory Critical Care Medicine* (Azoulay, 2005) stressed that exercising compassion was not enough. Providers must sharpen their communication skills, continuously evaluate their practices, identify their mistakes and inadequacies, and correct for them. Providing information and support to families and patients is the primary goal; however, this is inconsistently achieved in many settings, including critical care units. Tulsky (2005) explains that while patients have desires for information and we cannot always predict what they want to know, health providers do not sufficiently discuss the treatment options or quality of life or respond to emotional cues from patients and their families. Knauft, Nielsen, Engelberg, Patrick, and Curtis (2005) reported in their study of COPD patient care that when end-of-life discussions did occur, patients rated them as relatively high in quality. These authors concluded that the real issue may be addressing the barriers to these discussions because, once they happened, patients were highly satisfied with them. They identified two barriers that were endorsed by more than half of the patients: patients' desire to focus on staying alive rather than talk about death and not being sure which physician would be taking care of them when the time came. Thus, helping providers use suggestive empathetic techniques while acknowledging with the patient that it is difficult to talk about is an important, but difficult, task. The second issue addresses a healthcare delivery issue: continuity of care. If patients do not have a continuous source of care provider, then questions about who and when it is appropriate to discuss these important matters with is confusing as well as disturbing.

Still, providers can learn to communicate better through intensive course offerings. Today, a number of communication skill training programs have been developed to specifically address end-of-life care.

CONCLUSION

There is a growing need for advanced expertise in chronic and life-threatening disease management as conditions continue to significantly grow in numbers and proportions. In the case of the care of the chronically ill and those patients with life-threatening illnesses, the assault of these conditions on patients and their significant others is important. Managing the care of these patients requires not only knowledge of the specific disease processes but also basic principles related to the patient's process of adapting and coping. Providers must be aware of the cognitive and affective changes these patients experience so that they can communicate effectively with them. They must be able to conduct an evaluation of coping responses over time. The majority of these patients will receive their care almost exclusively in ambulatory care settings and in the home. Because of this, providers will be expected to comprehend patients' needs in a rich and diverse cultural, ethnic, social, and economic context.

A good deal of the care to these patients will consist of effectively communicating in order to identify risk factors and detect early signs of decline. Care to these patients involves managing symptoms collaboratively with patients and those in supportive roles around them.

The issues of chronic debilitating and/or life-threatening illness must be understood if providers are to effectively help patients and their families cope. Patients, themselves, need to understand how coping responses influence their current health and the progression of their disease. In cases of terminal illness, the communication capabilities of providers is extremely important. Providers must understand their own responses to patients' conditions, individual patients' desires for information, and how these factors influence the content of their discussions and what information they share or withhold from patients. While there are general guidelines regarding truth telling, each situation should be treated uniquely. Providers will generally lean toward truth telling for many reasons, including ethical imperatives and patients' preferences to be told. It is false to believe that patients know only what providers have explicitly told them. Under most circumstances, open, truthful disclosures best prepare patients and families to cope with the inevitabilities surrounding their illnesses. An estimated 50 million people die each year in the United States, many without access to sound palliative care (Paice, Ferrell, Coyle, Coyne, & Calloway, 2008). End-of-life care communications call for the removal of barriers because most patients value these discussions if they are encouraged to have them.

CHAPTER 15

Communicating with Patients in Crisis

Crisis may be considered an acute variant of stress that is so severe that the individual or group (family) reaches a state of disorganization in which ability to function deteriorates . . . crisis, which is a temporary state, can be a source of renewed strength when successfully negotiated.
—*Ellen H. Janosik*

CHAPTER OBJECTIVES

- Define crisis response.
- Describe both individuals in crisis and groups in crisis.
- Describe typical dysfunctional aspects of communication in times of crisis.
- Discuss the relevance of stress and adaptation to crisis responses.
- Distinguish between adaptive and maladaptive coping responses.
- Discuss stressors, coping resources, and stress resistance resources.
- Differentiate between situational and developmental crises.
- Identify the stages of crisis resolution.
- Identify interventions that are useful for managing highly anxious patients.
- Identify interventions that are useful for managing agitated and/or confused patients.

Providers in both acute care settings and primary care will be expected to help patients in crisis. Crisis can occur at time of diagnosis, when discharged from the hospital and the inevitability of facing illness without the intensive support of providers, or when the disease takes a turn for the worse. Some of these patients will be experiencing a medical crisis as well as a psychological crisis. Proper assessment and interventions are needed to assist the patient to cope.

How will we know whether the patient is facing a psychological crisis? People who experience severe disturbances in perception and in processing and expressing thoughts and feelings may be exhibiting what are called *crisis responses*. From a system's perspective, when the stimuli input and the demands for output exceed the capacity of the individual (i.e., a crisis is pending), then we are witnessing a deviation in communication that has clear implications for immediate intervention. Observing people's communication in a time of crisis shows not only the stress of the emergent situation but also their inherent (in)abilities to cope with challenges. People in crisis need special consideration because their abilities to receive, process, and respond will be altered by their crisis state. In sum, crisis occurs when the patient is presented with a critical incident or stressful event that is perceived as overwhelming and outside the individual's abilities to cope. Crisis impact relies heavily on the perception of the event (Kavan, Guck, & Barone, 2006).

What is "the straw that broke the camel's back?" As previously noted, in every crisis situation there is a precipitant (sometimes referred to as a stressor) that acts to offset whatever level of equilibrium existed. Precipitating or stressful events are change-producing events of special significance. These events are usually defined as accidental or situational, occurring without warning or occurring as ongoing events that are more or less anticipated. Individuals are vulnerable to a variety of both expected and unexpected events depending, in part, on their evaluation of these events. Illness and injury can fall into either category but are almost always events that result in imbalance.

DEFINITIONS OF CRISIS

Crisis occurs when more change or adjustment is required of an individual than he or she is capable of at the time. The first major false assumption about people in crisis is that they are always physically or mentally incapacitated. When we think of people whose tolerance has been exceeded and who become paralyzed, we are not talking about a simple stress response, we are talking about central nervous system overload. Crisis situations that produce less-severe responses are more common. These situations are characterized by their more temporary nature and by their tendency to leave individuals less physically and mentally incapacitated.

A second major assumption about people in crisis is that the people experience crisis alone. It is true that crises are felt by individuals and that these events affect their behavior and somatic and psychological responses. Individuals act out of crisis, and these actions are usually significantly different from their usual behaviors, which may be exaggerated as in a person with high excitability. A bombing, fire, shooting, flood, or hurricane is called a catastrophe, although the event itself is not a crisis—how individuals respond to the event will determine whether the situation is a crisis or not.

It is also true that groups, as well as individuals, experience crises together. The most obvious examples of group crises are situational events that lie outside the normal range of expectancy. These include situations like war, natural disasters, and witnessed violence. Not only do individuals who are experiencing crisis influence others with their emotions and behaviors, they are also affected by observing others who are sharing the same events. We know, for example, that mood states, such as fear, anxiety, and depression can be transmitted to others. We also know that the interactions of individuals in crisis may worsen or improve a particular individual's responses to the event. That is, parties to the same disaster may worsen each other's responses. For example, individuals running from a scene of violence will excite others and cause them to run as well. This is self-presentation. Family members also react to the patient's diagnosis as a crisis. They might elevate the fear and anxiety of the patient. Providers, then, need to be cognizant of group responses to crisis because treating a person may include sheltering the patient from highly anxious or distressed family members.

A third common misconception about crisis is that it leads to total psychological breakdown. We worry about how we will need to care for people in crisis because we think that they are incapable of good judgment. The idea that people in crisis are helpless is also erroneous. While it is possible that some persons would respond with helplessness, poor judgment, and cognitive distortions, many do not. Any temporary collapse is usually corrected, at least in the majority of instances. As providers, we learn to recognize the patient's weakness and strengths in coping with a crisis situation. The critical issue is to assess how and to what degree this functioning is limited.

A final common misconception is that crisis is the same as the stressor or stimulus-provoking response. While stressors or stimuli are always involved in crisis situations, these stimuli may not always cause a crisis. As previously indicated, the stimulus or catastrophic event may not elicit a crisis. In fact, there is a great deal of variability in individuals' responses to stress stimuli. This variation occurs within the same individual, over time, and across individuals when exposed to the same stimuli. What, then, explains dysfunctional responses when individuals are exposed to stressful or noxious stimuli?

Dysfunctional Aspects of Communication in Crisis Situations

People in crisis are affected on several levels. They may experience extreme disorganization, which has ramifications for somatic functioning. Anxiety, erratic behavior, and inadequate decision making may occur as well as a set of physical signs and symptoms that parallel these responses.

A major factor in the imbalance and disorganization that accompanies crisis is the presence of anxiety. Anxiety itself appears in varying amounts and with varying frequency. Even in a crisis situation, individuals' anxiety levels may fluctuate. *Anxiety* is characterized as a distressed state accompanied by diffuse feelings of uncertainty, apprehension, and sometimes imminent danger.

People in crisis also exhibit several forms of communication difficulties. They generally have difficulty perceiving accurately; their abilities to process information may be significantly impaired, and their ability to express ideas, thoughts, and emotions may be limited. They might be able to speak; to hear you; and, if they do hear you, to move. Awareness of their functional limitations and declined capacities may intensify their feelings of fear and anxiety as they sense their state of disorganization. Thus, persons in crisis may become even more dysfunctional as they observe their responses to the initial stimulus.

Disturbances in perception frequently occur as a direct result of overstimulation. *Overstimulation* includes rapid or excessive bombardment with stimuli or stimuli that exceeds the particular tolerance of the individual. Persons who are raped or tortured are known to endure multiple stimuli, and inherent in these situations is the fact that the stimuli exceed the tolerance level of the individual (and would do so for most people).

Although crisis is frequently associated with overload, there are circumstances where understimulation or stimulation with inappropriate noxious information also creates crisis. Is the prisoner who is in isolation experiencing crisis? When sensory deprivation is involuntary, the situation may exceed the tolerance level of the individual and therefore present a crisis to the individual.

Persons in crisis also experience the inability to process stimuli. The most common example is when recognition and memory fail, which is usually at the point of peak crisis stimuli. Memory fails for several reasons. First, there may be sensory overload. Flooding a person's awareness with stimuli can create problems in properly sorting and prioritizing data. A second way in which memories fail us in crisis is when information is constructed or reconstructed in faulty ways because we were not expecting or have no way of dealing with the new and different signals that we received. Our decision making can be affected by either sensory overload or memory impairment. Decision-making capabilities are also affected in that our usual ways of dealing with problems do not suffice in the new crisis situation.

Crises also affect individuals' expressive communication capabilities. Crises frequently affect our ability to sleep and concentrate as well as our ability to remember and process information appropriately. Disturbances in perception and the processing of stimuli will also affect individuals' capacities to express their thoughts, ideas, and feelings in a complete and coherent manner and even to recall prior ways of coping that might help them in the current situation.

In Exhibit 15–1, the various levels of anxiety are described along with their consequences for communications. The patient's ability to observe, focus, and learn in crisis situations is mitigated by the patient's level of anxiety at the time.

A crisis that affects groups reflects these problems in manifold proportions. Groups in crisis may behave like mobs or highly disorganized, chaotic gatherings. Additionally, groups in crisis will frequently exhibit a variety of internal changes. In response to crisis, they may change in size or composition, in reciprocity or mutuality of relationships, in symbolic or explicit goals and values, in the pattern in which information and messages flow between members and among the group, and even in how the group communicates with the external environment. For example, when observing crowds in crisis, it can be seen that as they respond they scatter to run from the stimuli. This includes whole families being separated.

Groups, including families in crisis, can be dysfunctional, though not all the time. Some groups that are experiencing crisis events operate at high levels of sophistication previously thought to be impossible. Catastrophic situations have shown that major threats to groups can actually improve group communication and functioning. Dysfunctional or disorganized family units, characterized by deficient and inappropriate relationships and role enactment, frequently exhibit crisis states because family resources are severely limited even in the pre-crisis stage. Marginally functional families are able to maintain minimal levels of functionality when no excessive stress is present but suffer significant disruption when demands on the family seriously exceed their resources.

STRESS THEORIES AND UNDERSTANDING CRISIS

Theories of stress and stress management provide us with a better understanding of crisis and responses to crisis.

Exhibit 15–1 Level of Anxiety and the Patient's Ability to Observe, Focus Attention, and Learn

Level of Anxiety	**Effects on Patients**
Mild (+)	Sensory perception and ability to focus are broad. The ability to observe oneself and what is going on is enhanced. Connections between events are made and verbalized. At this level, learning can take place. The individual at this level of anxiety is alert and able to function in emergencies.
Moderate (+ +)	Sensory perception is somewhat narrowed, but alertness continues to the extent that the individual is able to concentrate on a delineated focus. With some effort, concentration on relevant data is possible, and appropriate connections are made as long as the individual is able to shut out irrelevant data.
Severe (+ + +)	Sensory perception is greatly reduced. The person focuses on a small detail of an experience and is unable to make connections among scattered details. The individual is unable to get a total picture of an experience. Learning cannot take place.
Panic (+ + + +)	There is major dissociation of experience, and the person does not notice or remember major experiences. Details become enlarged and distorted. Communication is not understood by the listener, and personality disorganization is apparent. The individual is in a state of "terror." At this level of anxiety, learning cannot take place. The immediate goal is to get relief.

Source: Reprinted with permission from M. C. Smith, "The Client Who Is Anxious," in *The American Handbook of Psychiatric Nursing*, S. Lego, ed., p. 389, © 1984, J. B. Lippincott Company.

Stress and Adaptation

Lazarus and Folkman (1984, p. 3) define *stress* as the demands placed on us from either internal or external sources that are perceived as taxing or as exceeding the resources of the individual. Subsequently, researchers have operationalized stress not only as responses to stressful life events (discrete, episodic life events) but also as ongoing stressful conditions or chronic strain. As in the theory of Lazarus and Folkman, whenever stress is discussed, the basis for coping with stress is also addressed. In fact, a large part of what we know about stress and stressors comes from studies of coping and adaptation. Over the past two decades in particular, considerable evidence has accumulated to suggest that there is a link between levels of stress and maladaptive outcomes.

A large part of the research on stress has focused on stress that results from change, hypothesizing that any change—large or small—that requires readjustment in a person's life causes stress (Holmes & Masuda, 1974). Even seemingly benign changes such as starting a better job and forming a new friendship were believed to lead to stress and to its negative consequences. The extent of the change or change demand was viewed as important, and it was found that many people experienced elevated risks from many emotional and physical problems when they experienced either numerous life changes or several high-demand changes within a short time period. According to the original classic work of Holmes and Rahe (1967), a clustering of life events or a high level of change demand precedes such health problems as depression, psychosomatic conditions, and suicide attempts. Additionally, it was found that the demand of events accumulates over time.

The number of events that occur over a six-month or one-year period may significantly increase a person's risk for physical illness. One major criticism of this early research is that too much attention was given to events that were typical of middle-class people, to the neglect of things that happened to poor people. And although life events were viewed as important, once an analysis of these events was conducted, it was determined that the originally identified events had value, but so would have a number of other minor occurrences. Thus, being able to adjust to sporadic change was also seen as important. That is, the necessity of adjusting to unchanging (or slowly changing) conditions that must be endured daily are important sources of stress. This principle is important because it stimulated providers to conceptualize not only major events (e.g., acute illness or injury) as stressors but also chronic illnesses as legitimate stressors. Thus, conditions such as asthma, arthritis, emphysema, and many disabilities (including paralysis, loss of hearing, and loss of vision) are stressful from the standpoint of the strain, difficulties, and vulnerability associated with them.

Coping is a concept that is associated with the ways in which people deal with, adapt to, or adjust to stress. Coping has also been used to describe day-to-day problem solving as well as the strength of personality. Because coping is a general concept, there exists a broad range of domains that are considered relevant to it. These include behavioral, affective, and even physiologic response modes. What has been shown repeatedly is that coping has both immediate and long-ranging implications. That is, people try to cope with the immediate implications of a current situation and at the same time try to find meaning in the situation in order to integrate the occurrence into their ongoing lives. Additionally, the process of coping appears to be multiphasic; individuals seem to go through stages or phases in which they attempt to "digest" and manage the stress and the secondary implications of the stressful event.

Maladaptive and Adaptive Coping Responses

Traditionally, the literature on stress and coping tended to focus on coping strategies. The purpose of this research was to identify and evaluate strategies that individuals used to deal with certain stressors. The focus was twofold: (1) identify individual variance in strategies across situations, and (2) identify strategies used across individuals facing the same types of stressful conditions.

Earlier notions of stress and coping also implied that coping strategies were largely either adaptive or maladaptive. This basic premise predominates in current analyses as providers attempt to get patients to seek more adaptive coping strategies. Lazarus and Folkman (1984), for example, suggest that maladaptive responses are emotionally based, while adaptive responses are problem-solving based. The fate of any coping response is highly contingent on its ability to address stressful events and their symptoms.

When people are asked about the ways in which they cope with stress (and if they are honest), they may identify one predominant method or a specific series of actions. Some methods are used infrequently, others almost all the time. The following are responses that people identify when they describe the way they cope with stress:

- Seek comfort/help from my friends or family.
- Try to put my stress out of my mind.
- Try to get information that will make me less worried, less afraid.
- Tell myself things (self-talk) to help me feel better.
- Turn to my religious beliefs.
- Seek to be alone; withdraw; sleep.
- Cry; feel sad and depressed.
- Search for a solution to my problems.
- Drink alcohol; smoke; use drugs; eat more.
- Take out my tensions/anger on other people.
- Hope that things will get better.
- Seek out professional counseling.
- Use meditation, yoga, biofeedback, or other stress management programs.
- Exercise.
- Take more frequent breaks or vacations.

Before advancing this discussion of stress and crisis, it is important to explore the notion that some individuals are more crisis-prone than are others. Typically, the so-called crisis-prone individual is perceived as someone who cannot avail him- or herself of certain coping resources. These individuals, for example, lack the ability to use problem solving and social supports that help people deal effectively with crisis. These individuals also may be alienated or lack meaningful, continuous relationshps and usually exhibit a variety of the characteristics depicted in Exhibit 15–2.

Providers must be careful, however, in presuming that these deficits are solely a reflection of individual culpability because several of these factors depict certain socioeconomic conditions that place people at risk through no particular fault of their own. Studies of women in crisis have shown that low-income women with young children are at higher risk. Money stressors were correlated with several mental health indicators and with problems and feelings of stress in more areas of life than any other single variable (Belle, 1982). Studies of the coping experiences of low-income women suggest that chronic and unpredictable stressors, limited options for coping, and unreliable outcomes of coping efforts significantly affect the health and well-being of these women. It is suggested that any of these factors (alone or in some

Exhibit 15–2 Collective Ideas about Crisis-Prone Persons

- Difficulty in learning from previous experience.
- History of multiple crises, ineffectively resolved.
- History of mental disorder or emotional disturbance or developmental delay that make the individual particularly vulnerable.
- Low self-esteem, which may be masked by aggressive or provocative behavior.
- A tendency toward impulsive "acting out" (doing without thinking).
- Marginal income and employment, generally low socioeconomic status.
- Lack of meaningful, continuous social and/or family support.
- Alcohol or other substance abuse.
- History of numerous accidents and/or injuries, particularly within short periods of time.
- Frequent encounters with law-enforcement agencies, either as a victim or suspect.
- Multiple changes in address, including homelessness.

---

combination) can considerably erode an individual's beliefs that her world is consistent and can be effectively controlled. It is a sad commentary that we criticize individuals whose place in society puts them at continued risk for crisis.

Stressors, Coping, and Stress-Resistance Resources

Coping methods are significantly affected by people's actual and perceived coping resources such as the availability of social support. It has been shown, however, that the availability of resources is not always the critical factor in supporting people in stress and crisis. In actuality, people can have very extensive social support networks but experience those resources as deficient. Similarly, persons with small support systems—just one good friend—will evaluate their network as more than adequate despite the fact that there are fewer persons to turn to.

Factors that mediate emotional distress due to crisis are stress-resistance resources (e.g., social support and a tendency toward optimism and hopefulness). *Stress-resistance resources* refer to both the internal and the external elements that a person employs to deal with and resolve the problems that are creating stress. If coping fails to provide a solution to the problem, stress continues. It may even be heightened by the awareness of a failed capacity to handle the problem(s) or taken as perceived lack of control over an undesirable event such as in the case of incurable cancer (Abramson, Metalsky, & Alloy, 1989).

Many individuals use social support as a means to cope effectively with stress. In many instances, social support can moderate stress, and the mere perception that adequate support is available can serve to buffer situational stress as much as the actual support itself. Still, studies have shown that social support can be variable and may have a mixed influence in assisting the person with stress and crisis. Researchers have studied the effects of social support on psychological symptoms and have concluded that the stress-buffering influence of social support is, indeed, complex (Cohen & Wills, 1985).

Hope or hopefulness has also been addressed as an emotional prerequisite to overcoming major stressful events, especially those events outside the realm of expectancy. Herth (1989) found a significant relationship between the level of hope and the level of coping among cancer patients who were either in the hospital under outpatient care or in home-care settings. Herth suggested that mobilizing and supporting hope is important to the patient's overall coping response. While hopefulness generally refers to expectations that elicit a positive effect, hopelessness refers to low expectancies of success and, therefore, a negative effect. Vaillot (1970) speculated that when people find hope, meaning, purpose, and value in their existence, they are more effective and more capable of combating illness. Weisman and Worden (1976) found that patients lived significantly longer than expected if they had a desire to live (a positive outlook). Buchholz (1990) contends that the will to live is diminished in proportion to the degree of hopelessness.

Stress and crisis events may be more or less lethal to individuals. Research evidence strongly supports the need to evaluate specific features of the events in order to explain the individual variability in responses. Why do some people view getting a new job as very stressful and others meet this challenge with ease? The early research of Holmes and Rahe (1976) suggested that all life events, positive or negative, could be assigned units. These units were to identify the magnitude of change required of the average person. These researchers believed that all those events that an individual experienced within either a six-month duration or over a year could be identified and from their total unit score, a negative health outcome, injury, or accident could be predicted with some accuracy. Judge panels were asked to assign unit values to events. The idea was that greater numbers of events, and the more events requiring moderate to high levels of adaptation (with moderate to high unit values), placed the individual at greater risk.

More recent research suggests that negatively viewed events are more likely to predict stress. Therefore, it is important not only for providers to know about patients' recent life events, they need to understand whether the patient perceives the event as positive or negative. If positive or negative, what positive or negative valence do the patients assign to these events?

Researchers who have studied the quality of stressors have elucidated more specifically the link between events and stress. Those events, for example, that are perceived to be outside the individual's control, to be global (i.e., affecting many aspects of a person's life), and to be enduring (not likely to change), are viewed as more threatening and are more likely to yield high levels of stress. Consider, for example, a patient who has been told he will never walk again. This realization is likely to put this patient in a state of extreme distress. Never being able to walk again will affect many aspects of this individual's life. The ability to ambulate or move about is now outside this patient's control. And, the problem will endure. Because his condition is perceived as enduring, uncontrollable, and global, he experiences high-level stress. The anxiety, fear, and depression that result reflect the crisis he is facing. Usually, individuals are able to correct for most of the effects of crisis, at least over time. Three to six months post-event is sometimes used as a benchmark to separate those who have learned to adapt and those who have not. In truth, we see many deviations from this range and sometimes only partial adaptation, where one or more areas of personal and interpersonal functioning are affected. For example, in the case of grieving, the actual relief from distress can occur much later than a year from the event and can recur over several years.

TYPES OF CRISIS

In the literature on crisis, two types of crises have been identified: (1) developmental crises or (2) situational crises.

Developmental Crisis

Individual development requires that we pass successfully through certain psychosocial task developments that correspond to our physical potential. Erickson (1963) described these tasks; Duvall (1977) later enumerated the tasks that characterize the life span of families. To understand developmental tasks as crisis points, we must first accept the idea that each developmental task has a potential for crisis. Theorists did not adequately explain this phenomena, but the idea is that elements of growth are not givens. Just how successful we are in mastering these tasks depends on our own physical and mental capabilities and our psychosocial environment. If we do not derive a satisfactory outcome, we are set up for future problems because, in passing through developmental stages, previous mastery affects future abilities to adapt.

Situational Crisis

The type of crisis more familiar to most people is situational crisis, which includes assaults on physical and psychological health. Natural disasters (e.g., floods, fires, earthquakes, and hurricanes) are situational crises affecting not one, but many persons. An additional type of situational crisis is manmade and refers to bombings, attacks, assaults, and so forth.

Developmental and situational crises have similarities. There are precipitating events, responses, attempts to cope, and changes (temporary or more prolonged) in individuals' states of equilibrium that are of concern to providers. To some degree, crisis can be likened to an acute state of stress in which the individual or group of individuals reaches a state of disorganization wherein even minimal functioning is severely curtailed.

Phases of Crisis Resolution

The initial and most obvious sign that a patient presents in acute crisis is anxiety. Sometimes this anxiety is reflective of a severe state of disorganization. Anxiety may be accompanied by some level of physical exhaustion, particularly when the precipitating event(s) may have caused sleep deprivation. The thoughts, fears, and concerns of someone with a high level of anxiety are not repressed, however. In a state of hypervigilance, the patient is seeking optimum awareness to ward off perceived or actual threat.

Some clinicians view the course of response to crisis in a hierarchical manner whereby acute anxiety leads to withdrawal or other deviations in behavior that place the patient in danger. Responses to crisis (e.g., exhaustion, sleep deprivation, and possibly nutritional disturbances) signify a decline in individuals' abilities to protect and care for themselves. A variety of protective and injury-preventive interventions are needed to safeguard patients, their families, and others around them. At this stage, responses to crisis may have escalated to where the patient is a clear threat to him- or herself—refuses to eat, exhausts him- or herself, or injures him- or herself—or is a threat to others through physical assault. The escalation process of crisis is complex. It usually includes a pre-crisis state and also a precipitating event. While past experiences of patients may sensitize them to the situational stimuli, there is always a trigger that is found in the immediate situation.

Acute anxiety attacks are common outcomes of crisis. Newly diagnosed cancer patients are not able to tolerate the amount or magnitude of the stimuli. Initial hypervigilance is exhausting and further lowers the individual's tolerance. The patient becomes disorganized. Studies of persons who are reacting to natural catastrophes (e.g., bombing, floods, and earthquakes) have provided a great deal of information about human responses to crisis. With high-level anxiety, people may become silent and tense. They may also begin to sweat, feel weak, feel tightness in the chest, and hyperventilate. They may feel like they are going to have diarrhea and may exhibit urinary urgency and frequency. If they perceive the danger as imminent, they may shake or tremble, become pale, repeat themselves over and over again, or fail to put the most elementary messages into words. The physical paralysis that is first observed may quickly change to a state of excitation or defensive striking out. The urge to do something—the fright, fight, and flight response—overpowers them; they may run, release their temper on objects around them, or attack others.

The outcomes that occur in crisis situations are several. The aim is that the patient will, as quickly as possible, return, at the minimum, to the pre-crisis state and preferably to a much higher level of functioning. With preventive measures during the crisis experience, restoration can usually occur without severe levels of disorganization. However, when the crisis is prolonged and intervention is not available, the patients' perception of imminent threat can result in a more severe state of disorganization. Full recovery is still possible, but restoration may take longer.

MANAGING CRISIS BEHAVIORS

Early intervention in crisis situations has been effective in not only reducing the disorganization that individuals experience but also in fortifying individuals' abilities to cope effectively with the residual aspects of the initial crisis or subsequent crises. We know now that crisis intervention programs lead to both short-term and long-term positive outcomes.

An important, pervasive idea in counseling patients in crisis is that they will inevitably draw from the strength of the provider. Connecting emotionally with a patient in crisis will not only enable the provider to better predict the patient's subsequent reactions, it will allow the patient to take direction from the provider that, in many cases, may save the patient's life. Even from the standpoint of emotional and physical equilibrium, the provider's own organization in the presence of the patient's disorganization will restore to the patient some ability to hold together.

A supportive relationship with the provider during crisis has been likened to a symbiotic relationship that increases dependency on the stronger, reliable problem solver. The ability to connect in this way may help the patient repress or suppress the disconcerting or traumatizing perceptions and thoughts brought on by the crisis. Additionally, the partnership that the provider establishes with the patient tends to minimize the impending threat; the patient now has someone else who knows about the trauma and the threatening aspects of the crisis and feels that he or she has an ally. While the patient's fear may remain, generally, the experience of acute anxiety and alarm subsides. Patients do, however, also register the level of alarm that providers experience. When they see that the providers are not particularly threatened by the event, this acts to reduce feelings of panic and further relax their tendencies for fright, fight, and flight. Once patients have spent time with the provider, under the protective wing of professional involvement, they are able to begin to compare actual occurrences with anticipated, feared occurrences. It is the provider's role to activate and encourage this comparison. The inherent ability of patients to conduct this comparison enlists the patient's own therapeutic potential.

Many have addressed the therapeutic guidelines for helping patients in crises. These interventions sometimes parallel the hypothetical stages or phases of the crisis experience and are designated as primary, secondary, and tertiary interventions for people in crisis. In actuality, phase-based guidelines are usually most helpful in dealing with patients who are confronting situational or environmental crises.

All providers need to be aware of the General Adaptation Syndrome (GAS). Stress makes demands on individuals that are physiological, social, and psychological, and these occur singularly or in combination. In the mid-1950s, Selye described the stages of stress response that together constitute a syndrome (GAS); they include alarm, resistance, and exhaustion. Crisis, in this text, is regarded as a variant of stress that is so severe that it leads an individual or group to a state of disorganization in which one's ability to function is significantly affected. In Selye's (1976) description of crisis, the various stages of the stress response were paralleled with a corresponding level and type of disorganization. Exhibit 15–3 depicts this conceptualization.

Because crisis is also felt to be time limited, deterioration may be short-lived. Some theorists feel that it is the very severity of crisis that causes it to be temporary. This theory suggests that the subjective distress that accompanies crisis erodes the adaptational powers of the patient so much that a continued crisis state is incompatible with continued existence—life itself. At the same time, it is believed that the extreme distress that accompanies crisis makes individuals highly amenable to change. In this way, the distress that is

Exhibit 15–3 General Adaptation Syndrome (GAS)

Stage	**Behavioral Response**
1. Alarm	The mobilization of adaptive mechanisms occurs (e.g., with heightened awareness, perceptual acuity).
2. Resistance	The stressful event or stimuli require sustained, high-level use of adaptive mechanisms.
3. Exhaustion	Adaptive mechanisms are depleted through prolonged use; confusion, disorientation, lapse of consciousness may occur.

experienced is fought with survival instincts. Thus, the crisis event may actually act as a catalyst, stimulating adaptation to change. To clarify, then, prolonged adaptation to stressful life events or daily hassles tends to lead to pathological conditions, whereas crisis, which is more temporary, can lead to renewed strength and problem solving to address the need for behavioral change if addressed appropriately. A paradigm for viewing the elements of stress and coping is provided in Figure 15–1.

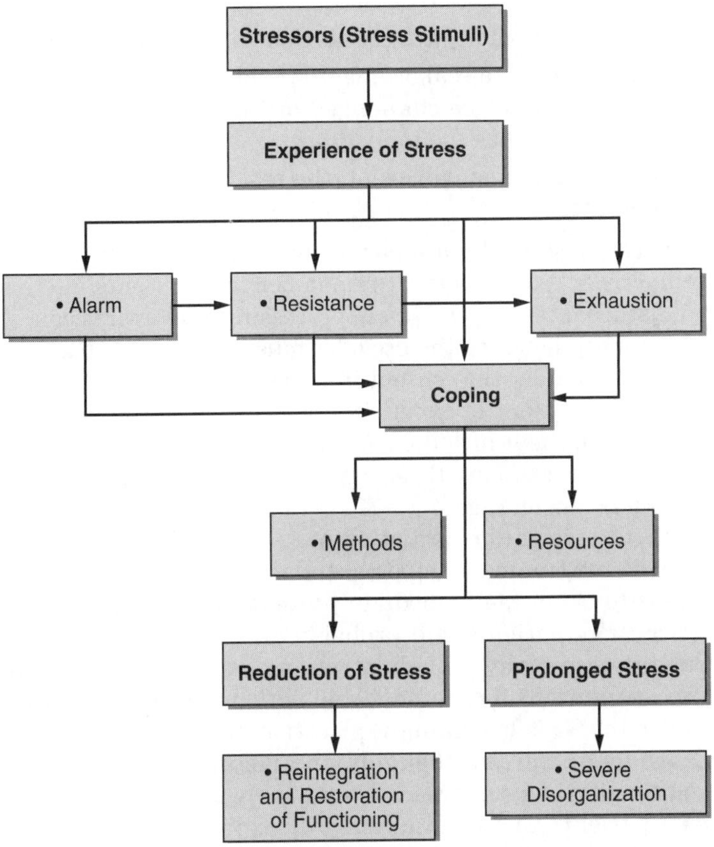

Figure 15–1 A Paradigm for Viewing Stress and Coping

Can you imagine making a choice between prolonged stress (e.g., driving long hours on the freeway for five years) or a temporary crisis (e.g., an abrupt unanticipated cut in pay)? Most people would approach this decision with caution because neither is desirable. Still, most of us would say that we would choose to avoid an emergency. Emergencies are immediate and the consequences are less foreseen (Janosik, 1984). Prolonged stress is generally less compelling than emergencies. There are certain events that do not bring on emergencies but do present challenges that could lead to a crisis. Some providers define emergencies as any event requiring immediate intervention. Thus, if a patient is in distress but can wait 24 hours to be seen, the situation is not an emergency. Nonetheless, the situation may still be a crisis for the patient and family. In most cases, crises are unlike emergencies because the situations leading to the crisis have been building over time. So, unlike emergencies that respond well to remedial measures, crises are generally more complex and may involve longer-term intervention. This intervention includes mobilizing a variety of coping strategies; active problem solving; and collaborative efforts among the patient, family, and healthcare team.

General guidelines are helpful in dealing with patients regardless of the type of crisis. These interventions can also be practiced by crisis workers who are not professional providers. Several basic principles are key:

1. Crisis victims should not be re-victimized in the process of being helped.
2. An emotional or psychological connection with the patient is critical.
3. Crises are responses to real or imagined threats—the validity of the crisis stimuli should not be challenged or underestimated in judging its potential to disorganize the individual.
4. Crisis is not merely a single event; the residual effects of crisis can continue indefinitely.

Therapeutic response modes are obviously important when communicating with people in crisis. Providers must remember that patients in crisis exhibit a number of disturbances in perception, processing, and expression.

First, and foremost, however, the provider must practice good active-listening skills. They must listen for the content in patients' messages as well as for the affective states the patient is experiencing. What does the patient say happened; What is the patient afraid of, What does the patient anticipate? What feelings and effects accompany these expressions (e.g., fear, pain, generalized anxiety, depression, anger, rage)?

Second, a direct, straightforward attempt to elicit information about the situation(s) causing the trauma is important. Rather than exploring past events, the focus needs to be on the immediate present. Due to their deficits in processing information, patients will probably do well with directives or commands. Explorations of why, including rationale and motives, are irrelevant and can even be injurious if communicated without compassion. The provider needs to realize that this beginning exploration helps a patient master his or her experience by organizing thoughts and feelings and that the patient's experience of the provider's approach is extremely important.

Sometimes patients and/or families will express attitudes, feelings, or thoughts that are difficult for providers to accept. These ideas or observations may conflict with their personal or professional values and standards. One family's statement that their son "deserved" to be injured—he was headed for trouble, it was a matter of time—may be difficult for providers to hear. Their immediate response may be to challenge, judge, or even condemn the family for such remarks. It should be remembered, though, that these remarks by family members are made under duress and are actually attempts to deal with the traumatic event. To argue with a parent at this point would deny the context of the parent's experience and own personal trauma.

Because patients in crisis are not focused or are not always clear in their verbalizations, they need to know that they are being heard and understood. Validating their experience, the pain and distress they must have, and expressing understanding about the impact of the event is extremely important.

Consider these two different responses toward a patient who has learned that his tumor is malignant. The physician is conversing with the patient's wife.

Provider #1: "We're not right all the time—guess this was one time when we were wrong."

Provider #2: "I know you didn't expect these results, I didn't either; I feel very badly about the outcome—I was hoping for the best."

Which of these responses validates the family member's experience and expresses understanding of the trauma? Obviously, the second disclosure demonstrates both active listening and empathetic responsiveness. The first response suggests that the physician is more concerned about being right diagnostically, and he dispassionately ignores how the news may be received by the patient's wife.

In every instance, for the patient and family in crisis, the provider needs to connect emotionally. However, connecting emotionally does not mean becoming overinvolved to the point that the provider loses his or her professional objectivity. The reader needs to recall the differences between sympathy and the therapeutic response mode, empathy. Avoiding feeling too much but at the same time clearly communicating support and caring with an understanding of the impact of the trauma is critical in managing the patient through the crisis experience and immediately thereafter.

Dealing with Highly Anxious Patients in Crisis

Sometimes patients in crisis might be on the edge of total physical and/or mental collapse or exhibit self-destructive tendencies. When this is the case, the situation becomes more urgent and there are few or no words directed at the patient after an assessment has been done. Generally, the approaches of choice are directive and commanding, clearly communicating the protective role the provider plays in the crisis. The provider must have a full command of the clues about acute reactions to crisis.

The primary task of dealing effectively with individuals in acute anxiety is one of regulating the intensity and flow of messages. This regulatory process has been described as changes as a function of the intensity of anxiety (Ruesch, 1961). According to Ruesch, in the acute or panic state, the knowledge that others are in control helps patients contain their feelings of fear and alarm. Sometimes the provider will deliberately separate the patient in crisis from environmental noise or others who are also experiencing high-level stress. The protective, supportive, and consoling attitudes of providers, who must have their own fear and anxiety under control, is essential.

After this initial phase of severe shock and when the patient is calmed through the use of medication and/or support, the provider must evaluate what information is needed and whether the patient has the capacity to give data. When able, patients should elaborate on what happened—their thoughts, fears, and feelings. Sometimes the patient will begin to show extreme physiologic effects of stress after the stage of panic has subsided. The patient may begin to shake, perspire, and falter, even though the provider initially assessed the patient as having regained control. This is because fear can sometimes have an incubation period; the full impact of the danger may be more obvious when the danger is over.

Frequently, family members who are alarmed by prognostic details will appear stunned but coherent. But, after the physician leaves the room, the nurse observes that the family exhibits signs of panic and high-level stress. Was the family saving their response until the physician left, or has the incubation factor played a significant role? Sometimes the exit of the physician stimulates heightened awareness of feelings of helplessness and powerlessness. The management of acute anxiety in patients or family members must always include close monitoring and follow-up. If the patient (or family member) is encouraged to depend on providers, and is allowed to lean on others, the patient and family will recover more quickly.

Dealing with Agitated and/or Confused Patients

A separate but important issue related to dealing adequately with people in acute crisis states is the appropriate response to disturbances in consciousness. These disturbances can range from simple intellectual impairment to total loss of consciousness.

There are several causes of lapses in intellectual capabilities. Brain disease, cerebral vascular accidents, brain injuries, alcohol and drug abuse, brain tumors or lesions, infectious diseases, toxins, and metabolic disturbances all contribute to altered consciousness. These conditions may be temporary and reversible, or they may reflect progressive and irreversible disturbances. In addition to judging potential causes and prognoses for these states, the depth of disturbance must be assessed because this will influence not only the patient's ability to cooperate and communicate but will also affect the level of appropriate response from the provider.

At one end of the continuum is simple reversible cognitive impairment. This condition may consist of minor disturbances in memory and poor judgment, but orientation and reality remains intact, and hallucinations and delusions are absent. When intellectual impairment is coupled with personality changes, the condition is regarded as more severe. Ideas of reference, mood swings, and even delusions may be present. In these instances, providers must compensate for minor cognitive impairment and provide frequent reality checks for the patient.

Confusion commonly occurs with patients in crisis. This is a condition that includes a disturbance in orientation as well as intellectual impairment. In rare cases, *delirium*, a state of confusion significantly more serious, can occur and is usually accompanied by a severe state of restlessness.

Fluctuating levels of consciousness can be seen in patients under severe anxiety; however, rarely will providers see patients in stuporous states. Although stuporous states are rare, they can occur and providers must always be alert for the possibility because patients in prolonged states of fear and anxiety who have become significantly confused sometimes present in stuporous conditions. Examples include emergency situations in which patients wander aimlessly, sometimes in mute states, bordering on drowsiness or potential lapse in consciousness.

CONCLUSION

In summary, both stress and crisis are becoming so predominant in our society that everywhere we turn we can witness their emergence and impact. Stress, and even crisis, is inevitable. With this recognition, we need not have to question the wisdom of teaching stress resistance and coping with crisis in our major institutions—schools, churches, and health and welfare programs. In contemporary society, although there are many sources of stress that predispose people to ill health, we pay relatively little attention to teaching crisis–stress coping skills.

Crisis theory suggests that crises are one of two types: situational (external) or developmental (maturational). Situational crises, including being party to a natural disaster, are usually highly unpredictable, affect many aspects of people's lives, and affect more than one person at a time. Developmental crises are usually predictable because they have a basis in the demands placed on individuals as they pass through sequential stages of development.

Patients may not always present in full-blown crisis situations. They may be acutely distressed, very worried, or experiencing chronic stressors. Providers help patients and their families weather many situations and life transitions. Just how well providers do this will influence not only the current strength of their patients to master their circumstances but also their ability to deal with crisis residuals and any future crisis or stressful life events they will encounter.

Individual differences in response to stress have long been recognized. More recent research suggests that individual variability in response to stress is affected by many factors, such as patients' attitudes and perceptions of stressors, perceptions of risk and danger, and perceived self-efficacy. Ongoing life strains and daily hassles are now being recognized for their potential to be disruptive. Previously, the burden of proof rested with how many stressful life events the patient experienced within a particular time span. Providers' communications will vary, depending on the patient's responses to stressful life events and whether it is a medical, situational, or developmental crisis. Empathy, assessment of the severity of the crisis response, ensuring patient safety, stabilizing the patient's emotional responses, drawing on their present cognitive strengths, and following up on crisis situations with post-crisis assessment to deter problem, post-urgent situations are critical in the provider's approach to these patients and their families.

CHAPTER 16

Communicating Effectively with Patients Displaying Significant Negative or Resistive Coping Responses

Staying grounded in emotionally charged situations is an essential aspect in working with difficult patients and families.
—Judy Bluhm

CHAPTER OBJECTIVES

- Describe how situations may be multidimensional—difficult patients, difficult tasks, and difficult care contexts.
- Discuss types of difficult patient behaviors and underlying communications.
- Discuss ways in which the provider can both monitor responses to difficult patient behaviors and apply specific guidelines.
- Identify several selected patient encounters that would be difficult and identify corresponding therapeutic communication responses.

Every provider will come in contact with challenging encounters involving a number of patient situations. "Staying grounded" in these exchanges depends a great deal on the behavioral and social science content that providers have learned in the course of their educational programs. As stressed by the Institute of Medicine's 2004 report, *Improving Medical Education: Enhancing the Behavioral and Social Science Content of Medical School Curriculum*, it is through this knowledge that providers will be able to strengthen their therapeutic alliance with patients and increase the likelihood that patients will follow their advice.

Along these lines, it is thought that most of what is deemed "difficult" will, at least in part, be resolved. In situations with "difficult patients" some aspect of the patient's physical or mental health, personality conflicts and control struggles, or a critical transition in care is influencing the encounter with the provider. Frequently, systems of care delivery will affect both the origin and resolution of encounter difficulties. Because these situations are frequently anxiety ridden on the part of patient and provider, they are worthy of in-depth focus.

It has been estimated that at least 50% of the provider's time with patients is spent in communicating. These verbal encounters include taking a history, teaching, answering questions, counseling, ensuring compliance, and achieving satisfaction with care. Health providers mainly engage patients in discussions on a variety of subjects that are organized around major categories of dialogue, but there are other times when contacts are less structured. In truth, the provider is heavily influenced by the patient's condition and any dialogue during the encounter.

Patterns of healthcare provider dialogue with patients vary, and thus there are differences in what providers will accept, how much irrelevant information they will permit, and how they will respond to patients they regard as "difficult."

DIFFICULT PATIENTS, TASKS, AND CARE CONTEXTS

The label of difficult patient is assigned to those patients whose behaviors evoke distress in the provider that exceeds that which is either expected or accepted. Hull and Broquet (2007) paraphrasing Jackson and Kroenke (1999) suggest that up to 15% of patient–physician encounters are rated as "difficult" by their physicians. Hahn (2001) stated that 10% to 20% of patient consultations are with patients of this type. It should be noted that the term *difficult patient* should be expanded to consider difficult tasks and difficult care contexts. For example, some instances of difficult patient encounters should be viewed in the context of the relationship (difficult relations or tasks), while others should be viewed as difficult encounters due to the context of care. Some providers would argue that this percentage is probably higher and that there is a certain level of challenge and difficulty presented in managing care to all patients in the typical day-to-day practice of the profession. The following scenario illustrates this point.

Before the provider begins his shift, he reviews his patients and makes the observation that some of his patients are disagreeable, one is dying, two want to change to another medication, one wants to be discharged early, and one patient is not getting better despite several changes. The unit clerk gives him a message from a disgruntled family member, and the charge nurse reminds him that the quality improvement meeting is in five minutes and he is going to chair the meeting this month.

Most providers would comment that this is pretty typical of their workday. Otherwise, they are usually facing a number of challenges predating any specific encounters with their patients. The purpose of this chapter is not to discuss the average day-to-day occurrence but to focus on more challenging encounters, although these situations set the stage for the impact of patient responses and challenges.

In this chapter, a substantial proportion of the discussion focuses on how certain so-called difficult behaviors may be appropriately addressed (see Table 16–1). Sufficient discussion of the underlying meaning of difficult behaviors is provided so that the rationale behind the recommended responses is clear. Some of these behaviors are atypical (e.g., aggressive and condescending behaviors). Still others (e.g., outbursts of crying and denial) are common but nonetheless difficult for some providers. In this chapter, the concept of the "difficult" patient is differentiated from "difficult care context" and "difficult tasks."

Patients who are receiving end-of-life care may be difficult to encounter because they are dying. This is a difficult encounter because the context is uncomfortable for all involved. Sometimes the patient's behavior is easier to address than the context in which it is displayed. Such is the case, for example, of the young burn patient who cries and screams during her debridement. The patient's behavior may be difficult to encounter; however, the task of wit-

Table 16–1 Common Negative Behaviors: Underlying Meanings and Therapeutic Responses

Behavior Type	*Specific Manifestations of Behavior Type*	*Innermost Feelings / Underlying Meaning*
Dependent-manipulative	Controlling Passive-aggressive	Loss of control Frustration
Aggressive	Attacking Blaming	Low self-esteem Feelings of inferiority
Condescending	Critical Belittling	Low self-esteem Fear of rejection Frustration
Self-pitying	Self-centered	Low self-esteem Fear of disapproval or rejection
Complaining	Rejecting of assistance, unrealistic expectations	Fear and anxiety Frustration Feelings of futility
Demanding	Frequent requests that may also be unrealistic	Threats of loss of control Feelings of inadequacy

Source: Courtesy of Judy Bluhm, Phoenix, Arizona (1991b).

nessing the debridement of the wound may be equally or more distressful to the provider. At other times, the context does not arouse uncomfortable feelings, but the patient's behavior does. This would be the case if the provider encountered a patient who had come for an appointment or to get a prescription and complained profusely about the service he received. Dissatisfied patients, who actually feel insecure, can be perceived by providers as being uncooperative, noncompliant, and unpopular (Raatikainen, 1991).

Hypertension patients, for example, were found to have patterns of self-presentation that could present an obstacle to effective communication with providers (physicians). And this difficulty may be amplified by providers' (physicians') disinclination to probe for psychosocial concerns (Roter & Ewart, 1992). The event is common, but the behavior arouses irritation and defensiveness in the provider. The fact that the provider did not anticipate the patient's response further aggravates the provider.

Good communication with all patients—regardless of whether they are difficult or not—is important. Increasingly, the patient–consumer will be heard and heeded, and providers will have to learn how to communicate more successfully with a broader range of patient behaviors, particularly with those that elicit disturbing thoughts and feelings.

Students will find that encounters with difficult patients will evoke more learning if they use audiotape recordings and/or written process recordings. Audiotapes capture verbal and some nonverbal aspects of the encounter. Usherwood (1993) found that students' audiotape recordings were extremely useful in changing students' communication styles: 85% of the students felt that their interview skills had been improved, and 68% said that listening to their own recordings had been the most helpful aspect of their course. In interviews with patients recorded at the end of the course, students asked more open-ended questions; fewer questions referring to physical symptoms; more questions referring to feelings, beliefs, or behavior; and fewer questions of a checklist type than during interviews recorded at the beginning of their course. Process recordings or sequential accounts of what the provider and patient said and did are the most traditional forms of learning to improve communication under difficult circumstances. Audiotapes can also be used to construct process recordings and help re-create encounters as they actually occurred.

Types of Difficult Behaviors and Their Underlying Meanings

The Nonadherent Patient

If there was a vote tomorrow about what kind of patient provokes the most distress in providers, many would answer, "patients who don't adhere to their treatment." In fact, one of the most frustrating aspects of provider–patient relationships is learning how to deal with *nonadherence*. Patients can passively or actively refuse to follow doctors' recommendations or orders. This is also true in nursing when patients refuse medication or explain that they did not read the written material outlining what they should do because "they just didn't have time to get to it," in dentistry when patients fail to comply with oral hygiene instructions, and in pharmacy when patients do not read the cautionary comments on prescription labels.

Providers react with dismay and frustration when patients ignore professional recommendations. By being nonadherent, patients can cause providers to feel disconfirmed. Additionally, the provider might feel that he or she knows little about what the patient is really doing, and this places the patient at risk as well as devalues the expertise of the provider. At a personal level, these patient behaviors can trigger more deep-seated issues relating to the provider's sense of self-worth. When deep-seated issues surface, providers are more likely to make additional mistakes (e.g., unleashing their frustration on the patient, inducing guilt, withdrawing or moralizing, and preaching to the patient). Recognizing that these are less than desired responses, providers can experience even greater levels of frustration. These unhelpful responses also affect the patient, whose ability to trust providers is initially tentative at best.

It is one thing to experience defeat at the hands of disease or inadequate technology, but another to experience defeat at the hands of the patient. Breaking down barriers to treatment including dealing effectively with patient resistance is as germane as establishing a medication dose and schedule that will successfully treat infection. Nonetheless, providers are not prepared to deal with patients who are, themselves, barriers to better care.

There are many reasons for nonadherence (Exhibit 16–1). Patients may not fully understand a medical order or they may not fully comprehend the consequences of refusing to follow the order. Pharmacists now elicit from patients their signature when they pick up medications. These signatures attest to the fact that the patient received or refused to receive counseling about these prescriptions. Why should such details be documented? Obviously, these pro-

Exhibit 16–1 Establishing Reasons for Nonadherence

Patient Barriers
- Beliefs and perceptions of treatment (unconvinced of need for treatment).
- Cultural and religious beliefs surrounding disease and treatment.
- Language barriers that affect patients' understanding and acceptance.
- Perceptions that interventions are too costly in patient's time or resources.
- Illiteracy and cognitive deficits.

Treatment and Disease Barriers
- Serious side effects of treatment/medication.
- Complicated and burdensome medication regimen.
- Functional deficits related to disease.

Patient–Provider Relationship and System Barriers
- Lack of trust and satisfaction in relationships with health provider(s).
- Poor continuity in treatment relationship to establish adequate therapeutic alliance and follow-up.

---

viders want some record, if things go wrong, that instruction either took place or was refused.

In addition to not fully understanding a health care recommendation, patients may fear or mistrust the provider and the treatment. If they fear it, for whatever reason, they are not likely to abide by the provider's advice. Still another cause for nonadherence is a unique pattern of reasoning that results in a patient's judging the steps to be unreasonable, impractical, too costly, or in competition with another cherished need or goal. Time and time again the literature documents that one reason patients do not adhere to their treatment regimen is that they do not want to bother their provider with things that will embarrass them, elicit provider disapproval, or just take up the time of the busy provider.

Recent research in persuading people to practice safe sex, stop smoking, or adapt healthy behaviors indicate that if the behavior change results in the loss of a perceived positive experience (in the case of sex, loss of enjoyment; in the case of smoking, relaxation; and in the case of drugs, an altered emotional state), the behavior is not likely to be adopted. This is true even if the risk of continuing the behavior is known. Risky behaviors have also been associated with group conformity—peers influence both substance abuse and risky sexual practices. Despite the fact that noncompliance or lack of adherence has been an issue since the advent of medicine and health care, providers frequently lack the skill to address this problem. The advent of motivational interviewing gives the provider a structured program to follow that seems to result in greater commitment on the part of the patient to change his behavior.

The Manipulative-Dependent Patient

Patients who are *manipulative* frequently display a number of behaviors where they test the interest of others, invoking guilt. They also may threaten angry outbursts or even legal action. Manipulative patients are frequently viewed as "dependent" patients, inclined to get things the way they want. A few patients may appear as "frequent fliers," signs of which are the thickness of their medical record. They may be lonely, dependent, or fearful. They may have perfectly rational questions or may engage providers just for the sake of the attention. Some providers argue that with the exception of the noncompliant patient, the dependent-manipulative patient is the most frustrating of all personality types. They may be difficult to distinguish from borderline personality disorder patients that actively "split" the staff creating the "good" providers from the "bad" ones. The good providers understand them better and will do what they want.

While these types of patients are frequently thought to be of certain genders and socioeconomic status, the fact is that manipulative behaviors can be found in patients of all ages, genders, ethnicities, and socioeconomic classes. Unlike patients who are exhibiting dependent behaviors consistent with their disease stage and level of impairment, patients with dependent personalities exhibit this behavior in routine situations and in most of their human interactions and personal relationships. What is occurring dynamically is that these patients attempt to establish control of the provider–patient relationship, usually by playing the role of a helpless, powerless patient. Their weak and passive presentation usually suggests a lack of power. It is clear, however, that the patients, through this passive role, are exercising a great deal of control, and when the provider responds in a complimentary fashion to this helplessness, the patients have actually succeeded in getting the additional needed attention. This process is marked, however, by the distinct conclusion that no intervention seems to work completely; the provider has two choices: (1) to admit defeat or (2) to keep trying to find ways to meet these patients' needs.

Dependent-manipulative patients tend to reinforce the authority-subordinate aspects of provider–patient relationships; some providers liken this to a parent–child relationship. When providers recognize that they are caught in a parent–child relationship, they feel used and become angry. The patients in these instances usually assume no real responsibility for maintaining their health and combating the effects of their illnesses. Patients who have negotiated this role with providers are often experts in their ploy. To behave in this manner with providers is almost second nature to them. Providers who need patients to participate actively in their treatment (e.g., to follow nutritional guidelines, resume physical activity cautiously, or evaluate their own responses to medications) are understandably distressed by this type of patient. Characteristically, when something goes wrong, these patients are likely to make it appear that it was due to some deficit in the delivery of care.

Consider the following dialogue between a physician and a 56-year-old female who has been hospitalized for infectious hepatitis.

Provider: "You know you're going to have to be on bedrest for some time. You'll need to notify your work."

Patient: "Yes . . . doctor will you call them? I know they'll listen to you."

Provider: "This is something you're going to have to do; if they want a letter—and you permit it —I'll write one."

Patient: "But what if they ask me questions I can't answer. Oh boy, my back hurts (grimacing, shifting positions)."
Provider: "What could they ask?"
Patient: "I don't know . . . anything. Could you, please? It would be better if you called. I don't think I'm up to it, anyway."
Provider: "I'm sorry, I don't have the time."
Patient: "Well, if I tell them to call you, then you don't have to call them. OK?"
Provider: "All right." (Leaves the room somewhat frustrated by the conversation.)

In keeping with the style of most dependent-manipulative patients, this patient asks the provider to go "beyond the call of duty," which comes as second nature to the patient, who seems not to question the appropriateness of this request. While the physician seems to agree with her request, clearly he agrees out of duress. The request is not appropriate, is something he does not customarily do for patients, and puts him in an awkward position with the employer. He may be anticipating a scenario where he is asked questions that he cannot rightfully answer. Dependent-manipulative patients frequently ask favors and demand more than other patients. They may threaten that they will leave if they do not get their way. Although the requests are novel and it would seem that responding affirmatively would be OK (at least once), this is usually not the case. For this type of patient, there may be a series of such requests or demands. Frequently, this behavioral pattern is a learned response, reflecting primitive ways of coping with basic needs for attention, love, and affection.

Dependent patients who suffer acute and chronic illnesses present a particular challenge to providers. Continued reliance on medical care is needed; however, self-care and individual patient responsibility for symptom management is also essential. This case is complex because providers struggle with the "right" amount of dependence. Patients such as those with asthma, hypertension, arthritis, pulmonary disease, congestive heart failure, and many major mental illnesses require a high level of compliance to keep the disease under control. Those patients with chronic, life-threatening diseases (e.g., advanced cancer and AIDS) are a subset of patients, where medical treatment is critical to patients' quality of life. Many times providers feel that they are in a double-bind where they want to avoid infantilizing patients, yet they cannot leave patients on their own to follow even the simplest directions. Providers—nurses, physicians, pharmacists, and many paraprofessionals—are not equipped to take care of patients around the clock. Many patients, particularly the elderly and the socially disenfranchised, may not have adequate support. Under these conditions, the question of whether the patient's dependency on providers is appropriate is indeed difficult to answer.

Frequently, a critical deciding factor is whether the problem or need of the patient is judged to be authentic or fabricated. Some patients seek out providers because they need human contact and attention, not because they have legitimate somatic complaints. Patients may invent complaints, call at unusual hours, or call frequently with "important" or "urgent" messages. These patients can react negatively to providers who are too busy to respond and become extremely upset by providers taking holidays. They also tend to worship their providers and expect the same level of commitment in return. They act as if the provider has no other competing commitments but to care for them.

Providers need to recognize that passive-dependent behavior is sometimes indicative of patients with defined clinical syndromes. In the Diagnostic Statistical Manual of Mental Disorders (DSM-IV) of the American Psychiatric Association (APA, 2000) dependent personality disorders are diagnosed as legitimate medical conditions requiring professional counseling.

Persons who are considered to have dependent personalities will exhibit the following behaviors:

- Allow others to assume responsibility for major areas of life.
- Lack self-confidence; perceive self as helpless, inadequate, or stupid.
- Be unable to make decisions.
- Possess fears of being alone or abandoned.
- Seek constant reassurance and approval from others.

If providers have such patients, special precautions are necessary to avoid patient entanglements. Above all else, the provider must be aware of his or her own emotions and feelings. Providers must also try to understand why the patient is making these demands because some of them might be reasonable. Improvement in the patient's medical condition may be highly contingent upon the dynamics of the patient–provider encounters. A cycle of ineffective contacts is worrisome to the provider. The provision of unending advice, opportunities for ventilation, parental guidance, and "free" counseling and education often fatigue the provider. The following steps are helpful in responding to these patients:

1. A thorough assessment of the character and appropriateness of dependent behaviors is needed.
2. Inappropriate and manipulative behaviors can be recognized and differentiated from appropriate dependency.
3. Providers need to set limits on the demands and requests of the patient. It is important that the provider learn to say no.
4. In assertive ways, providers need to establish the goals of treatment and expected patient behaviors. Aggressive responses fueled by frustration, anger, and resentment can be avoided.

Precautions against entanglements can include avoiding the following:

- Socializing with the patient.
- Honoring special privileges.
- Accepting patients' exaggerations of their conditions and symptoms.
- Allowing the patient to bargain with providers for special treatment.
- Encouraging the patients' desires in choosing or designing their treatment.
- Accepting flattery or positive reinforcement.
- Allowing the patient to manipulate time, frequency, and duration of contacts.

Providers who are able to analyze their personal responses to dependent-manipulative patients and check nontherapeutic replies are more likely to succeed in managing these patients appropriately. Major feelings of tension, frustration, or anxiety are clues to the provider. These feelings may be followed by feelings of dread or resistance in seeing the patient again. Frequently, providers make derogatory remarks to other members of the team before, after, or even during an encounter with the patient. And these discussions, while they help diffuse the tension that has accumulated, will not solve the problem.

The provider may view these situations as hopeless and consequently respond in a passive-aggressive manner. Their responses can include limiting lengths or numbers of contacts or simply ignoring what the patient says or asks. Another response that is very common is for the provider to go along with the requests or demands, thinking that the requests will not be that much trouble or will soon cease. Finally, the provider may overreact with hostility and overt aggression. Expressions of anger can be overt, such as losing one's temper or more covert, including allowing the patient to experience some uncertainty. These nontherapeutic responses do not address the problem and therefore contribute to rising tensions. The only viable solution at this point is to remove oneself from the situation in order to evaluate one's responses and regain a therapeutic perspective on these interactions.

The Aggressive Patient

Although less common than either nonadherent or dependent-manipulative behaviors, *aggression* expressed by the patient toward a provider or the healthcare team is troublesome. Caring for angry patients in intense encounters can be threatening for all healthcare professionals, especially when the patient is threatening physical harm. In a classic study of the reactions of physicians and nurses, Smith and Hart (1994) discovered that nurses reacted differently than expected. When the perceived threat to self was high, nurses managed the patient's anger by disconnecting from the patient. Low or controllable threats were generally managed by connecting empathically with the angry patient.

The attitude communicated by the aggressor is one of hostility. Behaviors that are demonstrated are usually ones of condescending, blaming, attacking, or criticizing. Sometimes these behaviors take the form of insults and sarcasm; less often, patients may exhibit aggression through physical attacks, including hitting, pinching, biting, spitting, and pushing. Perhaps it seems strange that patients would respond in these ways; still, these reactions do occur. Although they are abusive, they are often not intended as such. Most of the time they are results of unabated frustration that might culminate in blind rage. Either patients have not assessed the consequences, or they anticipated counteraggression, which will justify their rage. It is important to recognize that aggression is a sign of unhealthy coping. Sometimes in unfamiliar, frightening, and threatening circumstances, patients' usual ways of coping may not suffice. Patients who react aggressively indicate that they are feeling overwhelmed; thus, anger and aggression are secondary responses resulting from feelings of being overwhelmed or out of control.

There are times when aggression is rooted in a patient's experience of his or her illness and disease. Anger, for example, is cited as one phase of the grief response. Once denial has diminished, other primary feelings surface, and before patients reach a level of acceptance of their disease and its consequences, a state of "Not me!" occurs. This stage of adaptation is in essence a protest against the illness. Patients who fall victim to life-threatening illnesses or injuries experience a reduced ability to cope and therefore sometimes project their anger and rage (surrounding their illnesses or injuries) onto their healthcare providers. Ironically, those individuals most capable of helping and of understanding the patient become targets of the patient's rage. In these cases, small problems or unexpected events can trigger the patient to "let go" a barrage of feelings and accusations. Witnessing these behaviors can be like observing a volcanic eruption: a powerful, forceful barrage of words—perhaps accompanied by movements and gestures—gush to the top, displaying intensity far beyond anything anticipated. Usually patients' angry, aggressive outbursts do not last long. While providers may fear that the patient will harm someone or damage objects in the immediate environment, this rarely happens.

When patients become agitated and potentially assaultive, avoiding direct confrontation is important. Providers can learn to recognize signs of escalated agitation, can practice presenting oneself as a calm, caring professional, and maintaining control even when facing a potentially violent patient. Stevenson (1991) states that every effort should be made to provide opportunities for patients to be in control of their own behavior. Physically apprehending the patient should be used as a last resort only when there is a clear danger of immediate physical harm. It may be that the use of force is an encouragement to aggressive behavior and a hindrance to treatment. Effective use of therapeutic communication encourages patients to express their feelings and become cooperative partners in their treatment (Stevenson, 1991). While these guidelines apply particularly to hospitalized psychiatric patients, they have relevance to all patients, regardless of the setting (see Exhibit 16–2).

Consider the following dialogue between provider and patient in an inpatient encounter. The patient has a history of substance abuse but is hospitalized for symptoms related to HIV and his current opportunistic infection. The patient exhibits provocative behaviors; hostile, threatening gestures; and verbalizations. He appears suspicious of his caregivers.

Provider: "Edward, I hear you're having trouble with the food. We need to get you to eat better."
Patient: "Don't force me to eat!"
Provider: "We don't want to force you, but we need to supplement your diet. That's how we are going to get you better."
Patient: (Emphatically) "What good is it? I'm going to die anyway!"
Provider: "We're all going to die someday, Edward."
Patient: "That's bull s___, what does it matter?"
Provider: "It matters because we can get you better. We can't cure you of AIDS, but we can certainly get you over this disease (PCP)."
Patient: "Where the h___ did they get you? You must be new!"
Provider: "So, what would you like to eat? Whatever, we'll try to get it."
Patient: "McDonald's."
Provider: "OK. Hamburger, fries? . . . anything else?"

Patient: "A prostitute!"
Provider: (Jumps to respond) "I'm not talking about extracurricular activities, Edward!"
Patient: (Coughs several times; silent; looks at provider) "What if I spit in your eye? . . . Would you get AIDS? (menacingly looks at the provider)."
Provider: "No."
Patient: "Would you be scared? (laughs)"
Provider: "No . . . (pause). Edward, we're really here to get you better; there's nothing more to it—that's what we're here for."

This patient's responses were very provocative and explicitly hostile. There is a good chance that his anger toward the provider includes displaced feelings about his illness, particularly his prognosis. In attempting to set limits rather than to quiet the patients' agitation, this provider's response tends to increase the patient's agitation and induce aggressive outbursts such as the patient's threat that he will spit in the provider's eye. Had the provider slowed his own reaction time and avoided response-matching the tone of the patient's replies, a somewhat different outcome may have resulted. Still, the wisdom of afterthought is not always available to us, and we say and do what first occurs to us. The provider's expression of acceptance despite the patient's unacceptable behavior is what seemed to turn this encounter toward a better course. Still, when dealing with patients who are clearly and presently abusing a substance or whose history includes violence, the provider needs to always be cautious about presuming too much about the patient's own internal controls. With persons prone to violent, angry outbursts, certain things are unknown, including:

- How patients perceive others.
- How the environment stimulates patients, increasing their agitation.
- The ability of patients to control their emotional and physical outbursts.
- The extent to which patients are able to rechannel hostility into socially acceptable behaviors.
- Patients' level of tolerance for frustration.

Because these aspects are unknown and/or difficult to judge, any behaviors that suggest aggression should not be underestimated. Providers who recognize the potential for every patient to respond angrily or aggressively at some

---

Exhibit 16–2 Nonverbal and Verbal Signs of Anger and Potential for Violence

- Body language: clenched fists, facial expressions, rigid posture.
- Hostile threatening verbalizations; boasts about prior abuse of others.
- Overt aggressive acts (e.g., destruction of objects in the environment).
- Increased motor activity (e.g., pacing, agitated movements, excitement, and irritability).
- Provocative behavior (e.g., hypersensitivity, argumentative, overreactive responses).

point will anticipate how to minimize this possibility. Provider attitudes of acceptance (of the person, not the behavior), maintaining low levels of stimuli, and encouraging patients to verbalize feelings of frustration and to explore alternative ways of coping will assist many patients in controlling their levels of anger and hostility. In cases of potential violent outbursts, prevention is always the strategy of choice. And when prevention is not possible, securing one's physical safety and removing dangerous objects is paramount.

Complaining and Demanding Patient

The patient who complains about the care, the cost, the providers, and the treatment regimen is clearly difficult to encounter and deal with over time. Many times this patient is demanding as well. *Complaining* is the expression of negativity that implies that the patient is difficult to please. This patient is thought to have unrealistic expectations, and if providers judge this patient's expectations as unrealistic, they are likely to resist any requests that seem to be out of the usual or outside what is acceptable. Ignoring this patient, though, may increase the level of demand that ensues because the patient's perception is that the provider has not heard or does not understand the importance of the request.

The feeling of loss of control triggers hostility and the need to intensify demands. Under the surface, the complainer is feeling fear and anxiety, coupled with frustration. This patient views situations as undesirable or threatening and judges that no other rational discussion of the problem will work. And, demands become expressed concerns about the lack of control. By the time the patient issues commands or demands, feelings of loss of control are usually compounded with feelings of inadequacy. As one would expect, this patient might be experiencing multiple feelings that need to be addressed separately. Unfortunately, these concerns do not elicit analytical replies. Unless a provider is astute and is capable of examining the underlying feelings, this patient's inner feelings will go unaddressed. A worst-case scenario is that the patient's behavior is needlessly exaggerated because the provider withdraws, tunes out, or otherwise avoids this patient. Avoidance and withdrawal responses tend to increase the patient's feelings of fear, anxiety, and concerns about rejection. This awareness serves to escalate patient demands.

A subcategory of the complaining patient has been identified as one of a provider's most trying patients. This is the hypochondriacal patient. *Hypochondriasis* is an official psychiatric disorder (APA, 2000). This disorder is distinguished by the presence of physical symptoms for which there are no demonstrable organic findings or known physiologic mechanisms. Additionally, there is positive evidence, or at least a strong presumption, that the symptoms are linked to psychological or psychiatric factors. Hypochondriacal patients unrealistically interpret physical signs or sensations as evidence of physical illness. These patients are usually preoccupied with the fear or belief of having not just a disease, but a serious disease. Unlike people who periodically wonder about small changes that they observe or experience, these patients have enduring concerns that they have a serious disease. They tend to be chronic complainers, unrelentingly complaining of physical problems. Typically, these patients will shop for a doctor or clinic who will believe them. During this search they can become virtual invalids, impairing their social and occupational functioning and interpersonal relationships. There is excessive preoccupation with the symptom(s) that are usually exaggerated out of proportion. For these patients, hardly one social encounter will occur without them focusing on the symptom. Most have a history of seeking assistance from numerous health care providers. Excessive use of analgesics with minimal relief of pain may be reported, and this person is vulnerable to addiction. Unmet dependency needs, anxiety, and the tendency to shop for cures while engaging many physicians, each responding to the anxiety with prescriptions of anxiolytic medications, increases the risk of drug dependency. As these patients cling to their symptoms, a pattern of broken provider–patient relationships characterize their history.

Providers often face a double-bind situation with these patients. Denying the patient's symptoms and their seriousness can hinder the development of a therapeutic relationship, yet not telling the patient that the symptoms have no basis communicates to the patient that they do have medical meaning and it is appropriate to consider medications, treatment, and even surgery. In fact, the more that providers seem to try to help these patients, the more important the symptoms become. The irritation that providers feel is understandable. They tend to reflect on the fact that there are so many people with real problems who are truly fighting for life, while hypochondriacal patients seem to revel in the diseases they think they have. Encouraging patients to focus on the stressors in their lives as well as their fears of not being cared for may provide the foundation for the patient to accept a psychological or psychiatric basis for these symptoms. However, if there are powerful secondary gains associated with the patient's experience of symptoms (e.g., a reprieve from work, child care, or the demands of a significant other), patients can exhibit prolonged use of symptoms despite beginning awareness that there is no real physiological explanation for them.

Not all functional bodily complaints are hypochondriacal. There are many reasons some symptoms for some patients are experienced. For example, patients who are depressed, grief stricken, or delusional or who are experiencing conversion reactions may amplify their experiences of backaches, headaches, stomach ailments, and a variety of other minor aches and pains.

Providers' responses should not cause the patient to be defensive. Focusing on the patient's life situations and current feelings, including feelings the patient has toward the provider, are usually helpful. Arguing or debating a symptom usually results in the patient leaving the provider's care. Consider the following dialogue between an obese 35-year-old male and his physician.

Provider: "Your hand is just fine. I don't see any reason why you can't go back to work."

Patient: "But it still hurts, and it swells up on me."

Provider: "Well J____, I might say you are not really interested in returning to work."

Patient: "What if I injure it again? Then it would really be bad."

Provider: "Well, we don't know for sure. J____, what's going on at work? How's work?"

Patient: "Work s____. If I don't find a better job, I'm going to be put in some institution!"

Provider: "So maybe your job is the problem—not your hand."

In this dialogue the physician reframed the problem, which was not the injured hand, but the problem of going back to work. Resuming activities means going back to a job this patient dislikes. Mistakes that the provider could have made would have been to (1) focus needlessly on the hand, (2) challenge the patient to prove the problem existed, and (3) engage in a power struggle over who knew the most. The value of this provider's response lies in the fact that the physician did not support the patient's unrealistic view of his hand. By establishing an interested, concerned tone, the physician actually met the patient's needs for support and caring.

The Patient in Denial

Prolonged stages of denial are usually, but not always, indicative of maladaptive coping. Authors who address the various stages of adaptation to disease, illness, and injury describe denial as an early stage of eventual resolution and acceptance of one's diagnosis and prognosis. *Denial* is a self-protective mechanism. It defends against underlying threats that would ordinarily overwhelm the patient. Because of this, providers are always cautioned to treat denial with respect.

Problems can occur, however, when patients exhibit prolonged periods of denial or when, in denial, they avoid actions or treatments that are absolutely necessary for full recovery. Denial can sometimes be constructed so elaborately that to maintain their denial, patients process information to negate substantial aspects of their experience. This may include denial of pain (or minimization of its intensity), fatigue, stress, and impaired functioning related to vision, hearing, or motor-sensory abilities. Patients who minimize flu symptoms, pain from an injury, a prolonged cough, the stress on the job, or their inability to accurately read street signs due to impaired vision are very common.

Patients who use denial are unable at the time to deal successfully with the reality of their condition. Although they may in fact be assisted to cope effectively, their anticipation that they will not is sufficient to cause them to deny problems that are obvious to others. Denial may be accompanied by other defenses (e.g., rationalization and blocking). Rationalization is the process of justifying or rejecting feedback that would cause the patient to acknowledge reality. Thus, a patient may deny the risk of exposure to HIV and at the same time rationalize the process of denying. AIDS, as everyone knows, is a problem, yet a patient can translate it in the following way: "It is not a real problem and certainly not a problem that should impinge on me (my health-related behaviors). Therefore, the threat of AIDS is not something to worry about because it is not significant (denial). If it is not significant, no real changes are needed (rationalization)."

Patients who use denial to cope may also use "blocking." *Blocking* is thought to be an unconscious defensive mechanism. It operates by not allowing certain facts into one's awareness. Patients who block awareness of new or different data may interrupt the provider, become inattentive in conversations, and change the subject. This occurs when they anticipate painful awareness of facts and prognoses.

Denial, as was previously mentioned, may initially be adaptive. We know that future successful adaptation may occur if people are allowed an initial period of denial and inactivity. This period protects the individual from stress and sometimes the many responsibilities and activities that are required as one actively deals with illness, disease, and injury. Denial that is adaptive can be likened to a stage of respite, a period of "calm before the storm."

Denial is maladaptive when it interferes with appropriate treatment. Health care providers must always assess whether the patient's denial is interfering with care and placing the patient in additional jeopardy. While some providers would argue that denial, by definition, suggests the patient is not ready to deal with realities and cannot be pushed quickly into facing the primary and secondary consequences of one's illness, other providers will argue the contrary. Arguments that denial should be addressed early are usually supported by the following reasoning:

- The patient's fear of the reality may be exaggerated (i.e., the real facts are less threatening than the patient's anticipation of them).
- Prolonged denial contributes to unrealistic estimates of the disease and one's ability to cope.
- Providers can successfully address most threatening aspects of injury or illness.
- Future collaborative efforts between provider and patient require a level of reality-based problem solving that is not forthcoming if denial is permitted to continue.

Dealing effectively with a patient in denial is complex because it is intimately linked with a level of hope and hopefulness. Experts suggest that if denial is reduced, the patient's level of hope may also be diminished. It is unwise to be so confrontational as to bankrupt the patient's ability to be hopeful; hopefulness is recognized as integral to the process of fortifying patients' abilities to tolerate stress and pain, including negative prognoses and loss of functional abilities. Providers who are attempting to alter patient denial for the purpose of achieving better adherence or better collaborative encounters with the patient must appreciate this phenomena and balance their approach. Providers need to move patients closer to reality while preserving their spirit and optimism about their quality of life and their ability to manage their illnesses, disabilities, or impairments. Consider the following dialogue between a patient diagnosed with advanced metastatic cancer of the colon and a healthcare provider.

Provider: "The tests don't look good, Tina."
Patient: "Well, they couldn't be too bad. I've been feeling OK, really."
Provider: "I'd like to tell you that things are OK, but they're not."
Patient: "How long do I have?"
Provider: "I can't be sure."
Patient: "A year, two years?"
Provider: "We need to think in terms of six months."
Patient: (Silence) "Six months?" (Silence, begins to cry.)
Provider: "I know this is hard; you wanted more time." (Reaches out to touch patient's hand.)

As providers, we might question commissions and omissions in this scenario. Should the physician (1) have been so blunt?, (2) have said something else (e.g., "We can keep your pain under control")?, (3) have asked more about her feelings? The issues are multiple. The main idea here is that the physician presented the reality of a shortened life span to the patient in concrete, simple-to-understand terms. The patient may have anticipated a more negative outcome—some patients admit that they "know" in advance. Nonetheless, the patient needed to be told and was perceived by the physician as able to tolerate the announcement. Additionally, other aspects of care were in place that were potentially supportive to this patient. First, the physician and patient have had a continuous, ongoing relationship. Second, they have had previous discussions of the gravity of the illness. Third, the patient trusts the physician's ability to empathize and understand the unique implications of declining health. It is these elements that bolster the patient's ability to manage the trauma of being told a negative prognosis.

The Depressed or Anxious Patient

There is every reason to believe that healthcare providers, no matter the treatment setting (hospital, clinic, or hospice setting), will repeatedly encounter people in distress who are experiencing significant degrees of anxiety and/or depression. In the context of any one day, providers can encounter up to 50% of patients in a primary care setting who have anxiety and depression and will require specific intervention to provide support and treatment. Either depressed or anxious patients are frequently seen in primary care settings. And, we know in fact that feelings of depression frequently coexist with those of anxiety. There are multiple levels of each state, which compels us to not only assess the presence of anxiety and depression but to identify its severity. These conditions may be reactions to stress, particularly to the stressful life event of an illness or injury. Depression has been associated with many medical co-morbidities, including cardiac illness. It can be secondary to many medical conditions: metabolic disturbances (e.g., hypercalcemia), endocrine disorders (e.g., diabetes), neurological diseases (e.g., Parkinson's), cancers (especially pancreatic cancer), bacterial and virus infections (e.g., influenza) and others.

The anxiety and/or depression the patient exhibits may be mild and time limited or may reflect a clinical psychiatric condition. Clinical anxiety can appear as panic disorder, agoraphobia, social phobia, obsessive-compulsive disorder, post-traumatic stress disorder (PTSD), and generalized anxiety disorder (APA, 2000). For example, those patients seen in emergency rooms for gunshot wounds, rape, or other forms of physical assault may be experiencing initial signs of post-traumatic stress that are related to how they were injured. When the condition does not subside, a syndromic condition will result. But for many, the signs and symptoms are indicative of less serious prognoses. The uncertainties surrounding who, what, and when the patient will get medical attention may be important, but the driving force behind the patient's experience of emotional distress may be the recollections of events leading to the injury. Emergency room staff are aware of the effect of such trauma and monitor the patient's distress with mild to moderate tranquilizers if the patient's condition permits. PTSD is a more severe condition, warranting additional attention and is characterized by the development of physiologic and/or behavioral symptoms following the psychological trauma that occurred. A PTSD-inducing event would be considered markedly stressful to almost anyone and has usually been experienced with intense feelings of fear, "terror," helplessness, and powerlessness. While many patients experience this phenomena long after the event (referred to as PTSD with delayed onset), most patients show signs early after the trauma as the shock of the event subsides.

It is understandable that all occurrences of illness or injury are events that carry anxiety for all patients. And this anxiety may be evidenced in behavioral dimensions (e.g., expectant apprehension), vigilance (e.g., about medications and disease signs and symptoms), or perceptual scanning of the environment. Young children do not understand a hospital environment, and when combined with loss of a parent's support, are prime candidates for considerable anxiety. All patients who are subjected to hospitalization where control is lost and routines are disrupted experience some level of uncertainty and anxiety. Particular treatments can also create anticipatory anxiety. Families are vulnerable to anxiety surrounding the diagnosis, treatment, and prognosis of their significant others. Anxiety is so omnipresent in the healthcare delivery system that it behooves providers to be very adept at recognizing, differentiating, and intervening effectively to minimize this condition.

Like all conditions, anxiety is best addressed when the provider is more fully cognizant of the sources of anxiety, can understand both real and perceived threats from the patient's perspective, and can judge the level and magnitude of the condition. Is anxiety the predominant condition or is other distress (e.g., depression) also occurring? Do certain stimuli expose the patient to elevated levels of anxiety? Is ritualistic or compulsive behavior involved in patients' attempts to curb fear and tension? Answers to these questions will help providers assess the magnitude and complexity of the patient's emotional state.

There are clear behavioral responses that indicate that the patient is anxious. *Anxiety*, usually defined as a vague uneasy feeling, is different from fear, where there is a specific situation or thing that is feared. Patients who are feeling anxious will not be able to state or specify the source of their discomfort. The following signs suggest that the patient is suffering anxiety: dyspnea, palpitations, choking or smothering sensations, dizziness or unsteadiness, chest pains, feeling of losing contact with reality, hot and cold flashes, sweating, trembling, shaking, restlessness, hyperattentiveness, recurrent and intrusive fearful thoughts, and abdominal discomfort. Any combination of these signs suggests that the patient is experiencing significant anxiety and this recognition might alter provider communication.

The highly anxious patient can only comprehend the most elemental communication. In giving these patients orders or directions, clear, simple, and brief commands will often be reassuring. The patient's immediate environment is usually perceived as overwhelming; therefore, it is important to remain calm, restore quiet, and speak slowly. Patients with very high levels of anxiety will lack the usual abilities to care for themselves, at least temporarily. Some patients may even significantly regress for a period of time. While it is important for providers to encourage these patients to take care of their own activities of daily living, they may initially need additional assistance from staff and family members.

Depressed patients are usually thought to be difficult to care for because they are experienced as "draining" and "time consuming." Some providers admit that caring for depressed patients makes them feel depressed. Of all emotional disorders that require psychiatric labels, *depression* is the most common condition that providers are likely to confront. The American Psychiatric Association (2000) states that 20% to 25% of individuals with certain medical conditions (e.g., diabetes, cancer, strokes, and myocardial infarctions) will develop a major depressive disorder during the course of their general medical condition. And patients who do experience these depressive episodes present with complex treatment conditions and suffer poor prognoses. Major depressive disorder, however, is only one class of depressive conditions that a provider may observe. There are other less severe conditions. Depression is generally viewed on a continuum from low levels (sometimes referred to as "the blues") to more enduring episodes that fit the diagnostic criteria of a syndrome or disorder.

In responding to patients who are anxious and/or depressed, communications that provide information, show empathy, respond to non-verbal clues, listen attentively, and avoids close-ended questions are critical to establishing a therapeutic alliance. Providers sometimes justify that under the circumstances, anxiety or depression are understandable. However, if this conclusion presents a barrier to treatment, it must be seriously questioned. Some providers feel uncomfortable dealing with anxiety and depression due to lack of training or feeling that they might be alienating patients and subsequently avoid tackling these important behaviors and conditions.

MONITORING AND MASTERING REACTIONS TO DIFFICULT PATIENT BEHAVIORS

All providers need to be aware of their emotional reactions to patients whose behaviors are difficult for them. A primary point of departure is that providers need to respond, not react. To respond means to thoughtfully consider the patient's communications and to formulate a careful return. To react, on the other hand, means to move quickly without forethought and sometimes in opposition to what the patient is saying or trying to say.

The primary process of responding, not reacting, to patients' communications is the process of thoughtful consideration. This consideration aims to answer the questions: What is the patient really saying? Why is the patient saying it? Otherwise, the provider is looking for the underlying meaning of the patient's communication. It is easier, for example, to communicate with a demanding patient when the provider understands that this behavior is triggered by his or her feelings of losing control. It is easier, as well, to communicate general acceptance of aggressive patients if the provider understands that patients' behavior is a result of their feeling inferior or frustrated. Therefore, from the standpoint of increasing responsive statements and decreasing reactive responses, it is critical that providers look inward to their own emotions and outward to the underlying meaning behind patients' expressed behaviors.

Part of the task of looking inward is to identify personal "triggers." Most responses to difficult patients will be positive if the underlying motives are addressed and providers can control their own fears and concerns. But providers who are upset with, or angry at, patients will fail even if they do address underlying motives. Patients need to feel that providers' responses are, in a sense, "neutralized." Neutrality will encourage patients to response-match with their emotions more under control. Assisting oneself and the patient to remain grounded in emotionally charged situations will help the provider gain further insight into the patient's situation while engaging the patient in useful self-disclosure. The delicate healing relationship then has a chance to develop and move in directions that are helpful to the patient.

What to Do about Feelings

The area most confusing to providers in the majority of encounters with difficult patients is the *feeling dimension* of emotions. Feelings are one of the most important ingredients in the relationship between patients and providers, and the degree to which feelings should be controlled or expressed is not always clear. Patients look for warmth, friendliness, and understanding under all conditions, even when their behavior is offensive. They become concerned when providers appear cold, aloof, withdrawn, or critical. The reasons for this usually involve the patient's anxiety that these more negative expressions indicate that the provider does not care and will not give them good enough care. For some, the fear of "divorce" or referral out to another provider is behind their apprehension, especially if this has happened before. A simple referral to a specialist can be interpreted as a gesture of rejection even though there is a clear rationale for the referral.

There are specific instances in which feelings toward difficult patients can be problematic; these include providers' (1) lack of, or withholding of, feelings and (2) expression of too much feeling (e.g., elevated feelings of agitation, frustration, and anger). In all but a few patient encounters, human drama, and sometimes great tragedy, unfolds before the provider's eyes. The expression of no feeling tends to minimize the reality of the circumstances and the patient's experience. Demonstration of lack of feeling or "stoicism," may be due to the provider repressing very strong feelings. Patients have absolutely no way of knowing whether they are getting through to the provider or whether the provider does not care enough. If patients think that they are not getting through to the provider, they will repeat or accentuate their behavior. Whether the behavior is repeated or accentuated, the provider is still subjected to difficult behaviors that now occur on a larger scale. In short, a vicious cycle is occurring.

The expression of too much feeling or strong feelings can be problematic as well. Expressing too much feeling can heighten conflict when there are differences of thought or opinion. Anger matched by anger (and irritation matched by irritation) can threaten the strength of the therapeutic alliance and derail open communication. One of the best means of dealing with the provider's feelings toward difficult patient behaviors is to conduct a self-examination, which can include reflection and conversations with a counselor. When providers are able to understand their own feelings and control them, they will be better able to meet the needs of their patients and deal effectively with the patient's difficult behavior.

General Guidelines to Follow with Difficult Patients

While the following discussion can apply to all provider–patient relationships, the concepts and principles discussed are particularly helpful reminders when it comes to communicating with difficult patient behaviors.

Show Respect

Although the idea of showing respect seems obvious, it is probably one of the most seriously violated principles in health care delivery systems when difficulties are surfacing. Delivery systems might violate patients' rights for respectful treatment. This occurs, for example, when patients are left waiting for long periods, are not told what and when to expect procedures or tests, and are treated as if they are mere clogs in the wheel rather than human beings. Some providers who show disrespect display personal problems indicative of the personality of the provider. When providers treat any patient with disrespect, these insults affect the formation and maintenance of the therapeutic alliance. Ignoring, avoiding, and depersonalizing difficult patients all tend to escalate the conflict situation to the point where communication is blocked and/or a third person, usually another provider (but possibly the patient's significant other or family) is drawn into the interaction.

Practice "Unconditional Positive Regard"

Unconditional positive regard or acceptance means acknowledging the patient as a person of worth no matter what the patient says or does. However, although it means acceptance of the patient's way of thinking, believing, and behaving, it does not mean acceptance of destructive impulses, gestures, or actions. In many small ways, patients measure the level of provider acceptance. Providers are deeply committed to sound health care practices, and patients who test providers can use this fact as the major weapon in dealing with diagnosis and treatment. For example, "If you accept me, you will accept the fact that I prefer to eat foods that are bad for me," is a challenge for the provider. The question is: How can the provider show acceptance but disapprove of the behavior? Still, if acceptance is the issue that leads to adherence, the provider never wants to win the battle just to lose the war. Sometimes, bargaining for change involves persuading the patient to alter patterns, with the understanding that the provider unconditionally accepts the patient.

Show Concern and Interest

The therapeutic alliance between provider and patient is based on concern and interest. Caring, a feeling state related to concern, can be an underdeveloped skill in a high-tech environment. It is important that providers care about patients and nurture this feeling with even the most difficult of patients, showing concern and interest as an expression of preparing to help the patient. Patients view providers who do not have an attitude of concern as ill-equipped, not because of their competency but because they do not have the patient's interests in mind (i.e., they cannot be trusted). Spoken or unspoken, it is the feeling of concern and interest that patients look for when choosing a provider. It is also the basis for dissatisfaction with providers and their care when it is absent.

Practice Objectivity

Just as the show of concern is critical, the practice of objectivity is also essential. Providers' feelings cannot obscure reason and good judgment. Objectivity means that the provider can stand outside the immediate situation and evaluate it from all directions. The ability to look at an encounter from all sides before responding or taking action requires awareness of self, self-discipline, and practice.

Beginning providers usually have a great deal of difficulty stepping outside the uncomfortable encounters with difficult patients while remaining engaged. When faced with abusive remarks, they may take the criticism personally. They might experience hurt and rejection, and these feelings may immobilize them. Standing apart from the encounter and viewing the situation from different vantage points usually has the effect of increasing providers' insights while at the same time neutralizing the feelings they have about how they are being treated.

The process of establishing objectivity is similar to that of the role of investigator on a research project or a detective at a crime scene. It is important to assemble all factual information before making a conclusion. Any conclusions must be weighed against competing theories that would prove the results invalid. Incomplete data will always hide the truth, and it is the provider's job to uncover as many plausible reasons as possible. If providers, especially inexperienced providers, take this position with regard to difficult patient behaviors, they will be able to maintain their objectivity. When they maintain objectivity, they will be in better positions to respond, not react, to these patients. Objectivity, however, does not mean being aloof and noncaring. Withholding concern for a patient or patient's family while trying to maintain objectivity is both unnecessary and problematic. The skill is to show concern but remain detached enough to establish the facts as they relate to the encounter.

Enhance Awareness and Observation Skills

Being consciously aware of the patient's circumstances, including his or her state of wellness—symptoms and any changes—is the bare minimum. It is safe to say that a majority of difficult patient encounters are due to inadequate awareness on the part of the provider. Providers come across insensitively when they are not aware of patients' conditions and their responses to their changed conditions. Being unaware and approaching a potentially difficult patient or patient's family is like walking into a minefield. The risk of unsatisfactory communication is extremely high. Therefore, the provider has set him- or herself up for difficulty and the provider's failure to become aware is clearly the provider's fault—not the patient's.

In addition to being aware of the patient's condition, both physical and psychological symptoms and changes in the symptom picture, providers must be cognizant of the special caring needs that patients have. Does the patient want tenderness or detachment? Does he or she want to be informed about everything or just told the essential facts? Does he or she want to be alone or does he or she want to talk? Every patient has unique needs, and these needs change as his health and condition changes. Sometimes these needs are communicated clearly and directly; more often than not, they go misunderstood. In the case of difficult patient behaviors, these needs may be very obscure, and this obscurity must be matched with high levels of awareness on the part of the provider.

CASE STUDY

The Aggressive and Abusive Patient
Name: Edward S.
Age: 30 years
Occupation: Sales—unemployed
Marital Status: Single
Diagnosis: PCP—one week ago diagnosed HIV+
IV Drug Abuse History
Hospitalization: To control infection
Treatment: Includes supplemental feedings, nonroutine sedative and sleeping medications, O_2 PRN by mask

This patient has been a substance abuser and is suspected of continued illicit drug use. He is hospitalized for symptoms related to his HIV and his current opportunistic infection. The patient exhibits provocative behaviors, hostile threatening gestures, and verbalizations as well as suspicion of his caregivers.

Provider: "Edward, I hear you're having trouble with the food. We need to get you to eat better."
Patient: "Don't force me to eat."
Provider: "We don't want to force you, but we need to supplement your diet. That's how we are going to get you better."
Patient: (Emphatically) "What good is it? I'm going to die anyway!"
Provider: "We're all going to die someday, Edward."
Patient: "That's bull s___, what does it matter?"
Provider: "It matters because we can get you better. We can't cure you of AIDS, but we can certainly get you over this disease (PCP)."
Patient: "Where the h___ did they get you? You must be new!"
Provider: "So, what would you like to eat? Whatever, we'll try to get it."
Patient: "McDonald's."
Provider: "OK. Hamburger, fries? Anything else?"
Patient: "A prostitute!"
Provider: "I'm not talking about extracurricular activities, Edward."
Patient: (Coughs several times; silent; looks at provider) "What if I spit in your eye . . . Would you get AIDS?"
Provider: "No."
Patient: "Would you be scared? (laughs)"
Provider: "No . . . Edward, we're really here to get you better; there's nothing more to it—that's what we're here for."
Patient: "Ha, ha, ha." (Coughing uncontrollably)
Provider: "You know we're here because we care. I'm offering to help you. Do you need help to the bathroom?"
Patient: "No! I don't need help. I'm a man—f___, s___."
Provider: "I know you're a man, but you need help. I didn't say you weren't a man."
Patient: "Don't get smart with me—or I'll . . . I'll slap you!"
Provider: "You need help, Edward. Let me help you."
Patient: "I told you . . . I'm a man!"
Provider: "It takes a man to admit he needs help."
Patient: "Don't give me that phony psychology s___."
Provider: "Edward, do you need to go the bathroom?"
Patient: (Nods yes)
Provider: "OK, lie over on this side. Put your legs over the side. I'm going to help you get up so you can go to the bathroom."

Patient: (Silently responds to provider's directions, somewhat confused) "Which way are you going to sit me up?" (angrily)
Provider: "This way. How are you feeling now?"
Patient: "It's cold. Why don't they turn up the heat? If they really cared, they would turn on the heat."
Provider: "The heat is on, Edward. Are you dizzy?"
Patient: "I'm dizzy and I'm cold. If the heat's on, then why am I cold?!"
Provider: "You have a fever, Edward. You've got a major infection. Are you still dizzy?"
Patient: "I'm dizzy and cold!"
Provider: "If you're dizzy, I want you to lie down. Lie back down, Edward."
Patient: (Complies and is silent)
Provider: (Pulls up a chair by Edward's bed) "What's going on?"
Patient: (Silent, curled up in bed)
Provider: "Obviously something is bothering you a whole lot."
Patient: (Mumbles) "They won't let me see my son."
Provider: "They won't let you see him? Is that because of your drug problems or your diagnosis?"
Patient: "Both. I'm just tired."
Provider: "We talked before about your eating better, getting rest."
Patient: "I used to be able to jump out of bed—get going."
Provider: "You'll regain your strength once we get you over this infection. Then we can see about getting your family involved."
Patient: "What do you mean? What can you do?"
Provider: "We'll talk to the social worker—you have every right to see your son."
Patient: "I'm so tired."
Provider: "Do you still have to go to the bathroom?"
Patient: "I can't go by myself."
Provider: "I'll take you now."

(Provider successfully gains patient's cooperation and escorts him to the bathroom.)

ANALYSIS

This aggressive, verbally abusive, and threatening patient is experiencing a great deal of distress—not only about his illness (and prognosis) but also about the functional decline that he feels is linked with his masculinity. It is manly to take yourself to the bathroom when necessary, to jump up and get going, to get your own food—to provide for yourself. His symptoms and acute infection noticeably force him into unaccustomed dependency. He does not think that the provider understands or appreciates these aspects, and he does not want to be treated as an invalid. Unfortunately, the provider, at more anxious moments, feeds into this patient's concerns by becoming directive and authoritative, perhaps making the patient feel even more infantile. The patient, facing the threat of his own loss of power, challenges the competency and sincerity of his provider. He insists on being treated respectfully but treats the provider abusively.

Abandoning the task—getting the patient to the bathroom—was needed. Focusing on feelings, "What's going on—obviously something is bothering you a whole lot," was the primary therapeutic shift in this encounter. This intervention was punctuated by pausing. The open-ended question, "What's going on?" altered the style of communication and expressed the provider's concern and readiness to be open and receptive to the patient. The reflection, "Obviously something is bothering you a whole lot," expressed empathy and a desire to become more aware of the patient's situation as he experiences it. The fact that the provider did not reject this patient by leaving the room communicated a level of acceptance that the patient needed before trusting the provider with more intimate and painful details. The provider displayed respect for both the patient's identification of his problems and his inherent rights as a parent. Much of the dialogue that had occurred up to this point was affected by the provider's own reactions to the patient's accusatory and belittling comments. The provider communicated somewhat defensively to threats, e.g., "If I spit in your eye . . . would you be scared," and "don't give me that psychological s___." At either of these points, the provider could have attempted to refocus the patient on what was really bothering him. However, several factors may have prevented earlier attempts from working; this includes both the provider's and patient's awareness that a lot is going on here—this is not just a simple task of changing the patient's eating patterns or assisting him to the bathroom. Awareness of the complexity of the situation increased the provider's level of empathy.

What is also noteworthy is that the provider's effectiveness increased with the use of various therapeutic responses. Reflection, open-ended questions, expression of concern, showing acceptance, and enhancing one's objectivity and awareness were used effectively. They assisted the provider in this difficult encounter to compose a more therapeutic intervention.

CASE STUDY

The Demanding, Self-Pitying, Dependent Patient
Name: Marcia Y.
Age: 56 years
Occupation: Secretary, law firm
Marital Status: Divorced
Diagnosis: Acute bacterial intestinal infection acquired on vacation to the West Indies approximately two weeks ago. No other diagnosable problems.
Outpatient treatment: Antibiotics to control infection. Lomotil to control diarrhea. Encourage bed rest and adequate diet.

This 56-year-old legal secretary is off work and on bed rest for an acute intestinal infection acquired during a vacation to the West Indies approximately two weeks ago. Although she has no other diagnosable problems, she complains of a variety of aches and pains and seeks reassurance that these signs are benign. She is being followed-up in the outpatient clinic for this infection.

Provider: "Hello, Marcia. I don't think I've met you yet. Dr. S____ and I practice together."
Patient: "Oh, yes, Dr. R____, I've heard of you. Where is Dr. S____?"
Provider: "He's out of the office today. So, how have you been doing?"
Patient: "I guess OK. I don't feel well though."
Provider: "What's going on?"
Patient: "I feel weak, tired. Sometimes I have pains . . . you know, last time Dr. S____ thought I might have something wrong with my back. I get pains between my shoulders. And . . ."
Provider: (Interrupts patient) "Nothing in your chart about back pain, though. Let's see how you are doing with this infection you have."
Patient: "I've been feeling really guilty."
Provider: "About what?"
Patient: "Being off work for so long. Everything is piling up at the office. I've worked really hard to get the job I have now, and now I can't do it."
Provider: "I think in another week you'll feel well enough to go back to work."

Patient: "I don't know . . . do you really think so? What if this infection goes on longer than seven more days? This is serious—I thought I was going to die."

Provider: "You were pretty sick in the beginning. Seven more days though and you'll be able to get up and feel good about going back to work."

Patient: "I guess I worry too much. There is so much to worry about . . . You know I'm not 20 anymore. I'm weaker than I used to be."

Provider: "How do you mean, weaker?"

Patient: "I can't do that much. I sleep more. When I go home, I'll probably sleep for two days."

Provider: "Two days? Don't think so." (pats patient on arm) "I'm going to have the nurse come in to talk to you about your diet."

Patient: "You've been so kind, doctor. I guess I need reassurance. Other doctors don't take me seriously."

Provider: "We take you seriously."

Patient: "Yes . . . Before you go, do you think I should have X-rays of my spine? Maybe this infection will aggravate that back problem I have. It's probably a good idea, don't you think? Women my age have bone problems, and I'm worried that I could fall down and break a hip. That's all I need—an infection and broken hip at the same time."

Provider: "Marcia, I've got to see my next patient. Let's concentrate on getting you over this infection right now. I want you to come back in a week."

Patient: "OK Doctor, thank you. You're a good doctor, too. Will I see you next time?"

(Physician exits room and does not respond to patient's last question. It is not clear whether he simply didn't hear the patient's question or whether he chose to ignore it.)

ANALYSIS

This patient's general presentation was friendly and appreciative. She appeared eager to cooperate. Less obvious are this patient's multiple requests that resulted in the physician's spending more time on fictitious problems than expected. This patient wanted attention and was able to hold the physician's focus through a series of pleas to consider and reconsider potential somatic ailments. It is true that most of the symptoms she addressed were legitimate, with the exception of back pains, but she was not totally convinced that the back pains were insignificant. She used these problems to hold the attention of this physician. Her expressed reluctance to return to work raised the possibility that her current illness had some secondary gain. That is, she did not want to return to work, and because she was feeling guilty about not being at work, her symptoms and delayed recovery could function to legitimize her absence. Her response to the physician's reassurance that she could return to work soon was more of disappointment than relief. This patient's last request for attention, namely, her question about whether she would see this physician again, reflected her potential to engage the doctor in a special relationship not enjoyed by most patients.

This physician's responses were very typical. Initially, the physician attempted to meet the patient's need for attention. As the encounter progressed, however, he became aware that he would fail to provide the level of support she was asking for and that her medical needs, as she described them, were a result of her strong dependency needs. It became clear that reassurance about recovery was not what the patient sought. As the physician became progressively aware of this patient's dependent personality, he began to withdraw. His response on departure was to virtually ignore her last attempt to engage him in further discussions. Although one can only guess, this physician's thoughts and feelings upon leaving the room ("Will I see you next time?") may have included "I sure hope not!" "Sorry I can't tell you that you have another problem—I know that's what you want to hear!" The end result reinforces the patient's fear, that the provider will reject her, and any continuation of a helpful, supportive relationship is unlikely. That is, what the patient feared—rejection—is what she managed to achieve through her demanding, self-pitying interaction with the provider.

This provider showed respect for the patient's experience and exhibited high levels of patience in soliciting from the patient descriptions about her various concerns. Even when the patient clearly held onto false beliefs, the provider did not challenge her, express intolerance, or show irritation. Rather, reality was presented firmly, and her cooperation to work on getting better from the acute infection was presented as the appropriate objective. This focus set limits on the patient's attempts to distract the provider. Not responding to the expressed compliments in ways that would encourage a special relationship was also appropriate here.

The remaining issue here is how the provider could avert the ultimate outcome: irritation and rejection of the patient's pleas for attention. The answer to this dilemma is in his reflecting exactly what seems to be going on. Initially an open-ended question may be helpful: "Marcia, what's going on? You are continuing to talk about your back pain even after I told you there is no problem." This is a reflection about the process, not the content, of the encounter. These kinds of questions generally get through to patients at deeper levels. What will probably be discovered is that the patient's view of life is that small events can be overlooked and result in tragic outcomes; therefore, her need to dwell on what seem to be insignificant issues is understandable. Using an open-ended question actually invites the patient to talk about world views and basic premises underlying her life events. It also allows the provider an opening to discuss the differences in the patient's views (fears) and the reality of the situation. Had this conversation actually occurred, the provider may have felt more in control and less a victim of the patient's strong dependency needs.

CASE STUDY

The Complaining, Manipulative Patient
Name: Howard R.
Age: 48 years
Occupation: Institutional stockbroker
Marital Status: Separated
Diagnosis: Diagnostic screening, possible MI
Hospitalization: Bed rest, diagnostic work-up

This 48-year-old institutional stockbroker is hospitalized with a possible myocardial infarction. He is on bed rest and undergoing several diagnostic tests. The provider in this case is a nurse who is caring for this patient and supervising the care of 16 patients on this unit.

Provider: "Well, Mr. R____—it looks like you can get out of bed today. The doctor wrote orders for you to get up and begin to ambulate."

Patient: "Well, tell the doctor I'll get up later." (smiles at nurse)

Provider: "Because I need to help you, it's better we do it now."

Patient: "What's the results of all those tests?"

Provider: "I don't know. I have a big assignment today—it's hard to keep up on everything. . . Anyway, it's your doctor who will let you know."

Patient: "And who knows when that will be! Well, what about that blood test? It has something to do with my heart—what's the results of that test?"

Provider: "I know you want to hear about the results. It just isn't my place to tell you, even if I did know."

Patient: "Well what is your 'place'? Who are you, just the bath lady? I'll get up when I know the results of my test."

Provider: "I'm not the 'bath lady,' I'm a nurse. I guess you think that if you hold out in bed here you'll get what you want, but really, Mr. R____, I need to get you up."

Patient: "It doesn't make sense—how do I know it's OK when I don't know how my tests turned out? If I ran my business like they run this hospital, I'd be bankrupt in six months! Angiogram—that's what it was they did, an angiogram—how did that turn out?"

Provider: "Yes, you had an angiogram. Remember, your doctor will tell you."

Patient: "You know something—you've got to. You're not a robot . . . even though you act like one. How can you work in a place like this without knowing if it is safe to get a patient out of bed?"

Provider: "I know it is safe to get you out of bed, Mr. R____. Now let me help you . . . turn your legs around now . . . over the side of the bed."

Patient: (Sitting on the edge of the bed) "So, you do know the results. I hate to be difficult, but you know I need to know these things."

Provider: (Assisting patient to wheelchair) "I'm going to get a bath blanket to put across your legs—here . . ."

Patient: "I know you're trying to help . . . So my tests turned out OK, huh?"

Provider: "Yes . . . they're probably OK. As I said, I haven't looked at your chart yet this morning. Well, anyway, your doctor will be in to see you later this morning."

Patient: "He should have seen me before I was to get out of bed!"

ANALYSIS

It is obvious from an examination of this interaction that the patient was anxious about his test results and afraid of exciting himself in ways that would put him in jeopardy. It is also apparent that control is an issue for this man, who is accustomed to running a demanding and successful brokerage firm. He is sensitive to how work is organized and the way things should be done to maximize profits and production. He is also customarily in control as he directs the efforts of a staff of several people in his firm.

The overall presentation of the patient was hesitancy. He also attempted to "bargain" for information, implying that he would cooperate if he got what he wanted (test results). He paid little attention to the nurse's statements about the scope of her practice, suggesting that he did not believe her descriptions and did not really care about protocol. He used several responses to try to get what he wanted. He complained about not being informed. He challenged the basis of the nurse's actions. He bargained—"I'll get out of bed when I find out my test results." He attempted to get the nurse to elaborate by offering suspicions and waiting for the nurse to respond.

The issue in this case is not whether the patient is correct in his judgments, rather, it is the patient's need to trust providers and hospital procedures and comply with his treatment. Patients of this type can cause an uproar on a service very quickly because they seem to have legitimate complaints and they insist that procedures be done their way.

The provider responded appropriately in several ways. First, the nurse described the role of the physician and the nursing staff in his care. Limits were set on the patient's attempts to manipulate the nurse to tell him the test results. Further, reflective statements (e.g., "I know you want to hear about the results") were used instead of angry, hostile replies. The nurse redirected the patient to the task at hand (getting out of bed) rather than being entrapped in defensive replies to insulting remarks about, for example, being "the bath lady" or being just a "robot." The patient, however, got a partial answer by deducing that he must be "OK." And while the nurse could have expressed frustration, she conceded. Who won here? Did the patient get what he wanted? Did the nurse get what she wanted? And, at what lengths did both need to go to get these results? While it could be said that the patient won out over the nurse, in reality, the nurse won because she finally got the patient out of bed and into the wheelchair, thus fulfilling doctor's orders. It is likely that this patient will continue to want to direct his care and that he will utilize similar manipulative strategies to achieve this. And with other, more harried, nurses, the results may not turn out as they did in this case. Patients who complain and also manipulate providers can create a great deal of anger and resentment. Experience will show that angry or hostile remarks to these patients will likely result in battlefield conditions, wherein control is the central issue. Providers must remember to identify the underlying meaning before choosing an appropriate therapeutic response.

CONCLUSION

Of all the provider's communications, encounters that are with difficult patients, difficult tasks, and difficult care contexts are the most challenging. In the high-stress environment of health care delivery systems, the demands of providing care are complicated many times over by problems with difficult patients, families, and even difficult co-workers. These problems create feelings of frustration, tension, and sometimes stronger feelings of anger and disgust. The most critical skills are providers' capabilities in recognizing their own emotional responses and responding out of sensitivity and knowledge of the meaning of the behaviors presented.

Patients and their families are facing moderate-to-severe levels of distress due to the multiplicity of stressors that accompany illness and injury. They may respond in ways far removed from their customary reactions or more negative personality attributes, and even transient long-standing psychological or psychiatric problems could surface. A person who is usually cooperative, receptive, and responsible may present as complaining, demanding, and difficult to please. These individuals may actually feel frightened and helpless. Still other patients who are predisposed to reactions such as self-pity and dependency will manifest these personality tendencies in heightened ways. The behaviors that patients exhibit are frequently difficult for providers to deal with because they are outside what is generally accepted. Patient's responses may even surprise them, their family, and friends as well.

As previously indicated, the key to dealing with difficult behaviors in therapeutic ways lies in providers' abilities to respond, not react, to the communications of these patients. The crucial condition is engaging in an analysis of the patients' behavior wherein underlying meanings (hidden thoughts, feelings, and attitudes) are understood. Replies can then reflect both reluctance to response-match and thoughtful consideration of the patients' circumstances.

Perhaps the most difficult of all difficult patient behaviors are those that provoke providers to retaliate angrily or withdraw. Examples of these behaviors are aggression, demands, complaints, and/or manipulation. Therefore, it is important to anticipate such reactions and think intelligently and objectively about what choices a provider has in responding to these behaviors. Providers can prepare for these encounters by observing conversations between providers and patients and by identifying specific behaviors and attitudes that have a negative impact on them. Providers can expect fearful patients to behave in demanding ways, families to be critical of their relative's care, and co-workers to be on edge.

Expectations of patients, their families, and co-workers should be appropriately viewed in the context of difficult situations. Appropriate guidelines and the providers' use of therapeutic response modes will considerably decrease the toll that difficult behavioral responses have on provider encounters.

Beyond Patient–Provider Encounters: Managing Communications Within and Across Relevant Constituencies

The very dynamic that makes the healthcare system work is the very thing that can torpedo good communication. That is, a quality healthcare system is a series of layers—layers upon layers upon layers. The overwhelming number of constituents in any given case is mind-boggling.

The numbers, kinds, and levels of healthcare providers in managed care situations are almost beyond imagination. Each has a commitment and responsibility to serve the patient. Their service is complicated by the fact that they must have a common vocabulary and must view situations similarly. And, if that were not enough, they must design appropriate means or procedures for communicating among providers and for formulating and implementing decisions. In Chapter 17, Communications within and across Healthcare Provider Groups, group interpersonal communication skills are discussed. Because providers make decisions in the context of group dynamics, it is important to understand the development and character of healthy group communication. Because many providers will be both members of and leaders of these teams, skill at recognizing and averting dysfunctional group communication patterns is also important.

Chapter 18, Conflict in the Healthcare System: Understanding Communications and Resolving Dispute, describes the qualities of communication that are characterized by conflict. This communication includes interactions on a continuum from minimally helpful to disruptive. Negotiation and conflict resolution are discussed as potential solutions to conflicts and as restorative steps in cases where communication seems hopeless.

Finally, Chapter 19, Family Dynamics and Communications with Patients' Significant Others, addresses the constituency that rarely simply "sits on the sidelines." Families differ a great deal in their constellation, as do support networks in their complexity. Whatever the makeup, the "family" is a relevant constituency that must be considered. It is not simply another layer; rather, the family is pivotal in achieving successful medical outcomes. As such, we must concern ourselves with how the family adapts. Significant others, particularly families, have the power to represent the patient in affairs of health and illness. Communicating effectively with families, even beyond the immediate patient–provider encounter, is nonetheless critical to the outcome of care and the dynamics of the therapeutic alliance.

CHAPTER 17

Communications Within and Across Healthcare Provider Groups

United we stand, divided we fall.
—Aesop

CHAPTER OBJECTIVES

- Discuss the pervasiveness of group effort in healthcare delivery systems.
- Outline phases of the group process and corresponding communication patterns.
- Describe functional and dysfunctional communication patterns in groups, especially in problem-solving groups.
- Identify and describe common group communication problems (e.g., conflict and delays in solving problems).
- Identify at least one example of how problems in staff communications can result in poor patient care.
- Discuss several ways in which communications in groups can be improved.
- Discuss problems that occur across groups and how these impact patient care.

Solving work problems and resolving conflict in the healthcare workplace is critical. Reaching resolution can be both time-consuming and distressing as problems can spiral downward and manifest as minor disagreements or escalate to significant staff turnover and even litigation. Group conflict is conflict that occurs between professional groups (e.g., between physicians and pharmacists or between nurses and administrators). They may occur between families and physicians and nurses. Group conflicts have a way of affecting morale, productivity, and patient care. Providers interact in the context of group relationships. The substance of group relationships is human discourse. This includes the verbal and nonverbal transmission of both explicit and implicit messages. Human discourse is made up of a series of dynamic messages that characterize both a specific level of functioning and an evolving group process. Any work group has a defined content and process.

THE INTERPROFESSIONAL NATURE OF OUR WORK

In healthcare systems, we are always interacting in group contexts. These groups include peer, multidisciplinary, patient, and consumer groups. Some communications in groups are productive; they facilitate goal and task achievement, and they meet members' needs for a sense of belonging. Other group communications are nonproductive; they display an inability to define and/or achieve aims. Their communication is marked by conflict, apathy, and the inability to make decisions. A dysfunctional group frustrates its members and expends a great deal of energy in nonproductive communication. Providers should be able to diagnose group communication problems, interrupt dysfunctional interactions, and facilitate functional communication patterns. As health professionals, we do at times have a less than ideal collegial relationship with our health provider peers (Gadacz, 2003). As in any work group, a finely tuned team of providers can accomplish much more than the total individual efforts of its members. Professional work groups can be enjoyable and personally satisfying for most providers. The key is to better understand the nature of group relationships and avoid the traps of dysfunctional group interactions. Sound interprofessional communication is important in the care of our patients and their families, particularly those with many disorders, those who will have problems navigating the healthcare system, those with special health care needs (including children with disabilities), those who need different types of providers, those with life threatening illnesses, and those who might experience a greater risk of adverse events. As teams, we are responsible for discussing plans for treatment; for informing each other of changes in patients' health status, changes in treatment, and results of examinations and tests; and for ensuring that the records are up-to-date and that the records follow the patient through the healthcare system. When this happens smoothly, there is less trauma to the patient and family, less chance of repeated unnecessary tests, and less possibility for mistakes or omissions in care.

THE PERVASIVE NATURE OF GROUPS

Groups involve the interactions of three or more people. Typically, that which governs this interaction is the achievement of personal or commonly held objectives. The perception of interdependency among group members is the glue that keeps these individuals communicating with one another. Groups are, indeed, found everywhere. Human interaction is characterized by small-group constellations.

Types of Groups

We spend a significant proportion of our personal and work lives in groups. On the personal level, these include family, friends, neighborhoods, and communities. Reference groups are those groups to which we belong that typically represent an aspect of our personal lives. Reference groups include religious, ethnic, gender, and age groups. In our professional relationships, we belong to a number of professional task groups. Task groups include peer or multidisciplinary teams. Reference and task groups differ in that reference groups may not engage in specific tasks or goal achievement in the same way that task groups do. Task groups are work groups whose primary purpose is the completion of some objective or goal. They focus on the specifics of the task(s) at hand and on getting the job done. Task groups can serve as reference groups, but usually their affiliation is more transient. For example, we could say that we are members of a quality-improvement committee. We may identify with the objectives of the group and, in some arenas, reflect the goals and values of this committee. This task group serves as a reference group when we develop strong identification with the group. Such groups, however, rarely serve as permanent reference groups that constitute a standard against which we evaluate ourselves. We pay particular attention to our official reference groups (e.g., culture or religious groups) because of their universal and long-standing impact on our lives.

Another way of conceptualizing groups is through the designation of "formal" or "informal." *Formal groups* within an institutional setting are reflected in organizational charts, policies, and procedures. *Informal groups* function in more oblique ways such as those that influence needs, values, attitudes, expectations, traditions, group norms, and network communications (the grapevine).

Informal groups are made up of three or more individuals whose purpose is primarily to meet the affiliation needs of its members. The cliché, "people need people," describes the motivation behind the establishment of informal groups. Informal groups are always observed in organizations. If we were to study a formal organization such as a hospital or a large medical center, we would find a number of loosely formed social groups. Information, support, and a sense of belonging are generally the outcomes that motivate people to form informal groups. Within the formal structure of the organization, then, are a number of affiliations that create what has come to be known as the informal channels of communication. Informal groups can cross peer and professional lines. Because receiving and exchanging information for personal advantage is so key to these groups, informal groups rely heavily on face-to-face, regular encounters wherein they share the latest gossip, speculation about administrative decisions, and information that enhances personal influence and power. Some group theorists attribute a great deal of influence to informal groups and informal channels of communication and explain that if you really want to know what is going on, study the informal communication networks.

The second type of group is the formal group. Also known as task groups, these groups are organized around institutional aims, which include professional, moral, and ethical standards. More often than not, they have specific delineated objectives and procedures for reaching their goals, frequently articulated in mission statements and strategic plans. They possess authority, are accountable for their actions, and are generally regarded as having both official sanction and an area of recognized influence. They also display hierarchical arrangements, governing relationships, and influence within their membership.

Phases of Group Development

Some people find that the interactions that go on in groups are very mysterious. What makes groups decide what they decide, act as they do, come together and dissolve? The workings of groups are both complex and easily understood. An important way to understand groups is through the concepts of task, process, and stages of development. A group's task is an important feature. The *content* (task) that the group is working on is usually the explicit reason that the group exists, and this purpose should be readily discernible. The second aspect to understand is the *process* of the group, which refers to the manner in which the group works together. The process of the group may not be readily apparent, because it refers to the interpersonal relationships within the group and the sequential interaction as it unfolds from meeting to meeting. It is much more than what is recorded in meeting minutes.

It is commonly understood that groups proceed through various stages of development. Some theorists speak of phases and subphases, others of stages and substages. Inherent in this notion about groups is the observation that groups can vary a great deal, depending on how long the group has been in existence. This idea is not difficult to accept at face value. Most of us, even those who are not sophisticated in analyzing group process, would notice differences in communications. Those groups newly formed, we would note, remain relatively superficial in their discussions. Newly formed task groups may cling to the task, while established task groups are not threatened by an occasional deviation of the group's purpose.

In actuality, there are many theories that describe how groups develop over time. These theories range from complex mathematical models to theories that are grounded in the direct observation of group dynamics.

Whether we ascribe to a simple conceptual model or to a more complex model of how groups change over time, it is important, as healthcare providers working on teams and task groups, to understand that communication can differ a great deal depending on the developmental stage of the group.

Functional versus Dysfunctional Communication and Problem Solving in Groups

Groups, and particularly group communications, can be described as functional or dysfunctional.

In all likelihood, groups perform somewhere on a continuum of *functionality*. Usually if a group is proceeding smoothly toward its goals and if attendance and morale are high, the group is regarded as functional. Signs of functionality on a healthcare team would be working together to achieve common goals, recognition that each member is an essential member of the team, clear and fluid communication across and within channels, a cross section of skills and knowledge to achieve goals, and effective sharing of information to meet healthcare delivery goals and needs. In contrast, groups that appear to be *dysfunctional* would demonstrate difficulties in goal achievements, significant membership fluctuation (due to dissatisfaction, turnover), a tendency to miss deadlines, avoiding requests for information, absenteeism, passive-aggressive behavior, gossiping, complaining, and filing grievances. These may all be indicative of dysfunction. By definition, we know that if a task group is not successful, it is not a good working group. They are neither communicating collaboratively nor effectively. All of these indicators can be observed at some point in most groups, but it is the degree to which they are present that distinguishes a group's functionality.

Consider, for example, a team that is established to evaluate the cost-effectiveness of using nurses to perform minor suturing in the emergency room. The hospital's administration established a task force that consists of a variety of disciplines. Only one-third of the membership, however, is truly invested in the issue. The other two-thirds of the membership believe that a task force is not necessary, does not really care about the outcomes or decisions that are reached, do not have time to meet, and/or are not directly affected by the results of any decisions made by the task force. The group is dysfunctional because attendance is poor. It is not that the members are unable to make decisions or could not deliberate successfully and suggest a proposal, this same group of individuals may have worked extremely well together on other task forces. Nonetheless, we would judge the group to be dysfunctional.

To summarize, although that which comprises a healthy group is often unclear, organizational theorists generally agree that there are several attributes that are indicative of functional groups:

- Group processes encourage and enable work to be done; they do not prevent it.
- The individual knowledge and expertise of individuals and control and influence are equally distributed.
- Members of the group are clearly supportive of the group as a whole.
- Members come up with sufficient good and novel ideas and suggestions to keep the group working successfully toward its goals.
- Members evaluate their relationships in the group as supportive and constructive.
- Leaders take their roles and responsibilities seriously.
- Members know the goals and procedures that will meet group aims and have the resources to reach group goals.
- Members exercise and experience an appropriate level of feedback and rewards for goal attainment.
- Members' personal effectiveness is valued; individuals grow and develop as a result of their group involvement.

IDENTIFYING GROUP COMMUNICATION PROBLEMS

The ability to judge group effectiveness is critical to our roles on teams, particularly as we establish a leadership position within these work groups. Group problems have been described by many theorists. One classic conceptualization that continues to have practical relevance to work groups is described by Bradford, Stock, and Horowitz (1978, pp. 94–104). Essentially, the three common group communication problems are identified as conflicts or fights, apathy and nonparticipation, and inadequate decision making.

Conflicts, Fights, and Disagreements

In actuality, what is meant by conflict, fights, and disagreements is not shouting matches and fist fights; rather, it is the presence of disagreements, argumentation, nasty comments, and unresolved passive-aggressive displays of conflict. Member encounters are strained and uncomfortable, and usually the atmosphere is tense.

Bradford and colleagues (1978) enumerate 11 ways in which fighting occurs in groups.

1. Members behave impatiently toward others.
2. Ideas are criticized before they are even completely expressed.
3. Members polarize and take sides, refusing to compromise.
4. Members disagree openly on plans, objectives, and suggestions without resolving these disagreements.
5. Comments and suggestions are forcefully presented with a great deal of vehemence.
6. Members attack each other on a personal level and in subtle ways.
7. Members discredit the group (e.g., insisting that the group does not have the ability or knowledge to accomplish tasks).
8. Members feel that there is something about the group (e.g., its size) that keeps it from accomplishing tasks.
9. Members consistently disagree with the leader's ideas or suggestions.
10. Members are openly critical of one another, particularly of their inability to understand real issues.
11. Rather than hearing and understanding comments, members hear distorted fragments of other's communications.

As these authors suggest, there may be several reasons for group dysfunctional interaction. For example, the task group may have been given an impossible goal, and members are frustrated because they feel inadequate in meeting the demands of the task. Smaller groups such as committees within larger organizations may have this problem because they have too few members to accomplish the task(s) or the specifics of what they are to do have not been sufficiently made known to them. At other times, they may think they were given a task but do not have sufficient power or influence to implement their ideas. Any one of these predicaments can cause frustration and irritation and cause bickering and arguments within the group as well as between the group and administrators.

A second explanation is that the main purpose of members attending group meetings is not to work toward goals but to "flex some muscle." That is, the main concern for members is to establish their status in the group or the team. Consider, for example, a physician who is chief-of-staff and who is participating as a member of a multidisciplinary meeting. This physician feels the need to comment on every suggestion or issue before the group. It is as if the group cannot proceed toward closure on any issue before it hears from the chief-of-staff. This is an example of suppressing the power of others. Under these circumstances, members may disagree with each other or oppose a certain solution just to flex muscle. Once set in motion, this behavior may be seen in other members as well. Power struggles often predominate and stifle group movement. Group leaders are usually drawn into these power struggles, which sometimes are an attempt to dethrone the appointed group leader.

Sometimes groups are fraught with conflict because certain members are loyal to other groups that have conflicting points of view or interests. This might be the case, for example, if members of the multidisciplinary team on the emergency room task force have dual interests and are loyal to some other group. The most cost-effective solutions may not fit with the ideals and interests of the members' own professional group. If the nurses on the task force realize the best solution but evaluate it as opposing the best interests of nurses in the hospital, they may not know whether to respond as a committee member or in keeping with their professional alliance with other hospital nurses. In the group, these members may vacillate on issues or express confusing ideals. Occasionally, their expressed alliances to groups outside the task force may be made forcefully and they may be labeled as disruptive because of their irritation or stubbornness. Blatant opposition may be interspersed with expressions of passive resentment or refusals to cooperate. One response of the group may be to "blackball" these members, recognizing that it is difficult to work cooperatively alongside them.

Still, another explanation for conflict and disagreement is the honest, high-level involvement that members feel in relation to the task and their hard-working attempts to solve problems surrounding the task or goals. Rather than feeling uninvolved in the outcome, they feel that they have a really high stake in any solutions proposed by the group. Impatience, irritability, or disagreement may reflect their overinvolvement. Interestingly enough, their behavior may appear to others as disruptive of the goal. Others may come down "heavy" on their attitudes and outspokenness. To some extent, the group cannot handle emotions of these most dedicated and committed members. If other members engage these members in dialogue and the group moves further along in its goals, the group remains functional. If, however, interpersonal struggles take the place of needed problem solving, the group can fall prey to ongoing dysfunctional communication problems.

Imagine a group where some members are overinvolved and are expressing irritation in the group. And, suppose the leader or chairperson gets angry at those individuals and criticizes their behavior in the group. What might be the reaction of the group as a whole? Not only will these members be misunderstood, but it is very likely that the group will lose confidence in the leader. Rather than express criticism, it would be important to interpret the member's concerns with acknowledgment; for example, "Phil, I know you have a big investment in this issue—whatever we decide will affect just about everyone in your department." In this way, the leader addresses Phil's behavior with understanding and acceptance by engaging Phil in dialogue on the issues.

In assessing conflict and disagreement, leaders must decipher the underlying issues and motivation. It is these dynamics that should be addressed, not necessarily the behavioral symptoms of conflict.

Nonparticipation and Apathy

The opposite of overinvolvement in a group is, of course, underinvolvement. Underinvolvement can be evidenced as apathy, absenteeism, and nonparticipation. It is detrimental to group communication for many reasons. Frequently, dysfunctional groups are typified by high levels of apathy, and unfortunately, apathy occurs more often than we would like to think. Individual members, as well as entire groups, may suffer from apathy. However, functional groups can also go through "dry" periods in which productivity has slowed and the group lapses into periods of inactivity, and this would not be concerning. Taken at a different level, though, it is problematic. Apathy can appear as complete boredom or a lack of enthusiasm or a failure to mobilize energy toward the task. Some members may show a lack of consistent action; others will appear to be content with low-level performances.

If we were to walk into a multidisciplinary meeting at the medical center that we had never attended before, we might quickly observe the level of apathy in the group as a whole and the level of lack of enthusiasm in individual members. Verbal and nonverbal behaviors showing interest might include open exchanges between many members and attempts to clarify communication. On the other hand, verbal and nonverbal behaviors that might suggest apathy include silence, yawning or dozing off, distractibility, absences or lateness, restlessness, frivolous decision making, failure to follow through on decisions, early adjournment, and reluctance to take on more responsibility. These groups display low levels of decision making and responsibility. This group would probably be labeled as "deadbeat," "boring," or "going nowhere." It is true that apathy and boredom can overtake any group. Some groups, however, seem to be more apathetic than others. An apathetic group also reflects the quality of the group leadership. Generally speaking, groups need an upbeat, enthusiastic, inspirational leader—an individual with vision and direction—to establish and maintain interest and morale and to overcome periodic apathetic phases.

As with anger in the group, we should treat apathy as merely a symptom of an underlying problem. In their early work on apathy in the workplace, Bradford, Stock, and Horowitz (1978) identify several underlying causes for apathy: (1) lack of investment in the problem or task of the group, (2) barriers to arriving at solutions to the problem, (3) inadequate approaches or procedures to address the problem, (4) a sense of powerlessness over final decisions, and (5) prolonged conflict that has significantly affected the group over time. In many kinds of situations, members feel that they have had no part in initiating a program or project or in establishing its priority. Under these circumstances, members approach problems as if they were imposed on them. They may regard them and the group's activity as meaningless busy work. Apathy can be even more predominant if the tasks have little or no relationship to members' perceived needs or concerns. There may be members who are more immediately involved and committed, but a core of apathetic, disinterested members can bring the whole group to a standstill.

Sometimes members are given responsibilities but feel conflicted about fulfilling them. Sometimes this is a case of subordinates making decisions that they feel would be unpopular. Consider, for example, clerical staff who are asked to revise policies. If these policies are controversial, then any decision—one way or the other—will be met with disapproval from some professionals or administrators.

Groups rarely want to assume accountability for actions or decisions when the information or resources to solve the problem are inadequate. Group members usually see this as an inadvertent or deliberate set-up for failure. If, for example, a team of cardiologists interested in establishing an adequate teaching program for their post-surgery patients assigned the responsibility to their nursing staff but could not supply the task force with essential information as to the content that should be covered or who was available to help implement the program, the group would falter. The problem would be multiplied if the physician group did not communicate with the task force.

Most of the time, providers are assigned tasks they are capable of completing. However, sometimes they feel that they will make no real headway on the assigned problem. This may be because their recommendations are not really valued or because the real decisions have already been made. This happened to the staff on a geriatric inpatient and outpatient service. They were to establish a project for continued quality improvement. They met to deliberate but, over time, grew to realize that the supervisory group was really not invested in implementing their recommendations. They became suspicious that this assignment was a response to an anticipated review by the Joint Commission on Accreditation of Healthcare Organizations (JCAHO). They were expected to go through the motions, but no serious attempt to change patient care was intended.

Status and authority differences within a group can also create the feeling that whatever contributions members make will not be heard or heeded. On occasion, one member, and it may or may not be the officially appointed leader of the group, will dominate the group process. Sometimes, rather than a single dominant member, there will be a specific subgroup that monopolizes the group's meetings. In cases such as these, other members experience group communication as restricted because only the views of a select few will influence decisions.

In some cases, competition within the group can serve to provoke others to speak or may alienate quiet or passive members who may withdraw even further. Competition in a group can be healthy; however, when it is prolonged, it may cause a sense of helplessness and powerlessness that leads to significant disenchantment or apathy among noncompetitive members.

Inability to Make Decisions

Decision making in a group is not always easy because communication in groups can be quite complicated. Groups seem to have to progress through stages of development that correspond to members' interpersonal needs. Sometimes satisfactory decisions come easily; other times, especially early in the life of a group, they are hard to come by. Reasons for inadequate or incomplete decision making are many. Certainly problems such as anger and apathy influence decision-making capabilities in a group.

At other times groups are confronted with decisions that are too difficult (e.g., when members are pressured to make decisions too early or when the group has not jelled sufficiently to feel comfortable with the results of their deliberations). Certainly, no group of healthcare professionals wants to make what is deemed "a premature decision." Premature decision making is regarded as very risky. Therefore, asking a group of providers to come to a quick decision based on inadequate data stands in opposition to their customary approach to issues. These decisions may be perceived as potentially threatening. A fear of being wrong or of creating unclear and undesired consequences can be the result.

Signs that groups are manifesting an inability to make decisions include indecisiveness, repetitive discussions, or attempts to shift the decisions to some other group. The discussion may wander or be filled with hypothetical situations. Sometimes, just as the group appears to be reaching consensus, the group will argue that no real agreement exists or some members will disown responsibility for the decisions, and a new task group may be established.

IMPROVING COMMUNICATION IN HEALTHCARE WORK GROUPS

Fortunately, the number of conflict resolution programs and consultants have increased, and today, most providers are expected to be trained in conflict resolution and multidisciplinary collaboration. Several important factors contribute to successful communication in professional work groups. Among many there is an interpersonal awareness of self and others.

Understanding Self and Others

Self-awareness is not only extremely important in one-to-one encounters with patients, patients' families, and other providers, it is also essential to successful participation in health care professional work groups.

Becoming a valuable contributor to a work group is important; our leadership and membership capabilities determine the success of the group. We can actively influence movement in the group through our own self-awareness. Self-understanding includes our awareness of how we relate to others—the impact we have on others, our strengths and weaknesses, and how we use these in a group context. It is critical that we first understand our own personal reactions to key interpersonal issues. These are our feelings and reactions about needs to be interdependent, interpersonal intimacy, and authority. For example, how do we respond to having to work with peers that we feel are deficient in certain skills and knowledge? If others were to attempt to shape, direct, or control our attitudes and behavior, how would we respond? If we were asked to take on a leadership position in a group, necessitating that we direct others, how would we respond? Having been assigned to work cooperatively toward a group goal, what behaviors would we exhibit in collaborating with others?

One method of analyzing our current or potential behavior is to examine how we have responded in past relationships, particularly those within small groups. Our current behavior and ways of communicating in a group have indeed been influenced by our first primary group, our family. Depending on our birth order, role in the family, and experience in leadership positions, we may or may not exhibit leadership behavior. Still, the dynamics within our family contributed to our behavior; perhaps we learned to placate authority figures in order to get our needs met. Communication within our family may have been sparse, rigid, and guarded. Or, communication among members of our family was marked with openness, honesty, and trust. In either case, this experience in part shapes our current communication styles in groups, and we may not be totally aware of this fact or the ways in which we act on our early beginnings. One way of establishing self-awareness is to ask ourselves some very personal questions about early communication patterns within our families, both within the family as a whole and within specific dyadic relationships (e.g., between our self and an older sibling).

A second approach to self-awareness in groups is to assess our communication in relationship to role theory. Group roles have been the subject of a great deal of social science research. One model of viewing member roles is to classify these roles as either self-oriented or group-oriented.

Behaviors that primarily serve an individual's needs or interests without regard to the needs or interests of the group are *self-oriented* roles. The self-oriented member may communicate in a self-protective manner, which includes withholding data or communicating defensively. He or she may also manifest self-importance by establishing and proclaiming self-value at whatever cost. Self-adulation, then, is a predominate feature of this member's verbalizations.

In contrast to self-oriented communication styles are behaviors that are typically relevant to the fulfillment of the purpose of the group. These behaviors may be either group-maintenance or group-task focused. That is to say, both are group-oriented, but they differ in that group-maintenance roles tend to satisfy only the interpersonal needs of members. For example, rendering positive feedback is morale enhancing. It does not relate directly to goal or task achievement but is the important glue that keeps the group enthusiastically centered on its task. Behaviors such as initiating new topics, providing information, summarizing group opinion, and taking minutes are all directed at helping the group achieve its goal. Specifically, members who define problems; suggest procedures for solving problems; offer ideas, facts, or information to clarify ideas; explore alternatives; restate areas of consensus; and maintain a record of group ideas and suggestions move the group toward its ultimate goal. To what extent does a person choose behaviors or communications that maintain the group or move it toward its stated goals?

Another approach that we can use to analyze our own and others' behaviors in a work group is to examine our responses to group leadership. Whether our work groups are teams, committees, or ad-hoc task forces, the nature of leadership influences our communications within the group. The leadership may be democratic or autocratic, interactional or transformational. Despite common belief, not all members will prefer democratic-participative leadership styles over more autocratic ones. And some group tasks are more adequately addressed by autocratic styles. Generally speaking, the more dependent a person is on a leader's direction, rules, and disciplinary action, the more comfortable he or she will be with an autocratic leadership style. A very autocratic leader will make decisions and define rules; concomitantly, a member who is comfortable with an autocratic style finds it difficult to function without procedures and feedback from the leader. In contrast, a leader who encourages group decision making and simply acts as a coordinator will be most acceptable to members who tend to be self-starters and who do not need or seek close supervision.

Just how we respond to a leader's approach, as well as our own leadership styles will influence interaction within a group. There has been much attention placed on the leadership style and its ability to enhance participation and communication and correct for deficits in healthcare delivery and the retention of staff (Dunham-Taylor, 2000; Thyer, 2003). One such example is the relative value of "transformational" leadership over interactional leadership. The hallmarks of transformational leadership are its ability to influence, engage, challenge, and inspire. Transformational leadership appeals to a higher order of motivation. It seeks to raise the consciousness of members getting them to reach beyond problems of jealousy, need for control, and power plays.

Understanding others' responses includes knowing their value systems and personal goals, their relevant skills and past experiences, that which motivates them, and how they perceive others in the group. Understanding the group as a whole includes knowing the experience and capability of the members, the nature of the leadership, existing interpersonal relationships among team members, the cohesiveness and morale in the group, and the group's level of functioning.

Reflecting Observations and Assessments to the Group Members

Examining communication patterns within a work group is not only a common method that is used to study group behavior, it has potential positive effects on a group's process and sense that the information obtained can help the group move on. Just what is important to observe and reflect back to the group?

An assessment of how well a group is functioning is determined by gathering a variety of data about the verbal and nonverbal behavior that occurs in groups. These data include but are not limited to:

- Members' verbal and nonverbal communications.
- Spatial and seating arrangements that depict attitudes toward the group or selected members.
- Common themes expressed by the group (e.g., frustration with the task).
- The pattern of communication in the group and between individuals (e.g., who talks to whom and how frequently).
- The quality of listening that occurs: member to member and leader to member.
- The level and quality of problem solving that occurs in the group.

Through observing these aspects of the group's communication, we can identify interpersonal conflict and the quality of decision making. Additionally, these observations will give insight into dysfunctional communication patterns.

To effectively assess, monitor, and facilitate group members' communications, it is important to understand the roles that members assume. *Role* is the position a member takes with respect to the problem-solving process within the group. Each group role has certain expected behaviors and responsibilities. Much of what we report to a group is intimately linked with observations of role behavior. In addition to the identities that a member has outside the group, each member exhibits behavior that is typical of a group role. For example, a member may assume or be assigned the role of record keeper. Role selection and enactment are influenced by individual and group characteristics, such as the individual personality or character of the member, the specific task and size of the group, the character of group interaction, and the position or status of individuals in the group. These roles can be of three kinds: (1) group maintenance, (2) group-task roles, or (3) self-oriented individual roles not related to group functioning.

There are many ways in which data can be compiled. Different kinds of observations yield different kinds of information. For example, much can be gleamed from observing who talks to whom. It is possible to diagram interactions in a group over a given period and by this method, identify problems. Consider, for example, one 15-minute segment in which 45 statements were made, with the largest proportion being made by the leader of the group to the group as a whole. Few statements were made by members, and only one-eighth of the statements were members' comments to other members. Given this pattern, we might conclude that the group was in a beginning stage of development and functioning at a low level with an autocratic leadership style.

Additionally, we could study the kinds of contributions that were made by the leader and the members. Perhaps the majority of statements were made to challenge the advisability of the group's making a decision. Together with our appraisal of what happened in the group and our assessment of the quantity and quality of work that was accomplished, we have a pretty sound picture of the level of functioning in the group at this time (see Exhibit 17–1).

Groups need to include feedback mechanisms that evaluate and improve their effectiveness. This process of feedback is facilitated by directed observations. It is not enough just to make observations, the products of these observations must be fed back to the group. Frequently, either the leader or minute taker will contribute to the group's assessment of itself.

Certain guidelines are suggested for feeding information back to the group. It is important to realize that groups, like individuals, have a low tolerance for negative feedback. Also, like individuals, they may not be receptive to feedback at the time you are ready to share your observations. We should be sensitive to the kinds of information that the group is ready to hear and work with and to

---

Exhibit 17–1 Information Pertinent to Group Effectiveness

1. What is the group's goal? How successful is the group in keeping to the goals and/or aims of the group?
2. Where is the group in the process of decision making: the stage of discovery, analyzing, suggesting, or testing solutions?
3. What barriers and strengths are affecting the group's task performance? How severely is the group limited by these barriers and facilitated by these strengths?
4. Is the group using the most effective measures and/or procedures to accomplish its work?
5. Is the membership participating equally in accomplishing goals and in taking actions, or are a small number of individuals doing the majority of the work?
6. How are members getting along together? Are they resolving differences and disagreements?
7. What are members' opinions of and attitudes toward the group, its effectiveness, and the leadership?

assess what will be most helpful to the group now, rather than what is the most telling or interesting observation. It is important not to overload the group with observations. If too much information is presented, a group, like an individual, will not be able to put it to good use. Present one or two observations, and let the group assimilate this information. For example, it might be important to share an observation about the group's having difficulty in making a decision and the speculation that many facts are not yet known, which prevents the group from feeling confident about any chosen direction. Once this observation is brought to the group and discussed, members will better understand their barriers to decision making.

It is also important to gauge evaluative comments of a critical or rewarding nature. Critical, negative comments are usually received as judgments of below-standard performance. Sometimes those that make the comments are viewed as "superior" or "above it all," especially if delivered by someone with authority. It is also possible to praise the group so much that growth does not occur. When it comes to commenting on individuals' communication styles, it is better to discuss behaviors in general as they relate to goal attainment. It is too easy for members to perceive evaluative comments as individual attacks or favoritism; thus, placing the emphasis on behaviors to accomplish goals takes the emphasis off individual shortcomings or strengths.

Facilitating Group Performance Change

Early on we talked of leadership style, and the differences between types of leaders were addressed. While transformational leadership behaviors, for example, will be valued, it should be kept in mind that group changes are the business of the group members through their presentation of their views of group functioning. Once one or more members presents their views of the functional capacities of the group, thoughtful consideration of what the group should do can occur. But, for this to happen, a full discussion of group strengths and limitations must come first.

The group is no different from an individual who contemplates certain weaknesses in communicating. Members should review evaluations and determine the extent to which there is group consensus about barriers in communication. The group should also be encouraged to examine the reasons for poor communication behavior. As indicated previously, many group behaviors are symptoms of larger, more profound problems (e.g., organizational changes that are occurring in the institution). Finally, the group should move toward solutions. What corrective measures need to be taken, or what new directions should be sought? Unless the group can successfully utilize the feedback it has elicited through the observations of members, the overall functioning of the group will not improve. A point worth noting is that the process of members working on solutions together will increase satisfaction and motivation.

Modeling "Good" Group Communication Skills

What groups need most are members who can model functional communication. First and foremost, communicating effectively in groups in ways that will positively influence members depends on a particular style of interaction.

A variety of good group communication skills has already been suggested. In general, they include skills in the areas of receiving, processing, and sending. Sending clear messages, speaking clearly and thoughtfully, avoiding stereotyping, maintaining good listening posture, expressing oneself honestly, listening carefully, and qualifying or clarifying vague statements are important principles of effective communications in groups. It should be noted that climate or feeling tone in a group is extremely important because in general, supportive climates promote effective problem solving, while defensive or aggressive climates impede good problem solving.

The dominant motivation behind defensive communication is power and control. Defensive communication is easily recognized because it is often designed to persuade or sway the beliefs of others. Even if the member or leader appears to be friendly and open, the basic drive is to persuade or direct others. Strategy and superiority predominate.

Supportive communication, however, promotes group involvement in discussions and decision making. The dominant goal behind supportive communication is understanding. Contrasting positions on issues are not threatening because new and meaningful outcomes can be a result of different views. Members truly seek meaningful dialogue, to listen actively, and to explore and appreciate differences in opinion.

The results of supportive communication styles are very different from those of defensive styles. Rather than persuasion and control, members attempt to understand others' views. Empathy and mutual problem solving characterize members' statements. Supportive climates make room for the resolution of differences that are bound to exist in any group. Active listening in a climate of mutual trust and support not only yields good communication, it is necessary for high productivity and the achievement of group goals.

Although supportive communication styles seem straightforward and simple, they are often difficult to practice for many reasons. First, lack of cultural awareness and diversity training may be a major barrier. Second, emphasis on competition and individual achievement, reinforced by professional values, may inhibit abilities to establish supportive climates. As professional providers, and in our mainstream culture in general, we are rewarded for arriving at independent decisions. We are also rewarded for developing skills of persuasion. Although this varies across disciplines, less attention may have been given to teaching attitudes of acceptance and understanding. Therefore, it is important as healthcare providers that we nurture and protect our inherent abilities for supportive communication, and these should be present regardless of the discipline.

If, in fact, supportive communication occurred naturally and consistently, then we would not need to model these behaviors. In addition to our own inherent limitations, barriers exist in the context of our work environments. The chief and foremost barrier is lack of time or energy. Short-cuts (e.g., Internet and conference calls) have invaded our communication styles and, for the most part, work well in many cases. Creating and maintaining a positive milieu takes work. The team or work group must deliberately assume responsibility for developing an atmosphere that facilitates understanding because it is often easier to respond superficially or inappropriately to what is being said or discussed. At least one member must see to it that the group responds to what is actually being said. Supportive communication also includes some risk. To the extent that we are threatened by others' opinions and communications, we will not always perceive them accurately.

Finally, it is difficult to model supportive communications when we are not feeling good about ourselves. Feelings of anger, hostility, guilt, shame, insecurity, and self-consciousness will also affect our abilities to genuinely express and receive support. Our basic inclinations might be to response-match with criticism and negativity, which further limits mutual understanding.

There are five essentials to facilitating supportive communication:

1. An environment valuing mutual exchange must be established.
2. Active listening is important.
3. Grasping the full meaning (both fact and feelings) of what other members are saying, though not easy, must take place because discipline and role differences as well as status and authority discrepancies can create barriers to openness in provider groups.
4. Clarifying and checking out our perceptions of messages is essential.
5. By avoiding insecurities, we enhance better peer-to-peer exchange.

Dealing with Problem Group Members

Supportive communication is generally a sound technique in dealing with most group members. The idea is that supportive communications will facilitate group dialogue, and when response-matching occurs, supportive communication will form the basis of member-to-member encounters. There are some instances, however, in which supportive responses are inappropriate or not useful. When we think about members whose behavior is destructive in the group, we want to intervene to modify this behavior. Support in such cases may serve to reinforce behaviors that we really want to change.

Steps toward changing members' response patterns begin with a self-inventory. That is, as a witness to this behavior, how do you feel and what makes you feel this way? Examining your specific reactions will help define the problem behavior—is the member distracting the group from its purpose, challenging the authority of the leadership, seeking special attention, or resisting involvement? Also, what outcomes occur as a result? Is the member's behavior rewarded, punished, or simply ignored? How are other members responding to these behaviors? Are they reacting similarly or differently from you? And does the behavior warrant intervention, and if so, from whom?

As in dealing with specific problem behaviors in patients, there are also specific communications that are advisable in group settings with group member problems. In Exhibit 17–2, several problematic group behaviors are listed along with appropriate leadership responses. Problem behaviors included here are: (1) the aggressive, (2) the silent/withdrawn, (3) the shy to fragile, (4) the domineering/dominating, (5) the attention-getter/clown, and (6) the bored/detached member.

INTERGROUP PROBLEMS

While communication problems clearly appear, disappear, and reappear within a group, these problems transcend group boundaries. Intergroup com-

Exhibit 17–2 Problem Behaviors and Concomitant Leader Intervention

Problem Behavior	**Corrective Response**
Aggressive	Avoid negative confrontation. Encourage member to be concrete about personal feelings. Ask for a private conference, share feelings and ask for cooperation, point out harmful effects on others, or ask member to leave the group. Assign aggressor the helpee role on a "personally relevant" topic. (Look for clues to the aggression from the person's self-disclosure.)
Silent/withdrawn	Avoid negative confrontation. Invite responses. Assign nonthreatening roles that require responding but do not demand self-disclosure to the whole group.
Shy to fragile	Avoid negative confrontation. Reduce risk level by supervising one-on-one interactions and avoid group exposure. Arrange a private conference to investigate reasons for member's behavior.
Domineering/ dominating	Avoid negative confrontation. Avoid eye contact. Reward only very significant contributions. Ask for a private conference and assess person's sensitivity/awareness of the problem, ask for cooperation. Arrange for a presentation to the group that requires appropriate, extended verbalizing.
Attention getter/ clown	Avoid negative confrontation. Respond to insecure feelings if present. Assign serious roles. Ask for a private conference and assess reasons for the behavior. Assist members to identify inappropriate humor.
Bored/detached	Avoid negative confrontation. Assign responsible roles. Provide options for creative involvement. Support involvement.

munication difficulties are frequently reflected in intergroup problems. Sometimes the tension among staff on a treatment team (intragroup problems) mirrors communication difficulties elsewhere in the system or organization.

Organizations are composed of many groups; some are specific coalitions or alliances that compete with one another for resources. Discrepancies about goals and values, even ethics and morals, fuel a number of communication difficulties among groups as do issues of esteem, control, and affiliation previously mentioned in describing communications within groups. Consider, for example, a disagreement among a task force that has been assigned to choose a computer-based patient record system, the administrative group that will purchase the system, and the service center that will pilot the new system. The staff on the pilot unit wish to be recognized for their valuable practical ideas. The administrative group is concerned that the task force is exaggerating needs, which will drive costs too high, and the task force questions the sincerity of the administrative group, stating that the administrators do not have the real interests of quality-tracking systems in mind when they criticize the task force. Conflict and mistrust exist and are acted out in the relationships between the pilot group and the task force and between the administrative group and the task force.

The conflicts and disagreements between these groups may not be expressed openly. They may be acted out through various ambiguous communications and information exchange. Information from the task force to the administrative group may be withheld or may be rigidly guarded. The pilot unit staff may express their opinions obliquely, but at other times, aggressively, and all but boycott the decisions of the task force. The observable part of these intergroup conflicts is manifested in these communication responses.

Reflecting on this example, we can see that all the ingredients of conflict are present. First, an observable struggle exists in which opposing groups come together periodically to interact or do so through representatives. Second, there is a clear element of interdependence. The task force relies on the pilot unit, the pilot unit on the task force, and the administrative group on both the pilot unit and task force. Third, areas of contention arouse feelings. Because needs for control, affiliation, and esteem are involved, the arousal of strong feelings is inevitable. Finally, the differences felt between these groups are deemed incompatible or are feared to be incompatible. Incompatible beliefs, values, and goals form the content of these struggles. Desires for control and status, however, may also underlie the intergroup communication exchanges. Concerns about the unequal distribution of power among groups can affect many aspects of a provider's working life, including motivation, job satisfaction, absenteeism, stress, and turnover. It is understandable that these internal struggles may have significant effects on members.

Conflicts between groups can be avoided or resolved by the same interventions that are appropriate within groups. Supportive communication can replace defensive communication in these situations as well. In capacities of leadership, modeling supportive communication is essential but not enough. Recognition of the problems and their underlying dynamics, including the basis for contention, is paramount. It is important to understand the political struggles that also underlie intergroup communications. Recognizing and factoring in the feelings that are motivating intergroup communication will help tailor responses to the feelings of members within groups. Rather than focusing exclusively on superficial manifestations that are revealed in the content of disagreements, group leaders should also recognize and respond to the interpersonal struggles between groups. Finally, transformational leadership perspectives may enhance the groups' abilities to rise above smaller issues and pull together to arrive at the common good.

CONCLUSION

Whether they want to be or not, every health care provider is a member of different kinds of work groups. And whether they are aware of it or not, as group members, they have a significant impact on the functioning of these teams, teams that have the responsibility of delivering quality and safe care to a wide range of patients and families. The healthcare workforce is unique in that there is a wide disparity of knowledge, influence, and control among members. Conflicts and resolutions of problems are always executed in this context, which already assumes an uneven playing ground. By far, group dynamics are inherently important in understanding member communications, in judging functional and dysfunctional communications, and in coming to resolutions.

There are a variety of factors that predispose a group to communicate in a particular way. The type of group (formal or informal) and the maturity (stage of development) of a group are critical factors influencing the way a group communicates. The internal functioning within any group—and this is true of professional work groups—is a result of the dynamic interaction of all members. It also includes the relationship of the group within the context of the larger institutional setting because the goals and resources available to a group are contingent on this interdependency with the external work environment. Communication within groups can be said to be either functional or dysfunctional. In truth, most groups lie somewhere on the continuum of effective functionality.

Group communication problems are manifested in a variety of ways. Conflicts, arguments, disagreements, nonparticipation, apathy, and/or the inability to make decisions effectively are diagnosable features of poorly functioning groups.

Improving communications within groups not only includes knowing yourself and others but also reflecting knowledge and observations back to the group so that corrective processes can begin. Practicing and facilitating supportive communications is helpful not only in dysfunctional groups but also in maintaining a state of high-level functioning in work groups that are proceeding successfully toward their goals.

Intergroup communication problems are frequently reflective of communication problems in a larger context. Power differences, autonomy struggles, insufficient interprofessional understanding, unshared meanings, differences in perception, and interpretation of others' behavior contribute to intergroup conflict.

Inter- and intragroup communication difficulties are everyone's concerns. We must work together effectively in small groups if we are to provide both quality and safe care to patients and their families. The spirit and practice of collegiality makes quality care possible; without it, we are at risk of putting both patients and ourselves in jeopardy.

CHAPTER 18

Conflict in the Healthcare System: Understanding Communications and Resolving Dispute

Within discord there lies the dawning of harmony.
—George Leonard

CHAPTER OBJECTIVES

- Describe how conflict is reflected in interpersonal interaction.
- Define and differentiate among conflict, tension, and disputes.
- Identify signs and types of conflict.
- Analyze cases of poor resolution of communicated conflict.
- Describe the process of resolving interpersonal conflicts.
- Define the mediation process.
- Differentiate between positional bargaining and interest-based bargaining.
- Identify key factors in reaching resolutions (e.g., active listening and reframing).

Conflict is neither abnormal nor irreversible. That being said, the mere mention of the word strikes fear in the best of us. "Conflict!" and red lights flash. The English definition of the word means war, battle, or fight. In all instances it means that a struggle has ensued as a result of differences, usually incompatible needs, values, drives, wishes, or demands. The notion of conflict resulting in someone's getting hurt is vivid. There are needs for softer words and softer ways of framing the phenomena of conflict. This is the case in the healthcare arena as it is in most work environments.

It may help to know that conflict is inevitable. Conflict can occur within an individual (e.g., a conflict between wants and shoulds) or between individuals. It is predictable that two or more individuals will, at some point, express disagreement. In any one relationship, disagreements will recur, although they may differ in content. Some of these disagreements will go incompletely resolved. Conflicts that go unresolved lead individuals to a "deadlock" in decision making, and the quality of communications can be severely curtailed. Chronic communication difficulties between two or more individuals are usually evidence of unresolved conflict. In the patient–provider relationship, conflicts can result in patient dissatisfaction, the patient leaving treatment, and/or lack of adherence to treatment or impaired communications with patient and families about treatment dilemmas.

It is the purpose of this chapter to focus on several key concepts and principles that are used not only to describe conflict but also to describe the process of mediation that will resolve these communication difficulties. In some cases, providers will be a party in the dispute (e.g., between a patient and themselves or between a patient's family and themselves). At other times, they may not be one of the disputants, but they are intimately affected by the presence of the conflict. In some instances, they may have a role in mediating a dispute between others (e.g., between physicians and nurses, between physicians and pharmacists, or between teaching staff and administrators). Dealing successfully with conflict requires specific communication skills. Everyone needs to be familiar with the dynamics and skills of conflict resolution.

As previously stated, good or bad, in our society, conflict is inevitable. Disputes can happen at any time and are observed everywhere—in interpersonal relationships as well as in small and in large groups. Sometimes the disputes are quite apparent, but they can also be latent or emerging. In the workplace, disputes arise at all levels—between patients and providers; among co-workers, managers, and supervisors. On occasion, they involve many other departments directly or indirectly. Because the costs of unresolved conflicts are very high and result in potentially tremendous litigation expenses, more and more attention is placed on early resolution of conflicts, or better yet, on preventing them in the first place.

Certain work situations might appear to be "magnets" for conflict. Environments in which conflicts occur very frequently are those where major changes have occurred and where unclear or overlapping roles, ambiguous lines of authority, and inadequate communication occur. These conditions may produce conflict and/or worsen conflict that already exists. Issues of diversity (gender, age, status, ethnicity, and race) are sometimes at the base of the conflict. In other instances, these factors provide a unique context for the central issue around which conflict exists.

CONFLICTS AND COMMUNICATION

Conflict is omnipresent. Everywhere we turn, we can observe conflict in interpersonal relationships. We grow up witnessing and participating in conflict with siblings, parents, friends, and neighbors. When we enter the workplace with its pattern of rational responses, we might assume that these environments are without dispute and conflict. Or, if conflict does exist, it is circumspect and transient. In healthcare delivery systems, we expect this to be the case because clinical practice is an empirically defined practice and requires predictability and control. Yet, in healthcare delivery systems, disputes and conflicts arise regularly for different reasons. On occasion, these conflicts spill over to individuals or groups who are not parties in the dispute but who are affected directly or indirectly by the disputants. As in many other industries, healthcare systems become involved in large litigation suits between parties who cannot agree. Problems in the delivery of quality care may be a result of conflict; at other times, conflict results from perceptions that inadequate care was provided.

Consider the following event describing staff conflict. The nursing staff on a postpartum unit have felt long-standing tension toward the nursing staff in the neonatal-care division. Generally, the postpartum staff believe that the nursery department is staffed more generously and does not work as hard. One evening shift, a staff member from the postpartum staff observes that the nursery staff have left a newborn unattended. No one is around, and this staff member presumes that the nursery staff are on break. Angered at this apparent neglect, the nurse comments to her peers, "I'll show them." She proceeds to take the newborn from the nursery and hides the infant at the postpartum nursing station. The nursery staff return but do not find the baby where they left him. They realize that this is a retaliatory action and become enraged. Although the parents did not learn of this occurrence, we can imagine how they might have reacted—which would then have brought the parents into the conflict situation.

It is sometimes hard to believe that conflict and workplace aggression would escalate to these proportions in a health care agency bent on rational practices. But because providers are human, these episodes, though rare and quite dramatic, do happen. Regardless of whether you are directly involved in the dispute or indirectly affected (e.g., a member of the physician team or the administrator in this hospital), you will soon know about the incident. Likely, you will be somewhat confused about how to handle your relationships and communications with the at-war parties. Conflict and its behavioral and communicated aspects can affect the entire system, including the patients, patients' families, and legal department.

Historically, conflict and tension were viewed as inevitable, and as such, people just waited for resolution with expectations that in time, the tension would dissipate. Administrators would be called in to instruct staff and levy punitive responses if needed. With the escalation of potential conflict, multicultural work environments, and a new look at the costs of conflict, there has been renewed interest and commitment in attempting to prevent and control interpersonal conflict in the workplace. Studies have shown that the cost of replacing nurses lost to unresolved conflicts is far greater than training staff in crisis resolution. Healthcare institutions cannot afford to let conflict go without explicit intervention. Concomitantly, with various new approaches to conflict management, it has been shown that conflict and disputes can be resolved differently and, in some cases, better.

Differences Among Disagreements, Tensions, Disputes, and Conflict

The chief vehicle by which conflict is initiated, nurtured, and resolved is interpersonal communication. This does not mean that all conflicts or disputes are evidenced in verbal encounters. Many conflicts get played out nonverbally (e.g., in the deliberate absence of communication, in withdrawal and separation, and in posturing and facial expressions). Thus, two parties can be in conflict, but this may not be evident because many individuals hide or disguise their conflictual feelings, attitudes, and opinions. Conflict that has escalated out of control frequently gets played out in silence. "She or he is giving me the 'silent treatment' " means that the tension has escalated to the extent that an impasse has occurred and one or more parties is no longer sending or receiving verbal messages.

Disagreements and *tensions* are different from conflict. Although many conflicts might have started as disagreements, they may not always escalate to conflicts. *Disputes* are conflicts in which the parties have dealt directly with their differences but are unwilling or unable to resolve the issues. Usually these problems or disagreements move into a public forum, becoming the topic of a meeting, and frequently, they involve a third party. These third parties may simply observe and monitor the quality of communication or they may facilitate the resolution of problems through specific mediation and negotiation strategies.

Conflict arises when individuals (or groups of individuals) have incompatible, or seemingly incompatible, values, ideas, or interests. Conflict would not occur if these individuals or groups of individuals were separate, distinct systems and independent of one another. Individuals, groups, and even nations, can coexist without conflict, despite vast disparity in values and beliefs if they are not related in some way to one another. When the relationship changes, however, and these parties become reliant on one another, the potential for conflict surfaces when previously there was no basis for dispute. This principle is important to understand—conflicts are more likely to occur when there is interdependence.

The second basic principle is that conflict can be either positive or negative. Up to this point, we have illustrated the potentially negative results of conflict. Although we fear the destructive consequences of conflict (and there is good reason to do so), conflict does not always have a negative outcome. Advantageous outcomes can, and do occur, and they result in better communications, enhanced problem solving, and positive changes in the individuals involved. Still, the positive results of conflict are not necessarily forthcoming in a timely fashion. We take the position that conflict that is ignored will result in mostly negative outcomes. To keep conflict from having destructive consequences and to elicit positive outcomes from conflicts, deliberate strategies must be employed based on a thorough examination of the cause(s) of the conflict.

Tension and stress always accompany any kind of conflict. In fact, it is these emotional components that frequently produce the negative results of conflict. Tension and stress are the affective responses to conflict that are internalized as somatic and behavioral symptoms. They can manifest as headaches, backaches, or just heightened body sensitivity as well as job dissatisfaction. Left untreated, they tend to have direct and significant impacts on individual behavior. Poor abilities to concentrate as well as decreased abilities to express oneself and respond rationally can all occur as a result of the tension and stress of conflict. The staff's use of poor judgment in the scenario that was presented earlier in this chapter exemplifies how tension due to conflict can eventually erupt in exaggerated expressions of discontent. Incompatibilities, once present in chronic but latent proportions, escalated into the expression of one staff member's behavior toward the other parties.

Consider for a moment that you are either a hospital administrator or medical director and that you are responsible for addressing the dysfunctional communication on the postpartum and nursery units. The specific conflict issues are unknown, but disputes about staffing and cooperation between the units seem to be involved. These disputes have gone into the public forum in the shape of staff meetings but have not been resolved. While arbitration is a possibility, you prefer to facilitate the problem solving and closure without bringing in additional parties from outside the hospital. To skillfully handle this conflict and the underlying disputes, some of which may involve you directly, you must determine the distribution of staff per cost center and apply procedures that will maximize the probability of increasing both parties' willingness and abilities to resolve their differences. In essence, you attempt to modify the dispute, where possible, by providing facts and support so that the participating parties will negotiate a resolution within the ranks. You move a dispute toward successful resolution, maintaining the parties' faith in themselves that they have the power to resolve their differences.

Signs of Conflict

If we asked 100 people how they know someone was in conflict with them, at least 75% would mention anger or irritation as a sign. It stands to reason that in dealing with people under tense circumstances, when individuals are expected to cooperate but have conflicting values or beliefs, anger and frustration may result.

Consider, for example, the number and kinds of words we use to describe a situation where we are in conflict-fraught encounters:

- "He is upset with me."
- "She's hot about that!"
- "Let them 'cool off' for awhile."
- "Give them a 'time out' and they'll settle down."
- "He (She) is 'seeing red!'"
- "Blind rage—that's what it is."
- "He/She is 'psycho.'"

These descriptions suggest everything from mild irritation to irrational emotions of anger or rage. In conflict, as well as in other encounters where anger is displayed, the emotion of anger is secondary to other more basic emotions (e.g., disappointment, fear of loss of control, sadness, hurt, confusion, and guilt). It follows then that behavioral expressions of conflict may reflect either the primary feeling of anger or the secondary feelings of hurt and confusion that underlie anger.

What does anger look like? There are many verbal and nonverbal clues about anger and conflict. They include but are not limited to, verbal attacks, defensive responses, and even withdrawal into silence. They also include nonverbal defensive or aggressive posturing. What must also be recognized is that these clues may be complicated by expressions of other feelings (e.g., fear of lack of control). In fact, these primary feelings may predominate, but expressions of disappointment, sadness, hurt, confusion, and guilt may also be communicated. Part of the difficulty that parties have in responding to conflict is that they must sort through and prioritize among several affective states. If they choose to respond to one (e.g., anger), they may suppress their feelings of disappointment and confusion. While it is critical in conflict resolutions to appreciate all the facets of human experience, it becomes unwieldy to address every emotion. The tendency is to reduce the phenomena in order to make the situation resolvable. This tendency toward reductionism, however, is the very thing that can lead to negotiation failures.

Recognizing conflict through multiple cues about primary and secondary affective states and carefully registering verbal and nonverbal aspects of communication is only half the story. What we must remember is that individual parties will go to great lengths to hide their true feelings and reactions. Therefore, we must be cognizant of the fact that conflict is often masked, but individuals who are masking conflict will display a number of characteristics. They tend to avoid direct eye contact, to remain superficial or curt in their remarks, and to display politeness or courteous behaviors that are not really required. They appear "cool" or "cold" and mask their feelings for a variety of reasons. First, they may not want the opposing party to know that they are having any vulnerable feelings or reactions. Second, they want to hide the specific kinds of feelings they have (e.g., hurt or sadness). They may be willing to let the other party know that they are angry but not willing to let them know about hurt and sadness. The adage, "Don't get angry, just get revenge," implies that the better way to deal with conflict and betrayal is to hide or suppress feelings and take action that will ultimately hurt the other party. A third reason for suppressing feelings associated with conflict, especially if this is an administrative situation is the fear that revealing their true feelings will result in disfavor. For them, talking it out (e.g., sharing unmet expectations) is ill advised. The idea is to litigate versus resolve issues with the provider. So you may find that the individual will prepare a letter or memo to express a threat that their rights have been violated, the system is treating them unfairly, or there is prejudice in the decision making process.

Verbal and nonverbal masks of anger and conflict usually minimize or exaggerate. They minimize or exaggerate because the real stimulus, not the apparent stimulus, is what the individual keeps hidden. Therefore, being overly polite may actually express the fact that we do not feel like being polite; therefore, we will force it, and the other person will never know. This line of thinking is faulty because underlying feelings are always accessible, to some extent, to others. The other sees that the politeness is a feigned gesture. What is actually communicated is, "I don't feel like being nice, but I will be," and "you won't know" is the false assumption that we make.

Types of Conflict

The types of conflict reflect their source, which rests in differences in beliefs, attitudes, and values. These may be actual differences or merely perceived differences. Conflict need not reflect reality; there is usually a great deal of distortion in conflictual relationships.

These differences, however, do not need to result in intense conflict unless they are deemed to be in opposition. For example, if I want to ask the physician his opinion before I ambulate a patient, and you perceive that to be superfluous even though we depend on each other for help, we may experience conflict. If we perceive that our differences oppose one another, one approach may take precedence over the other. There are many options, and we come to terms with what we think is best.

While the most common conflict is relationship conflict—strong opposing emotions—there are many other types of conflict. Technologic conflicts are opposing ideas on how some aims—the procedures, steps, and equipment to be used—

should be achieved. They involve knowledge and perception of the scientific basis behind a situation and an awareness of the standards, policies, and capacities to apply technology to a given patient situation. Providers disagree frequently about the necessity of treatment, the best treatment, and the best surgical or medical intervention to achieve the desired results, although providers do not necessarily openly disagree. If one party, however, is more familiar or more knowledgeable and the less knowledgeable party does not yield, conflict can ensue.

Conflicts in life values, attitudes, and beliefs may stem from the disputants' inherent differences, yet these may be actual or perceived. Differences in values and beliefs, age, gender, race, ethnicity, political and religious persuasion, and education and socioeconomic status lay the foundation for opposing views on issues. One staff member may value small talk with patients' families based on the belief that families are important to patient care, and in the nurse's culture, that patients are treated as friends and members of a common community. Another staff member may believe that families are disruptive to patient care and that the patient's uninterrupted relationship with staff is essential. These individuals might behave in opposite ways toward families. Values and beliefs are highly influenced by an individual's personal characteristics. This is one reason it is believed that providers who come from the same ethnic or racial background as the patient deliver more compatible care. However, different values and belief systems do not have to result in conflict. There is one type of conflict that carries significant influence over staff decisions. That is moral conflict. In the context of care delivery today, staff are continually put in situations in which their values and morals are tested. Examples of this are issues of power of attorney and life support. Any one of these groups (family, physicians, and nursing staff) may be confronted with disagreements that represent larger legal issues and much more.

Relational and interaction conflicts are the most common type. Relationship conflicts frequently reveal differences in interests or needs. For instance, in the context of social relationships, one person may want a committed relationship, the other may not. For relationships to survive, both parties must perceive that a significant number of their personal interests are addressed in the relationship. This may be impossible if the real source of conflict is not an issue in the relationship (e.g., equality, authority, or superior/subordinate stances) but is actually a conflict stemming from ideological differences.

While conflicts may be technologic, ideological or relational, they can also have sources in one or more of these dimensions simultaneously. Sometimes issues have their origins in one source (e.g., technologic) and proceed to additional domains (e.g., relational). Additionally, relational conflicts can fuel conflicts in other areas (e.g., the ideological or technological areas). The cardinal rule is to analyze conflicts carefully, keeping in mind the various categories and origins of conflict.

Poor Resolution of Conflict

Most agree that there is a natural history to conflicts that are unresolved or underresolved and that this history can be analyzed in terms of frustration to destructive outcomes (Saltman, O'Dea, & Kidd, 2006). Saltman and colleagues suggest that there are four stages: frustration, conceptualization of the cause (an early attempt to clarify the cause of the problem), expressed solution where we direct a number of actions toward what we think is the problem, finally, destructive outcomes. It is usually not difficult to judge when conflicts are unresolved or underresolved because the tension that originally surfaced may be only somewhat alleviated or may erupt in significant ways without much provocation. Typically, communication styles remain the same. The disputants may exhibit evasive or avoidant gestures, express themselves rationally but also irrationally, use both direct and indirect messages, and display either rigidity or inconsistency.

Unresolved conflicts usually come about when the different parties have reached a stalemate or impasse. *Impasse*, synonymous with *stalemate*, suggests the inability of the parties to move forward and settle their differences. A characteristic common to many instances of unresolved conflict is that one or both parties is attempting to resolve issues through a series of positions that are presented as solutions to the issue. These positions may be presented sequentially—the first position is less demanding than the second, and so forth. If parties are fixed on one position and display rigidity in their ability to negotiate with respect to new data, then positional bargaining is a negative process. Stalemates connote inflexibility and rigidity with respect to positions on an issue is bound to lead to stalemate. Parties who participate in positional bargaining that has undesirable outcomes generally have a win–lose outcome. They perceive that the goal is "to win" and that they need to take a position. The only right solution is their solution, and conceding to the other person is a sign of weakness. For these parties, it is inconceivable that both parties can benefit because their goal is to come out on top.

Negotiations may worsen conflicts when the roles of each party are confusing. Sometimes third-party negotiators have a stake in the outcome. If this is the case, then the outcome will be generally unsatisfactory. Consider for a moment that you are the outside third party in a conflict between the nursery and the postpartum staff. Assume that you have also disliked members of the nursery staff and felt that they were not to be trusted. Your attitudes and previous history may have a significant impact on the process of resolving this conflict. If your job is to facilitate the negotiation, then you may be biased, and this will show. If your job is to decide for these groups what should be done, then your decisions will be suspect. Much will depend on your official power base, which you may or may not choose to use.

In healthcare delivery systems, the primary means for identifying unresolved conflict is to examine what went wrong. Because 85% of the time "what went wrong" is due to a fault in the system of care giving, a large part of the time the source of an error may originate in, or be complicated by, conflict. As previously stated, conflict is costly—the personal resources and energy devoted to conflict are high, and the costs of errors due to conflict are also high. So, when we establish the need to resolve conflicts, we must also recognize the costs of not resolving conflict (Ury, Brett, & Goldberg, 1988).

THE PROCESS OF RESOLUTION

Can you imagine a workplace that is totally conflict free? Most of us would agree that such a workplace does not exist and cannot be found. Certain environments may appear conflict free but, if there were an accurate appraisal of existing conditions, we would find that it is not likely to remain conflict free indefinitely. Understanding that conflict cannot be totally eradicated is important when we consider what we mean by resolution.

Resolution means to modify differences between individuals and bring disputes under control. Remember, these conflicts have surfaced in states of denial, accommodation, and competition (Saltman et al., 2006), so there is a history of some substance, which influences the resolution process. Modifying differences does not mean forcing one party's views on the other or even forcing a third party's view on the disputants. Resolution means facilitating parties to realize that their existing differences, which will not change, can coexist in harmony. This important principle—that incompatible values can coexist—underscores the work of many mediators or counselors who practice mediation.

When we speak specifically about conflict resolution, we are referring to the steps that are taken to bring disputes under control. While it is most important that individuals learn to deal successfully with conflict, they frequently need outside assistance. When they require outside assistance, a third party is brought into the interaction to either arbitrate or mediate the conflict. Successful negotiation involves a problem-solving process, requiring each party to discuss their differences and reach a joint decision about their common concerns.

Entering Disputes

There are various ways, then, of entering conflict situations. Most of us, if given a choice, will go out of our way to avoid being entangled in conflicts—and for good reason. Conflictual relationships produce a great deal of confusion and frustration, and they make our difficult jobs even more difficult.

Nonetheless, all of us at one time or another will be drawn into a dispute between ourselves and others or into a dispute where two or more parties are involved but we are, at least initially, only indirectly affected. It is important to differentiate roles in conflict situations—the disputants themselves, the third party who may be a "volunteer," and the officials who have been designated to mediate or arbitrate (see Figure 18–1). These groups function within the larger context of the particular healthcare arena.

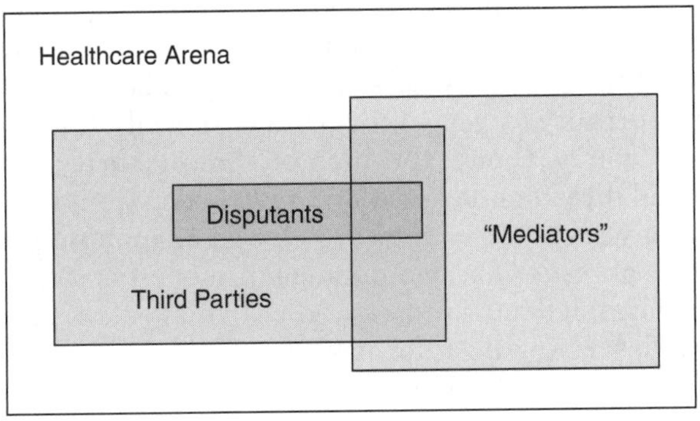

Figure 18–1 Roles in Conflicts/Disputes

Involuntary involvement in disputes is complicated. Because we would rather not have anything to do with the dispute, we have very strong feelings about our involvement, and our resentment and irritation tend to confuse the issues further. Examples of involuntary involvement in the health care workplace could include disputes between members of the staff and patients or between staff and patients' families. They may also include conflicts and disputes between staff as well as within and between disciplines or departments. Frequently outsiders become embroiled in the dispute or conflict. Not only is there anger when we are drawn in, but our tendency to withdraw from others' conflict may also play a role in the manifestation of the conflict or dispute and its resolution. The cost of merely witnessing conflict is sometimes just as frustrating. Silent witnesses suffer; the extent to which they suffer is intangible and difficult to assess, but it could lead to dissatisfaction in the workplace.

When providers enter a conflict or dispute voluntarily, they do so for several reasons. First, providers may understand that, quite unintentionally, they are a part of the problem. Second, providers may realize that their work and/or their personal lives are affected by the conflictual relationships and communications. They may perceive that quality and safe patient care are jeopardized by the conflict. A third compelling reason to enter a conflict or dispute is the personal investment an outsider has in the resolution of it. Just because we voluntarily involve ourselves in conflict or its resolution does not mean that we are the person(s) who can negotiate a compromise or arbitrate a solution. The skill of mediating disputes and conflicts requires both specialized skills and neutrality.

The Mediation Process

While it is hoped that disputing parties will resolve their own conflict or at least bring the conflict under control, the fact is that more often than not, specialized intervention will be needed. This fact reflects our lack of preparation in resolving conflicts, our tendency to avoid versus pursue resolution, and the overriding impact that our feelings and attitudes have on our communications and judgments.

Given this understanding, it will not be difficult to comprehend that the mediation process must be impartial. It stands to reason that successful mediators will not only be those who are skilled but also those who can maintain neutrality. One reason that authority figures are not regarded as effective in negotiation is that they have power that could be used to punish one or both disputants. Even if the authority person promises to be neutral and is capable of maintaining neutrality (a very difficult task indeed), the disputing parties may perceive (or worry about) the bias of the authority figure. Although administrators and directors have traditionally been viewed as good "referees" in disputes, in many cases today, they are viewed as inappropriate mediators.

When we speak of *mediation*, we may mean mediation with a small or big *m*—informal or formal. That is to say, when we speak of mediation with a small *m*, we are describing an informal process performed with and around people who are at an impasse. When we refer to mediation with a big *M*, we are describing a standardized formal approach to a dispute in which an official mediator is asked for or appointed to help the disputants overcome the stalemate. It is clear that when mediation at any level occurs, certain interpersonal and communication skills are necessary. These include nondefensive responses, active listening, and negotiation and/or bargaining skills (Lax & Sebenius, 1986). The need for these skills in formal mediation procedures remains the same. The difference is that formally appointed mediators have specialized training in negotiation, undergoing extensive education and receiving some form of certification.

In a classic statement about the process of mediation, Christopher W. Moore, with Communication/Decisions/Results (CDR) Associates (1986), defined the formal process of mediation as the intervention into a dispute wherein an acceptable, impartial, and neutral third party, who has no authoritative decision-making power, assists the disputants to voluntarily reach their own, mutually acceptable settlement. Each of these elements of mediation is necessary if the disputants are to arrive at an amicable resolution. *Acceptability* refers to the fact that both parties agree to the presence and even the choice of the mediator, which is important if the parties are to follow the mediator's direction and guidance. *Impartiality* and *neutrality*, referred to earlier as a critical element, means that one party will not be favored over the other. While it is not possible to be totally opinion free, mediators are expected to control their preferences, attitudes, and biases. Mediators do not have authority or power, so the tendency of disputants to feel threatened is lessened considerably. Mediators assist the parties in reaching mutually agreeable outcomes—neither the event of mediation nor a decision to resolve the issue are thrust upon the disputants. Mediation, whether informal or formal, is a valued process. It is expected that if the consequences of conflict can be better contained, settlements are reached more quickly, parties are more satisfied with the outcomes, and regardless of the agreement, compliance is more likely. Mediation is extremely important in situations where the parties are expected to have an ongoing working relationship.

Moore (1986) carefully outlines several conditions that have led to successful mediation. These conditions—or, in some cases, preconditions—make successful mediation more possible. Their absence does not make successful mediation impossible, but their absence and the number of unmet conditions will, however, considerably decrease the odds that positive outcomes will be reached. These conditions include:

- The parties have a history of cooperation and successful problem solving.
- The number of parties are limited.
- The parties have been able to agree on some issues.
- The parties have an ongoing relationship, and the hostility and anger toward each other is low to moderate.

Promoting Negotiation

Promoting negotiation and resolution of conflict in work settings is each and every co-worker's responsibility. Just how well we fulfill this responsibility for others varies and depends on several factors (e.g., our investment in the issue or potential solutions, our personal attitudes and opinions about the situation, and our beliefs about the disputing parties). Sometimes, personal characteristics will also influence us (such as our age, gender, discipline, race, or ethnicity—even our marital status).

What is also clear is that each one of us has a particular conflict management style that we resort to, particularly when we are under stress. We may be primarily collaborators, compromisers, accommodators, controllers, or avoiders. The point of becoming more aware of our inherent tendencies is to stimulate individuals to consider alternative styles. Conflict-management styles can be described on two continuums: one reflects the individual's concerns for relationships; the second reflects the individual's concern for personal goals.

For example, while avoidance would seem to be negative because issues may never get addressed, there are some potential uses for it. When arguments or demands get heated, avoidance sometimes provides the respite that everyone needs to reassemble their thoughts (and emotions) and come back together for more positive negotiation attempts. Similarly, compromising would seem to be a positive conflict-management style. Yet, compromising may lead to situations in which solutions do not please either party and the main issues lose their value and importance.

Changing Positional Bargaining to Interest-Based Negotiations

If we were to conduct an "autopsy" on those conflict situations in which no resolution was reached, we might discover an interesting phenomenon. Although there are many factors that influence whether positive outcomes emerge, there is one phenomenon that surfaces as a "vital sign" for diagnosing conflict-management failures. For the purposes of this discussion, we refer to this phenomenon as the balance between interest-based bargaining and position-based bargaining. These two distinctively different negotiation strategies produce significantly different outcomes most of the time (Moore, 1986).

Interest-based bargaining is a negotiation strategy that attempts to satisfy as many interests or needs of the disputing parties as possible. It is a problem-solving technique that is used to reach a mutually satisfying solution rather than to determine an outcome in a win–lose manner. Although compromise may occur, the intent is not to compromise but to construct a solution to address the specific needs and interests of both parties. When parties are cooperative problem solvers, they do not behave as opponents. In interest-based bargaining, win–win solutions are sought. This is very different from win–lose scenarios created by positional bargaining strategies.

Positional bargaining strategies are more familiar to us. They are, in essence, what we know. Classically, our view is that if we become assertive, we will be able to verbalize our position. And, verbalizing our position will increase the odds that we will have our needs met. Positional bargaining, like interest-based bargaining, is a strategy used by one or more parties in a dispute to maximize the gain he or she is likely to make. By stating a preferred outcome up-front, the parties hope to minimize concessions. Usually the parties view each other as opponents where a win is a loss for the other. Using positional bargaining strategies on the part of one party usually begets positional bargaining by the other party. The disadvantage of this mode is that compromise is not valued, and parties often reach a standoff, where no resolution is immediately foreseeable.

How do we change our patterns of negotiating, and how do we assist others to change from one strategy to another? We have already implied that interest-based bargaining is, in many ways, better. Stalemates, impasses, and deadlocks are less likely to occur with interest-based bargaining. The process of changing positional to interest-based bargaining includes a sophisticated analysis of situations. For example, in any potential conflict, three elements are always present. Although we tend to view situations from the positional vantage point (i.e., what a person's position is on the issue), there is more to it than mere proposals or solutions. Each conflict contains issues, interests, and positions. Dealing with positions alone decreases the potential for resolution because there is less to discuss and more temptation to polarize.

Consider the issue of assisted suicide. What is your position? Do you believe in it and support it? Or do you oppose it? If someone says, "I support the concept," the automatic response is to agree or disagree with the position—"I don't" or "I do support it, as well." However, if we discuss the situation from the standpoint of issues (e.g., "Is assisted suicide appropriate for only some medical cases?" or "How do we define assisted?"), we have much to discuss. Because we have more to discuss, there is a greater chance that we will arrive at a consensus.

Consider the issue of having fewer patients to care for. If this situation, a potential area of conflict among staff and administrators, stays at the position level, what becomes the issue of focus is whether fewer patients or better nurse–patient ratios are needed. However, if the discussion is expanded to include all of the issues behind patient–nurse ratios (e.g., acuity of patients, quality care, and cost constraints), there is a great deal to discuss. And, if the subject of personal interests are discussed in reference to the issue, the dialogue is not only expanded further but has more of a chance to satisfy the parties. Needs or interests of the staff may include fears that they will deliver unsafe care or that their patients may be harmed and that they will be held accountable. From the management or administrative side, the interests may include wanting staff to feel supported but knowing that an already out-of-control budget must be kept in line. Mediators will generally treat positions as incomplete. They may ignore them completely, and they will generally avoid coming to solutions too early. They tend to interrupt when positions form counter to other positions, or they will make the issue and interest elements in a dispute more explicit.

In successful negotiations, issues, interests, and positions are relevant. Arguments and compromises that adequately reflect these elements are more likely to be acceptable to both parties.

Reaching Resolutions

We make assumptions about coming to a resolution, and we may also harbor fantasies about it. In the workplace scenario presented earlier, we may have hopes that the postpartum and nursery staffs will come to realize how silly they have behaved and that each group is in some way responsible for the events; realizing all this and having compromised on other issues, we can hope that they will change and, in fact, be model communicators. Such a thought is more fantasy than reality. In truth, the potential for further problems is high. However, so is the potential for successful resolution if one was reached before.

In actuality, there are a host of potential resolution outcomes; in reality, however, more partial resolutions are reached. Settlements, compromises, and decisions to drop all or most of the issues are all possible products of resolution. The settlements or solutions may be partial or temporary. Sometimes disputing parties will just decide to drop the issue because the time, energy, and resources needed to face the issue are too overwhelming. In those instances, no resolution is perceived to be more advantageous than a partial resolution. And in those instances, stalemates may be initiated by one or more parties. Sometimes one party will initiate an impasse, hoping that time or resources will change things and that they will be at a better place down-the-line to compromise.

While the level of agreement or disagreement at resolution is important, of equal importance are the attitudes and feelings of both parties. Both sides must feel that they have had an adequate opportunity to explore their issues, interests, and positions. They also must believe that although they disagree with one another, they are better able to understand and to be understood by the other party. If this is not the case, whatever resolution occurs, partial or complete, the attitudes of participants are sufficiently problematic as to undermine any future cooperative activities.

Communication Guidelines in Conflict Resolution

To some extent, conflicts are synonymous with dysfunctional communication. Associations between communication responses and level of conflict are quite strong. Does faulty communication, however, lead to conflict, or does conflict lead to faulty communication? The answer is, both are true. In fact, we can significantly interrupt conflict by changing communication patterns. It is also true that by improving communication, we can avoid conflict, or at least, resolve it more quickly.

The following discussion describes three elements of interpersonal communication that are vital for avoiding conflict and resolving disputes: (1) active listening, (2) reframing, and (3) assertive versus aggressive styles.

Active Listening

Active listening is a strategy or technique that is very familiar to mental health professionals. A large part of what therapists do is engage in active listening with their patients. *Active listening* entails paying attention to all aspects and levels of communication—the verbal and nonverbal elements and the report and meta-communication aspects of messages. Active listeners not only perceive the explicit content of messages but also the implied emotions and views of how one individual sees his or her relationship with another.

Active listeners practice empathy. They are capable of reading beyond the expressed idea and into the feelings, attitudes, and beliefs of individuals. They are also able to articulate these perceptions in ways that increase the patient's learning and validate the patient's experience.

Because this strategy tends to legitimize the communication abilities of the other person, the process of active listening often encourages the sender to disclose more. With more disclosure comes better understanding, and better understanding minimizes the chance of conflict and controls the destruction that conflict can create in relationships.

Active listening includes a number of smaller steps to achieving more effective communication. These steps in the context of conflict resolution may include:

- Listening to and carefully observing the overt content of each party's message.
- Perceiving the feelings, beliefs, and attitudes behind the spoken messages.
- Placing both the verbal and meta-communication aspects within the personal or interpersonal context in which they occur.
- Placing oneself in each individual's shoes—noting discrepancies in messages, feelings, and context.
- Expressing your understanding in meaningful ways.
- Feeding back to the parties observations about the foregoing process.
- Listening for the parties' clarification and responses to your stated observations.
- Assisting parties in forming new conclusions based on the entire process.

Active listening, like most other strategies, can be both taught and learned with relatively high rates of success. Active listening reinforces this process and tends to increase the probability that it will be used repeatedly to facilitate successful communications.

Reframing

Reframing is a term that describes the strategy of redefining the issues, the importance of the issues, the investments of the parties in the issues, and the value of one or more perceived solutions. The act of reframing can redefine the issues and make them appear as if they are resolvable. It can also convince the disputants that they are capable of resolving the problems.

Reframing in conflict resolution occurs when an outside third party describes a problem or issue in a different manner from how the parties are accustomed to perceiving it. Cognitive behavioral theories suggest that the way in which we cognitively construct our situations constitutes our reality. Therefore, if we offer a revised definition of a problem or issue, we are actually offering disputants new realities. Sometimes the manner in which a conflict situation is described or defined is detrimental to our ability to negotiate solutions. For example, with the staff conflict raised earlier in this chapter, an attitude or conclusion detrimental to these parties' abilities to resolve their differences would be, "I'm not surprised; I expected something crazy would happen—they're 'psycho.' " This conceptualization of the problem is destructive, and no material that has been presented is worth discussing. Solutions to the conflict are deemed hopeless, and one has the feeling of "What's the use?"

When attitudes, beliefs, issues, or interests, or even the context of the conflict, interfere with conflict resolution, reframing must occur. Individuals and whole groups develop definitions and beliefs about situations according to their independent or collective realities. From earlier discussions of the principles of human communication, we know that people perceive based on need and thus do not always perceive accurately the stimulus that is presented. A part of managing conflict, then, is presenting a different reality, a reality that might more accurately reflect the stimuli and one that diminishes perceptions of competition, antagonism, and hopelessness.

A good deal of what occurs in teaching people motivational or remotivational skills is teaching them to redefine and reconceptualize the problem (Bandler & Grinder, 1982). Insurmountable problems are small glitches, and difficult people are people who are behaviorally compromised. Notice that when we describe the postpartum and nursery staffs as "energized" instead of "crazy," we have altogether different attitudes about their actions and the prospects of resolving conflicts.

Assertive versus Aggressive and Passive-Aggressive Stances

In the last quarter of a century, a good deal of literature has been produced to suggest that being assertive is good, being aggressive is not. Theorists have attempted to dichotomize these behaviors and project consequences if individuals behave in either manner. In truth, both aggressive and assertive behaviors make use of aggressive energy. It can be said that even passive responses are aggressive. This notion is borne out in descriptions of those behaviors that are labeled passive-aggressive.

At one level it was believed that individuals could be classified or typed according to certain personality attributes (i.e., they were either passive-aggressive or aggressive personalities). Assertive individuals were perceived to be healthy, well-adapted individuals taking advantage of life's challenges but never at the sake of another's interests.

The issue of assertive versus aggressive behavior and the relative preference for assertive communications over either passive-aggressive or overtly aggressive styles is still an issue today. When it comes to a discussion of conflict and negotiation of differences, it is generally believed that those who can express themselves assertively without being aggressive (disrespectful of others' needs), fare better than those individuals who are either passive-aggressive or openly aggressive (Bolton, 1979). Most theorists would agree, but why?

One reason is that *assertive* individuals bring their issues, interests, and positions to the bargaining table. They are open but not pushy, patient but not avoidant. Furthermore, *aggressive* individuals behave as if their issues, interests, or positions are the only ones or, at least, are the most important. For these reasons, they are not sufficiently open nor flexible enough to entertain alternatives and incorporate others' ideas.

Conflicts with a low probability of resolution generally involve one or more disputants who are either semi-aggressive or overtly aggressive. Also, resolution failures are frequently complementary where one party is aggressive and the other is passive-aggressive. Some authors argue that the symmetry or complementary nature of relationships and communications rules out the possibility of assertive behavior when one party is either overly aggressive or passive-aggressive. This idea underrates the human capacity to avoid dysfunctional patterns. We know from counseling victims of domestic violence, for example, that we can change the victim's responses even if we cannot change the perpetrator. That is, we can bolster the victim to the extent that he or she relinquishes the victim role, becomes assertive, and removes him- or herself from the perpetrator. The idea that aggressive or passive-aggressive styles once learned can never be altered is not true. These styles can be changed, and there are many training programs that prepare individuals to become assertive in both their personal relationships and their work settings. Needless to say, conflict mediators are very interested in the capacities of parties to relinquish aggressive and passive-aggressive styles and take on assertive, respectful responses.

CONCLUSION

Conflict is a growing concern among staff and administrators because of its negative impact on all involved and the consequences of low productivity, poor patient care, and staff dissatisfaction and turnover. Saltman and colleagues (2006) warn of the rise of workplace violence, which is at the extreme end of unresolved conflict. Communicating with people in conflict requires providers to have a sophisticated awareness of conflict as a human condition. This awareness includes knowing what spurs conflict and what resolves conflicts and disputes. Each provider will have his or her own unique conflict-management style. Whatever the style, there are always limitations and advantages in a given approach to managing conflict. Specific tactics to use in conflict situations are those that reframe situations in helpful ways and engage disputants in active listening. A general problem-solving process that encourages providers to stay grounded in the issues is important.

In sum, in the current healthcare climate, conflict is inevitable. These conflicts are played out in professional and bureaucratic differences, in differences in the perception of the goals of the institution, and in conflicts over roles and responsibilities (some of which may be competing). While it is possible that work conflict will reflect personality differences, there are many more potential sources of conflict. Usually, there are multiple causes behind a conflict, and a more complete understanding of its complexity increases the likelihood that any solutions that are reached will be more than just partial settlements resulting in underresolved conflicts.

CHAPTER 19

Family Dynamics and Communications with Patients' Significant Others

Current thought about the nature of comprehensive care would view blatant disregard of the patient's family or social networks as tantamount to health care neglect.
—*Gwen van Servellen*

CHAPTER OBJECTIVES

- Discuss how the family is a major dynamic constituency in health care.
- Differentiate between family and social networks.
- Discuss potential functional and dysfunctional characteristics of the family as a system.
- Identify traditional ideas about the impact of illness on families.
- List potential difficulties that providers may have in communicating with families or significant others.
- Describe the process that families experience in adapting to their member's injury or illness.
- Describe factors that affect family health and family relationships.
- Identify selected requests that patients may have regarding providers' communications with family members.
- Describe several types of difficult family responses, including provider responses that would be helpful.
- Discuss the concept of "caregiver burden" in a family coping with and communicating with an ill or injured member.

Providers cannot fully understand patients in isolation of their family unit however large or small. The family and significant others of the patient are the most important social network in patients'management of their illness and health care. The dominant ways in which families interact with healthcare providers and their sick family members are often unique but do show some common threads. Family goals are to maintain the equilibrium of the family system. The unity and viability of the family system is at stake with the advent of threats to health, illness, and injury that can appear unprecipitously.

It is important to recognize that patients are parts of family systems, despite the fact that they may be treated in isolation. A knowledge of family dynamics is critical to all providers before they enter practice.

Patients are members of *social units*, which are loosely referred to as social networks and more traditionally include formal and informal family systems. The importance of adequate patient–provider family communications is addressed extensively in the literature. Providers are sometimes accused of forgetting or ignoring the importance of family members in all phases of the caregiving process: as informants in the assessment phase, as decision makers in the planning phase, as caregivers in the implementation phase, and as reporters in the evaluation phase. Using family system theory, what happens to the patient happens to the family. The family may not feel the physical pain of the injury or disease but may suffer social, psychological, and financial consequences of significant magnitude. They become fearful, anxious, and frustrated as a result of witnessing the injury or disease that afflicts one of their members. They may understand the health risk but not how they can create healthy living for their family. If they adapt successfully with such issues, they are likely to be stronger for the experience. If they do not adapt, they experience prolonged and unnecessary helplessness and powerlessness, and their relationships and communications are characteristically dysfunctional. Providers can do much to alleviate the emotional pain and modify the communications of family members. Thus, it is important to learn to communicate compassionately and effectively with the family unit—the patient's major constituency.

The classical work of Miller (1992) maintains that provider–family encounters are of three different types, and thinking about family encounters in this way may help providers integrate family-system concepts into busy provider practices. These three encounters are: routines—clinical encounters that are simple, single, and brief; ceremonies—rituals that involve covenantal style; and dramas—a series of visits concerning situations of conflict and emotion that include families' psychosocial problems. These notions help us in shifting our focus from patient to whole family.

THE FAMILY—A MAJOR DYNAMIC CONSTITUENCY

It is our task to understand patients' experiences with their families and the dynamics of the family in general and in the specific context of the health problem. What is this thing called *family*? What real importance and meaning does this unit have in health care, and how best can we communicate with this unit, the patient's primary constituency?

Definitions of Family and Social Network

The concepts of *family* and *kinship* have been revised extensively in American society. It used to be that families were units comprised of children and biological parents living together under the same roof. Today, families are defined in a variety of ways to encompass many variations of the traditional family unit. We have single-parent, blended, nuclear, and three-generational household families. We have families not bound by any legal or blood ties that function in ways similar to traditional families and that are linked together in a system of exchange of resources and role reciprocity.

In addition to changes in notions of what constitutes a family, the family network has also been described as *fluid*. That is, it will change over time somewhat like an accordion; it may become expansive and then narrow and so on. Not only are individuals members of several types of family structures concurrently, some of these memberships change dramatically over the course of life. It is possible that one individual can be a child in a divorced family, grow up in a blended family, establish a nuclear family of her own and end up in a divorced-family situation. Adult members of a family are also members of their nuclear family of origin, which, in some cases, may itself be multiple units wherein child-rearing took place. Three generations of family form the structure of still another family system. Additionally, the in-law family is a family unit that influences its members. Culturally prescribed roles and social norms shape the nature of primary and collateral family units.

The complexity of kinship and family has been further described in the notion of *everyday family*, which may transcend households and extend to communities. Sussman (1982) explains that the everyday family is growing in incidence because of many factors, including lowered fertility rate and increased survival of persons over retirement age. The everyday family typically consists of persons who are not related by blood or marriage, who are of different ages, who live in the same neighborhood or community, and who trust one another as if they were family. These families provide varying degrees of contact and intimacy. Social networks are frequently comprised of loosely or tightly bonded everyday families who serve the functions of traditional, primary family units. Although these families are not bound legally or financially, they have a significant impact on their members and should be viewed similarly to flesh-and-blood systems. These groups influence the perceptions, feelings, attitudes, decisions, and behaviors of its members in everyday living and in other matters involving the members' quality of life and life transitions.

The structure of the American family unit both is and is not intimately linked with the roles and functions of contemporary families. That is to say, the structure reflects that which a family unit will and will not provide. Still, there are some traditional functions that do not seem to change, regardless of the nuclear, extended, or blended structure.

Functional and Dysfunctional Characteristics of the Family Unit

In the previous chapter, we looked at the unit (group), also using a system's perspective. Families act similar to groups. Families can be regarded as collections of individuals with subsystems. Families, like groups, are not just individuals, they are more or less cohesive systems organized for a specific purpose. Families are also affected by the supra-systems, culture, and genealogical structure in which they are imbedded. Thus, to understand the functional and dysfunctional aspects of families, we must first understand these rather basic principles. It is not the purpose of this text to delve deeply into theories of family pathology and teach about families from the perspective of family therapist. You can learn a great deal from current texts detailing the theories behind family psychotherapeutic interaction. If readers are so inclined, however, they may seek out such classic works as those of Satir and Whitaker (1967, 1996, respectively; communications in families), Haley and Haley (2000; strategic family therapy), and Minuchin (1974; structural therapy of families). These texts describe theories, each with a somewhat different interpretation, of family functioning. All tend to focus on how patterns of interaction within the family maintain the problem rather than trying to identify and solve the problems themselves. Whereas the family stress theory views the family in evolving stress encountering stressors throughout the lifetime, these stressors affect how a family will adapt to illness and disease. Unresolved stress over time produces chronic strain in a family that, in turn, causes undesirable characteristics in the family. A theory particularly useful in understanding the family's ability to adapt to illness in the family is the resiliency model (McMillan & Mahon, 1994). This model supports the idea that by intervening to help families, providers have positive impacts on the resilience of the family to regain homeostatic balance while decreasing the possibility of build up of unresolved stress.

A family's functioning can be, and has been, categorized to include various tasks that fulfill relational, communicative, and survival needs. Whenever the physical and emotional resources of the family are insufficient, the performance of critical family tasks and functions are threatened. When this occurs, families can become marginal or disorganized. Families who attempt to cope by appropriate but inadequate role enactment are labeled "marginal," while those that engage inappropriately are labeled "disorganized." In general, disorganized families tend to be more pathological and deviant than marginal families, who are functional but whose productivity is questionable and tenuous. Thus, one way families have been differentiated as healthy or unhealthy has been through the characteristics of their functioning.

Conceptual frameworks that have made significant contributions to understanding families facing illness are those utilized to analyze families' coping and adaptation to acute and chronic illness. Four different perspectives have been represented in the literature: (1) the resource perspective, (2) the deficit perspective, (3) the course perspective, and (4) the impact perspective (Steinglass & Horan, 1987). These perspectives are briefly summarized in Exhibit 19–1.

The Family as a Resource

The first perspective on family functioning conceptualizes the family as a resource to individuals who are coping with illness, particularly with chronic illness. Within this perspective is the notion that families are frequently the primary source of social support and comfort. As such, families serve a preventive, protective, and healing role. The family strengthens the patient's capacity to resist illness and is a major influence in patient adherence once the medical

---

Exhibit 19–1 Perspectives on the Family and Illness

- Family as a resource (protective)
- Family as a deficit (contributor to illness)
- Family and the course of illness (adaptive or maladaptive responses)
- Family and the impact of illness (burden and stress)

Source: Data from P. Steinglass and M. E. Horan, "Families and Chronic Medical Illness in Chronic Disorders and the Family." In *Chronic Disorders and the Family,* F. Walsh and C. M. Anderson, eds., pp. 128–135, © 1987, New York: Haworth Press.

regimen has been established. Families can act in tangible supportive roles to patients in reminding them to take their medications. They can monitor patients to see that the regimen is followed correctly and consistently. They can also give emotional support during the course of difficult times with medication side effects and weariness about long drawn-out treatment. Evidence for this aspect of the family's role comes from a series of studies indicating that family qualities such as empathy, as well as the family's own coping resources, have been associated with both improvements in the medical condition and in the patient's adherence with medical treatment.

Of significant importance to providers is the potential for the family or significant other to be supportive. Social support, typically derived from close social relationships, is felt to buffer or mediate the stress that is associated with chronic and/or life-threatening illness. Because most people use social support to cope with all kinds of stress, the mere perception that adequate support is available can be as important as the actual support itself (Sherbourne, Meredith, Rogers, & Ware, 1992).

The Family as a Deficit

The family as a deficit refers to the disabling role the family may play. In the classic work of Steinglass and Horan (1987), the idea that the family could be both a potential helpful resource but also a potential negative contributor was addressed. In this case, the main influence of the family is not its protective, buffering capability but rather its tendency to weaken the patient's coping and even increase the debilitating aspects of the health condition. This debilitation is believed to be a result of a dysfunctional, rigid, and/or very stressful family system that is incapable of meeting the patient's needs. In this instance, families share certain structural properties and response styles that render the patient vulnerable to their influence. We note that support systems might not always be supportive; thus, their impact can be of no value or negative value. Families might not always be supportive nor facilitate healing. Deliberately ignoring the low-fat diet prescription by the physician and fixing meals high in fat and sodium would be an example of how the support of a family could run counter to what is best for the patient.

Before leaving the topic of unhelpful aspects of the family, it is important to point out the fact that family members, particularly caregivers, may suffer their own health problems from the continuous demands that affect their care duty tasks. Several studies of caregiver strain and health have shown a relationship between health in the caregiver and consequences for the patient. Caregiver stress (e.g., overload) is found to be related to patient institutionalization in patients with Alzheimer's disease (Winslow, 1997); Schumacher, Dodd, and Paul (1993) found that there was a modest but significant relationship between caregiver strain and patient functional status in families where patients had received chemotherapy.

The Family and the Course of Illness

Families are also believed to influence the course of illness. This notion does not address the roles of families during the onset of illness, but it does focus on the ways families influence the course of illness. Because the course of chronic illness is observed to vary depending on the patient, some analyses of the differences in patients have attributed this fact to the family. The idea is that different illness consequences and phases of illness place different demands on the family unit. The manner in which families respond to these challenges, then, may have a substantial impact on the patient's adaptation to illness and its course. This perspective analyzes the interface between family behavior and illness characteristics; family and illness variables may mutually reinforce one another. Questions that often get asked are: "What aspects of family behavior serve to maintain symptomatic illness states?" "What illness factors provoke certain family behaviors?" For example, in the case previously described, family resistance to cooking low-fat meals might prolong disease; on the other hand, symptoms (e.g., uncontrolled diabetes) might put added stress on the family and their homeostatic balance.

The Family and the Impact of Illness

The fourth and final perspective described by Steinglass and Horan (1987) focuses less on the way families influence the onset or course of illness and more on the impact of the illness on the family. Chronic medical conditions, in particular, drain families of emotional and financial resources. These conditions can significantly divert the family from its usual operating agendas to deprive it of time and energy. Studies of the indirect costs of chronic debilitating disease address the significance of this burden.

One behavior associated with family burden is, for whatever reasons, overinvolvement. Overinvolvement is of concern because it threatens social resources. And the depletion of these resources may result in psychological states (e.g., suppressed anger, frustration, and guilt) that are ultimately communicated to and influence the patient in negative ways. Overinvolvement with the patient (or the treatment) can threaten the family's broader social life. Smith and Friedemann (1999) claim that social isolation from the community is a result of this threat and usually causes a loss of personal independence and autonomy. Also, when the patient's needs predominate over all else, someone else in the family may be neglected. In the case of an adult patient, a child or spouse may suffer, and in the case of a child patient, a parent or sibling may not have certain needs met.

Family burden has been linked with family perceptions of the seriousness of the illness, whether or not the illness is as bad as the family pictures it to be. Reactions such as worry, fatigue, guilt, anger, ambiguity, depression, alterations in eating and sleeping patterns, and decreased socialization can occur when families become preoccupied with their ill or potentially ill family member. Families will tell you that they do not have an appetite, do not feel like having a social life, and do not sleep well because they worry considerably about the health and welfare of their ill family member. Todres, Earle, and Jellinck (1994), in discussing how providers (internists) communicate with the parents of critically ill children, emphasize the importance of (1) the first meeting, (2) trust and understanding parental needs, and (3) coping mechanisms if they are to effectively assist families with the coping process and adaptation.

FAMILIES, ILLNESS, AND PROVIDERS

Notions of the Impact of the Family

Families, like patients, express changing needs, depending on the events that occur. Because family members influence patient recovery, failure to address their needs may hinder patient recovery (Bokinskie, 1992). One such need that is often expressed by family members of acutely ill patients is that of dealing with the anxiety that is generated by the hospital setting.

Originally, the stress of illness on the family was seen to be a by-product of the specific disease itself. That is, the stressors on the family when a member had cancer were unique to the disease and different from the stressors imposed by cardiovascular disease or diabetic conditions. The potential stressors were perceived to be a function of the specific disease. The underlying assumption was that the family lay victim to the demands and stresses associated with the particular illness, and health care providers tended to support this notion. As a result, there were separate family programs for renal failure, arthritis, diabetes, stroke, cancer, and AIDS within a single medical center.

A more recent approach to the study and design of support group programs for families is the development of typologies of illnesses based on the psychosocial challenges affecting families with ill members. That is, families might be grouped together based on the characteristics of the onset, course, or prognosis of the condition. Thus, terminal conditions based on acute onset that involve episodes of incapacitation, such as with AIDS and some cancers, have similar psychosocial challenges for the patient and the family. Epilepsy or asthma, however, have acute onsets but are not as incapacitating or as life threatening. Still other illnesses like Alzheimer's disease and late-onset multiple sclerosis, are characterized by a gradual onset and a progressive debilitating course. In sum, illnesses vary in type of onset (acute or gradual), course (progressive, constant, or episodic), and degree of incapacitation. The prognostic time frame (crisis, chronic, or terminal) is still another variable that differentiates illnesses from one another. Illnesses in turn differentially challenge families, requiring different resources, strengths, attitudes, and behavioral changes. The overall amount of readjustment may be similar, but the manner and pace of those adjustments can be quite different. Because family adaptation is fluid and dynamic, the degree to which the family meets these challenges can affect not only the patient's adjustment to illness but the strength of the psychosocial stressors that affect the family.

Much of this approach of looking at families presumes illness to have negative effects on families. We also know that illness can and does bring out the best in families. It has been reported that families sometimes grow closer, stronger, and more peaceful and even talk about more important things. Like individual patients, families can perceive the illness to be a challenge and then not only meet the challenge but even surpass expectations for coping. Just what makes the difference between high-level coping and low-level coping in families is not altogether clear but is probably accounted for by many factors relating to the family, the patient, the disease burden, and the demands of the treatment program.

General Difficulties Communicating with Families

With experience, providers learn about the different types of families that they may encounter, and they develop a communication style suited to each. Nonetheless, their comfort in initiating interaction with families may vary a great deal. Many providers avoid direct interaction with family members—at least, as much as possible. That there are those who do not feel at ease in communicating with families should not be surprising. There is a certain ambiguity related to encountering families. First, considering all the ways in which family members can or have participated in the illness process, they are the protector, the enemy, and/or the confounding variable in the onset and course of the illness. On the other hand, the family is as much the victim as is the patient. So, how is the provider to view the family, and how does the provider converse with such extreme possibilities?

In addition to this ambiguity about the effect of the family, there are other reasons communicating with the family is difficult. Some providers are not trained in communicating effectively with family members or with the family as a whole. Also, some providers feel threatened. They may feel outnumbered by people who may question their competency. They may feel that families will make requests that they found unable or unwilling to fulfill and that this could ultimately result in malpractice litigation. Other providers resent the time it takes to establish contact and talk with the family, especially if it is not altogether clear that this expenditure makes a difference. A final explanation for provider discomfort is that families may become another difficult variable with which to deal, and providers do not want to complicate an already challenging treatment situation. Is it plausible that some providers, on seeing the family from a distance, might feel like walking the other way to avoid them? Despite these fears and concerns that providers have, delivery systems do design, implement, and evaluate programs for families. Unfortunately, the families who need attention are not always those that are able or who choose to participate.

Families also express difficulty in communicating with providers. The classic work of Northouse and Northouse (1992) explains that families have traditionally faced two problems: (1) they have minimal or limited contact with providers, and (2) their access to information about the patient's health status is limited or controlled. And as these authors point out, in spite of these shortcomings and the stress they experience, families generally receive little support from providers. On the whole, providers generate strong feelings in family members. Providers are the source of help and hope, and when the patient gets worse or better, providers' behaviors or lack of response are considered to be the reason. When things go wrong, providers are safer to blame than the patient, and they are more tangible than the disease. Because family members are the patient's primary constituency, they feel compelled, in some cases, to fulfill the role of advocate to the maximum. The stress they experience in their advocate role can place additional strain on their communications with providers. Providers need to provide appropriate reassurance, referrals, and factual information in a caring manner with adequate follow-up in order for families to feel relief from the stress they experience (see Table 19–1).

Table 19–1 Family Communications, Underlying Meanings, and Needs

Selected Family Communications	*Request Value of Family Member's Statement*
"Is he/she OK?" "How is he/she doing?"	Reassure me; tell me he/she is OK.
"How did he/she get it?"	Educate me about this disease. Can I get it too?
"Will he/she die?"	Prepare me for what I have to face.
"Why hasn't his/her tray come/bath been given/medicines or treatments been started?"	Tell me I can trust you to do what needs to be done when it needs to happen.
"Can I talk to you for a minute?"	I really need more time. Can you talk to me? I need your input.
"I'm afraid I'll do/say the wrong thing."	Tell me how I should do this/tell me how I should conduct myself. Tell me I'm doing it OK.

Family Adaptation to Injury and Illness

The conditions that threaten the patient also threaten the family. As indicated previously, a number of illness- and treatment-related stressors affect families.

Families frequently experience crisis at the first sign of illness or injury. Principles that apply to working with patients in crisis, in large part, also apply to families. Families facing chronic, debilitating, or life-threatening illnesses are also believed to progress through grief-like stages in response to the illness. For a life-threatening condition, this may mean denial, anger, bargaining, depression, and acceptance. For chronic conditions, this may mean fear and anxiety, anger and hostility, depression, and resolution and acceptance.

The similarities in patient and family adaptive tasks are so great that the phenomena of adaptation is frequently attributed to both. The assumption here is that the patient and family progress through an illness process in a parallel fashion. Although this is generally the case, there are exceptions, and the gap between patient and family seems to widen with time. For example, an initial diagnosis may shock both the patient and the family, and the length of time it takes to move on may be similar. By the point of acceptance, however, the gap may have widened. The patient may have reached acceptance but the family, or selected members of the family, may not have. The reverse may also be true. That is, the family may be in resolution but the patient may be primarily angry or in the bargaining mode.

Assessing Family Health and Family Relationships

Taking a health history relies not only on the patient's self-report but also on the information that family members as informants give the provider. This information can be broken down into roughly three categories; the family's report of: (1) the patient's condition, (2) the health of its members, and (3) the nature of its roles and relationships. This information is gleaned from the patient because the patient is the first line of inquiry. Families, however, are often brought into the assessment process because patients cannot or will not report certain data. In other cases, patients have given their information, but they are judged to be poor historians so family members are utilized to clarify, extend, and corroborate data that have been previously derived directly from the patient or indirectly from records and charts.

The family's report on the patient's current condition reveals how the patient's illness or injury is perceived from the outside. This report may reveal the patient's tendency to minimize or exaggerate symptoms. It also reveals the family's level of awareness and their own tendencies to minimize or exaggerate changes in the patient's appearance, behavior, or demeanor. Essentially, the provider wants to know what the family member has observed—the nature of the signs and symptoms, the degree of disability or impaired functioning, and how the member has processed these data and been affected by the patient's condition and/or treatment.

Families are informants and can serve as a check on the reliability of the patient's report. Families are not necessarily better historians than patients, except in certain circumstances. Family members who are older, who have had recent experiences with illness, and who are (or have been) interested in health issues and familial problems are likely to be good historians. Some family members are hypervigilant about disease prevention and are able to report major illnesses (heart disease, cancer, strokes, etc.) three generations back. One by one, the provider progresses systematically through family members, accounting for major illnesses, injuries, and deaths. Where hereditary, infectious, or familial conditions are concerned, extending the list of significant others beyond the immediate family is important.

The third category of data that is the subject of family interviews is specific data related to the roles and relationships in the family support network. Providers need to identify which family members are most important to the patient, because their health and level of functioning will have the most bearing on the patient's current and future health status. (Is there a power of attorney? Who usually helps the patient in issues about health and disease treatment?) Inquiring, "Who lives with the patient?" and "Do they have health problems? If so, what kind?" generally picks up on nonfamilial relationships that the family member may have forgotten to mention. Full information about the patient's current life situation is important. There are several basic categories of information that are derived from these conversations with family members. They include:

- Factors that may inhibit communication in the family.
- Quality of communication between the patient and specific designated responsible parties.
- Patient's role in the family and alterations in role functioning as a result of the onset or progression of illness.
- Active or potential dysfunction in the family.

There are numerous strengths and problem areas that can be revealed from this dialogue. Evidence of social isolation or alienation may surface. Evidence of impaired verbal communication, altered family functioning, and compromised family and parental role performance can be determined. Beginning evidence of actual or potential violence directed toward family members may also surface. Additionally, family-role conflict, ambiguity, role reversal, and role overload may become apparent from these initial conversations.

It is expected that families can elaborate on details, especially in areas where the patient was vague or where independent corroboration is needed. It is not unusual that a provider will get more information from family members than from patients themselves, particularly in areas that the patient is unaware of or reluctant to expand. For example, patients may not be aware that they had a seizure or exactly how an accident occurred. They may not realize that their behavior was irrational or bizarre. Sometimes patients not only minimize or exaggerate symptoms, they distort them in other ways as well. Providers may find that the patient was more acutely ill than the patient reported. Families can also be helpful in understanding patients' reactions to treatment and hospitalization, because members have observed how patients have handled similar situations in the past. Sometimes providers will secure the entire history from a family member. This is the case if the patient is very critically ill, demented, delirious, unconscious, psychotic, cannot speak and/or hear, or for other reasons.

Repeated brief contacts with family members, particularly if they are assuming caregiving functions, is important. These contacts not only allow providers to follow the patient's disease course but also reveal more about their concerns. Throughout the course of illness, families' involvement can change—caregivers and their caregiving duties can change. For example, siblings may shift responsibilities for the care of their elder. Such information is essential in planning the patient's care and managing the patient's illness. On some occasions, providers will meet conjointly with family and patient to discuss the patient's condition and plan of care. These sessions can be very valuable but are not always possible unless the treatment program is specifically designed to actively involve family. A much more common occurrence is periodic family contact and very brief conjoint encounters, a structure that permits limited education and support.

The confidentiality of family communications is very important. Personal information about other family members is not communicated to the patient. Also, patients need to be protected from conflictual data that are obtained from the family unless their condition requires it.

Patients' Requests with Respect to Families

As if to make the process of communicating even more difficult than it inherently is, there are other circumstances that complicate the picture. These circumstances are defined by patients themselves and include formal and informal requests.

We understand that patients typically define their own family unit. They identify a responsible person, a next of kin, and/or a parent/guardian, but these individuals are not always the same person. These individuals may not even be those persons who actually and/or legally fill these roles.

In addition to this complexity, patients establish the boundaries of communication with either their significant others or their next of kin. These boundaries include what the patient wants and does not want the family member to know. "I don't want them to know," or "I don't want them to be told," is not a rare occurrence. In some cultures, however, the role of family prevails. Some patients, typically some Latino and Asian patients, expect the family to know everything and take a major role in decision making. To maintain the patients' trust, their requests to share or withhold data from family members must be respected. In some cases, the law or absence of laws will support the provider's decision to keep information from a family. In other cases, there may be legal grounds for suspending confidentiality (e.g., the risk of self-harm).

Professional judgment may override patient requests. Professional judgment can dictate the necessity of sharing information with family members if it relates directly to the well-being of the patient. For example, the family may be instrumental in helping the patient make a decision or obtain resources. Another reason professional judgment may prevail is that discussing the patient's condition with the family or a family representative may prevent reinforcing the patient's avoidance of health care problems. Providers should not support maladaptive coping strategies (e.g., by helping patients not face their condition), especially if it includes high levels of life-threatening nonadherence to treatment. Providers do not want to be placed in positions of conflict in their own clinical attempts to help patients acquire adaptive coping strategies.

For the provider to be released from the obligation of confidentiality, both patient and provider should negotiate compromises. Patients who openly express preferences do not make requests without reasons, and it is critical that providers understand the basis of the request. Providers cannot take these requests lightly. Still, by observing the patient with the family and by discussing the patient's reasoning, the consequences that are feared are usually clarified under most situations. Providers are not released from their promises of confidentiality until the patient has stated the circumstances (when and how) under which this confidence is to be suspended.

There are instances in which the patient's request becomes more imperative. Diagnoses and prognoses carry with them social consequences. A positive diagnosis of HIV infection, for example, produces stigma, fears, and responses that can lead to social isolation and even alienation and discrimination. While families may not, in reality, react negatively to information about the patient's diagnosis, the patient's concern may be deep-seated. Violation of the patient's confidence, even (or especially) with family, is prohibited in such cases.

If patients do not negotiate the release of confidentiality, the responsibility rests on the provider to determine if withholding information would jeopardize the patient's well-being. Sometimes these decisions are exceedingly complex. Consider, for example, the issue of teen pregnancy. If the teen patient requests that her next of kin (mother) not be told of her pregnancy, her well-being may be jeopardized. Also, withholding information about current or potential conditions from the patient's mother would be a violation of the mother's parental rights because it would significantly hinder her from fulfilling her parental responsibilities.

There are other instances in which the interface between patient and family becomes complicated. This problem is mentioned in instances of caring for terminal patients. As Cable (1991) describes, it is generally felt that caring for terminally ill patients requires effective communication with the families. Effective communication must become a regular part of the treatment. Decisions to support patients do not always have equally good outcomes for families, and conversely, decisions favoring families may not be good for the patient. Providers find themselves in a dilemma. If they, on the one hand, do what appears to be best for the family, they may violate rights or ignore the needs of the patient. On the other hand, if they address specific needs of individual patients, they may weaken the family unit. Examples of these dilemmas also include acting on the information that patients report about the alleged abuse they have experienced at the hands of a family member or significant other. Note that both child and elder abuse are instances of mandatory reporting regardless of what the patient, caregiver, or family members wish.

Difficult Families and Provider Responses

Families bring with them certain characteristic ways of responding that may make providers' roles more difficult. Frequently, families who have high stress levels also have difficulty communicating.

The following review highlights several types of families whom providers find difficult. Similar to dealing with patients who are difficult, it is important to understand the dynamics behind the family's communications and respond to these underlying issues, not just to the manifest expressions. For example, a family member who anxiously questions "Is he or she going to be OK?" is generally concerned, worried, and afraid. The underlying request to the provider may be interpreted as "Reassure me; tell me he/she is, in fact, OK." Questions like "How did he or she get it?" implies confusion and concern. The request behind the question is "Educate me about the disease." "Can I get it, too?" "Did I do anything to cause it?" Communications that express concern, fear, guilt, depression, and frustration are commonplace with family members who are or are not deemed to be difficult. Most providers will observe that if they try to understand the family dynamics, they will personally experience less stress and more satisfaction, will achieve better overall treatment outcomes, and will lower the potential for conflicts and disputes.

In Howell and Schroeder's (1984) work to analyze family responses to disease and illness, nine separate categories of difficult families were identified with the caveat that these categories are not mutually exclusive. Some families exhibit one or more categories or features from more than one categorical group.

1. Chaotic family
2. Family in crisis
3. Anxiety-ridden family
4. Guilt-ridden family
5. Enmeshed family
6. Intimidating family
7. "Split" family
8. Psychosomatic family
9. Uncooperative or abusive family

The following discussion highlights basic principles and concepts that are important in communicating with these selected categories of difficult families.

The Chaotic Family

According to Howell and Schroeder (1984), chaotic families are usually characterized by having multiple problems, and they might also have multiple caregivers. They may appear to lack structure, to have no goals, and to have no designated person in authority. In neuroscience terms, they seem to lack executive functioning. Their communication is confused and poor. This family looks to providers for guidance and structure but is uncertain about its needs. Because of the continuous chaotic lines of communication and members' self-defeating encounters with each other, it appears that little effective problem solving will take place. And while the provider may diligently seek the origin of each problem and offer suggestions, the family has a temporary plan and structure to follow but will be nonadherent to the plan laid out for them. Providers must recognize the character of these families and set limited and realistic goals. Guidelines to structure communications with the chaotic family in conjoint sessions would be to (1) structure the topics, direction, and duration of the interview; (2) speak clearly and gain and maintain control within the family; (3) appeal to the designated leaders to follow up on recommendations; and (4) establish definite timelines for follow-up.

The Family in Crisis

The family in crisis is experiencing incapacitating trauma. Like chaotic families, those in crisis also appear to have altered executive functioning. The major reason that providers have difficulty communicating with these families is that communication is boundless. Typically, they do not synthesize instruction or information in a rational manner (Howell & Schroeder, 1984). And because family members vary in their responses, providers may have multiple responses to deal with simultaneously. These include anger, rage, fear, panic, blame, and guilt. The provider can be flooded by the number of responses as well as by their intensity from a variety of family members. The primary therapeutic response is to allow family members time to express their emotions. A central organizing figure must be assigned to deal with this family's responses and needs, and feedback needs to be provided in an empathic, supportive manner.

The Anxiety-Ridden and Guilt-Ridden Families

Families who are in crisis over illness or who are facing uncertainties that accompany the illness process may be anxiety ridden or guilt ridden. Typically, the anxiety-ridden family is extremely tense, is upset about the status of the patient, and is frequently overinvolved in the patient's care. These families may be awaiting test results or the outcome of treatment or surgery. They have many questions and are not always certain that they have heard all that they should know. They are frequently anxious because they lack information that would calm them down or at least limit their worst fears. They also seek reassurance and information but utilize information poorly. It is important to be clear, to say the same things to all family members, and to avoid false reassurance. It is important to assure them what they can do if they have additional questions.

Guilt-ridden families can be draining. This family's communications are motivated by the desperate need to seek amends or reconciliation (Howell & Schroeder, 1984). Some guilt may be internally generated because a family wants to know that they did all they could do. These families may become desperate when they realize that the patient may be so incapacitated (or may die) that their desires for restitution will be thwarted. Whether their guilt is justified or not, if it is exaggerated out of proportion, they can become difficult to converse with. The consequence of this is that they may project their guilt onto someone else, typically the provider(s). Unreasonable demands made of providers are often a reflection of the guilt the family experiences. In other words, "it is not us (the family) who have failed," they want to establish "it is the providers who have failed."

The Enmeshed or Disengaged Family

Enmeshment and disengagement refer to distinctly different structural properties of families (Howell & Schroeder, 1984). Enmeshed families appear to be overinvolved, and individual member autonomy is either severely limited or nonexistent. It appears as if no boundaries exist in this family and whatever happens to the patient happens to them. Married elders sometimes exhibit these strong ties. While anxiety and guilt may account for these behaviors, some families have long histories of relating as enmeshed units.

In contrast, disengaged families have rigid boundaries; the experiences of one member seem to cause no response in others. These family members may be incapable of feeling or sensing the needs of the patient. Structurally, they may also have minimal contact and minimal interactions with the patient. An example of this would be encounters with primary relatives who know little of what is going on and little about the patient's needs or preferences.

Responses to enmeshed families include setting limits and clarifying boundaries. These families may not respect provider boundaries. Therefore, clarifying professional roles and expectations and maintaining autonomy for the provider's own clinical decision making are important. In contrast to the enmeshed family, the disengaged family typically must be brought closer together. Projecting feelings and discussing typical responses to injury or illness also help to encourage a revelation of feelings that can make these families more empathic toward the patient.

The Intimidating and Uncooperative Family

Two additional family types that providers find difficult to encounter are the intimidating and the uncooperative family (Howell & Schroeder, 1984). The intimidating family can be one of the most distressing types because there is an element of threat that looms in the background. These families' communications may be even characterized as abusive toward the provider. By putting providers down, by making providers feel that their actions could be questioned, and by alluding to the fact that complaints or litigation may be forthcoming, they become threatening. Some families ask for extensive details about treatment and question providers' judgments; when they do not get the response that they need, they become rude or belligerent. Guidelines for communicating with this family include establishing a clear treatment plan that is constructed similarly to a contract. Providers must also resist the anger these families provoke in them and focus on the underlying dynamics that explain the power struggles that these families tend to evoke.

Uncooperative families who clearly are problematic are those who exhibit very little or no real concern for the patient. They may also be very resistant to speaking with providers as well as carrying out any suggestions or recommendations. Some families in this category abandon the patient, leaving the patient to fend for him- or herself. This type of family may also not be helpful in the assessment and history-taking process. They may even be secretive and somewhat paranoid about being addressed in an official capacity. Establishing communication with these families requires careful analysis of underlying issues and assessment of how the family responses will affect the outcome of the patients' care and treatment. Establishing an alliance, communicating fully what care is planned, and how the family may be helpful are constructive measures.

The Phenomena of Caregiver Burden

The stress of professional caregiving has been reported in a wide variety of literature addressing the professional stress syndrome and burnout. An increasing emphasis has been placed on the stress of caregivers who are not professionals. With the advent of changes in the healthcare delivery system, including more care being carried out at home by family members, caregiver burden is growing significantly. Becoming more concerned about caregivers is appropriate because their health has been linked to the health, welfare, and successful rehabilitation of persons, especially those with chronic illness (Han & Haley, 1999). The problems of informal caregivers are not the same as those for the professional. Professional caregivers have been educated and trained, and it is presumed this knowledge and skill helps them cope with the stresses of caregiving. Informal family caregivers typically lack the skill, knowledge, and experience that providers have. Still, the number of informal caregivers is increasing significantly. These informal caregivers receive variable amounts of support and education with which to accomplish similar tasks. While their responsibilities are typically limited to one patient, these responsibilities can be 24 hours a day, seven days a week. This may be in the context, however, of caring for two children under age 5 and a nephew age 16. Professional and informal caregivers experience stress and burnout, perhaps for different reasons, but the expressions of stress are similar.

First, families experience stressors unrelated to specific caregiving tasks. Some of the most compassionate reports of caregiver stress have appeared in the last decade and come from family members of cardiac, cancer, HIV, and Alzheimer's disease patients. These family stressors are many and occur in significant magnitude to place the family at high risk for further problems and afflictions. These include social and emotional costs, physical exhaustion, financial drain, and, in some cases, stigma and alienation.

In most cases, the stressors related to the patient's illness and treatment are also many. But, among those that are of most concern to families who are giving care are the cognitive and emotional changes both in the patient and, potentially, in themselves.

Cognitive impairment in patients can include memory loss, disorientation, impaired concentration and judgment, impaired perception, confusion, mental slowing, and the inability to engage in abstract thinking. These problems can occur in patients with senile dementia, HIV, depression, and in patients with mental and addictive disorders. In addition to cognitive impairment, emotional changes and disturbances occur in patients who have mental illness, the elderly, persons with HIV, substance abusers, and with patients with medical illnesses such as cardiac disease and cancer. Patients who experience these disturbances can be bothered by sleep and eating disturbances, fatigue, generalized apathy, irritability, low self-worth, hopelessness, and even suicidal or homicidal ideation and/or risk.

Typically, the informal caregiver is faced with the same situations that confront the professional, but he or she may lack sufficient respite. That is, the informal caregiver must learn to give instrumental care (administer medications, treatments, etc.) and emotional support, and these must be accomplished in cases where the patient's ability to cooperate or render self-care may be minimal and variable. The difference is that informal caregivers must organize these responsibilities in and around their own activities. Thus, the social and occupational lives of informal family caregivers are threatened, sometimes considerably.

Informal caregivers' reports of emotional exhaustion indicate that the burdens that they experience are significant and not easily modified. To understand the informal family member's experience of emotional exhaustion, a list of potential reactions are provided in Exhibit 19–2.

CONCLUSION

There is no knowledge of a patient without knowing the family unit and its functioning. Dealing with families during illness implies a challenge to patient and family by an altered set of circumstances for which adaptive resources may not readily be available (Kercher, 1991). Adequate intervention implies an evaluation of the resources within the individual and an evaluation of the

---

Exhibit 19–2 Caregiver Burden: Emotional Exhaustion in Family Caregivers

- Physically and emotionally drained from caring for the patient.
- Angry and frustrated by the prospect of endless caregiving responsibilities.
- Frustrated about the program of caregiving and the numerous demands without clear signs of improvement or progress.
- Powerlessness over the disease, its course, and their ability to make changes for the better.
- Angry at the patient for significantly altering their personal independence and autonomy and, therefore, quality of life.

resources among those who surround the individual in the family and the community.

Families are not just "those people" who "ask stupid questions" or "get in the way"; they are special patient constituencies who significantly affect and are affected by the patient, the treatment, the provider–patient relationship, and the treatment setting. Providers need to enlist families in formal and informal ways. Because of their importance, it is critical that providers understand family communications and how best to converse with family members. A small part of this time will be spent in taking a social or family history; the much larger portion of the investment will be how to effectively engage the family in meeting the needs of the patient.

Families have been associated with the onset and outcome of diseases, particularly chronic conditions, in a number of ways. Research has focused on the protective role of families, particularly in their ability to buffer illness-related stressors. Studies have also isolated instances in which families may contribute to the progression of disease and worsening of the patient's quality of life. More recent research has addressed the interdependent nature of the patient's illness and the adaptive capabilities of the family. Finally, we discussed a model that addresses the significant burden that families endure as a result of an ill family member. Within the broad range of possibilities—to help or to hinder and sometimes both simultaneously—the family will need to be approached with appropriate respect and caution.

Families who are most difficult to communicate with (e.g., the anxiety-ridden, guilt-ridden, or uncooperative families) can be managed. The key is to understand that the behavior is amenable to change if the underlying issues are approached and resolved.

Families are currently faced with burdens of caregiving that they never before expected to see. This is, in part, an outcome of the many delivery-system changes that have moved caregiving from inpatient intensive care settings to outpatient facilities and the home. In a study by Davis-Martin (1994), it was found that the needs of long-term, critical care patients' families do not subside. The desire for information remained the number-one need. This is not the time to abandon the family because it is difficult to communicate with family members or the unit as a whole. Rather, as providers, we must embrace the family with all its rough edges, strengths, and limitations. Next of kin, parents or guardians, responsible persons, and everyday families (broader social units acting like families) are a part of the picture. Patients may need to rely on these constituencies for extended periods. Some, but not all, will deliver aspects of care. As such, they constitute the greatest potential health care resource that we have today and that we will have in the future.

In spite of the growing recognition of the influence of interactions with healthcare providers on how patients and family members respond to illness, the level of research about families and their roles is deficient (Knafl, Breitmayer, Gallo, & Zoeller, 1992). More research is needed.

PART V

Ethics and Communications in Health Care

Instruction in the skills and concepts of applied communication in health care would be incomplete without a discussion of the important ethical and legal concepts that shape and limit providers' communications with patients and families. Stipulations about the nature of the professional patient–provider communications underscore a good deal of what is considered ethical. Some rules and norms are not only standards of professional practice, they are displayed in statements of patient rights, in statutes, and in laws. It is important to understand the issue of patient rights in its fullest. Patient rights govern what patients have a right to know and what protection they have against others' knowing, that is, what will be communicated to them, but not to others.

In Chapter 20, The Privileged Nature of Patient and Provider Communications: The Issue of Patients' Rights, the concepts of informed consent and informed choice are discussed. These concepts are applied to research- and non–research-based clinical practice. They are basic in intent, but their assurance is far from simple; thus problems in securing informed consent and informed choice are identified and discussed.

In addition to patients' basic rights to informed consent and informed choice, there are specific stipulations that protect patients from exposure. One such stipulation governs issues of confidentiality—that which providers can ethically and legally divulge, to whom, and under what conditions. In Chapter 21, The Privileged Nature of Patient and Provider Communications: Issues of Confidentiality, Anonymity, and Privacy, the rules around confidentiality are presented. Two related concepts, that of anonymity and privacy, are also discussed.

It has been said that today we need to be more concerned than ever before with the ethical and legal foundations of health care communications. The U.S. Department of Health and Human Services established the Health Insurance Portability and Accountability Act of 1996 (HIPAA) to protect the use and disclosure of individuals' health information The flagrant abuse of patients' rights can be observed in many arenas and in many different ways. Certainly, the flippant disrespect of patient confidentiality is among the most serious. Policies that protect patient rights and afford patient control must be uppermost in our minds. Providers' commitment to ethical practices in the realm of written and verbal communications to and about patients must be fostered and reinforced.

CHAPTER 20

The Privileged Nature of Patient and Provider Communications: The Issue of Patients' Rights

This declaration of patient rights [AHA Patient's Bill of Rights] is even more important in today's health care environment, in which cost containment efforts so often seem to be driving most organizational decision-making, including patient care decisions.
—*Anne J. Davis and Mila A. Aroskar*

CHAPTER OBJECTIVES

- Define the principle of patient-informed choice.
- Describe the process of obtaining patient-informed consent.
- Discuss providers' legal duty to care for patients.
- Discuss dynamics under which providers refuse to provide care and identify how they communicate refusal to patients.
- Identify selected times in which patients do not have personal choices about communication.
- Identify which factors make informed consent difficult to obtain.
- Identify various patient groups for which informed choice and informed consent are especially difficult to obtain, and identify alternatives.

The privileged nature of patient–provider communications is played out in the specific encounters we have with patients and patients' families. It is understood that patients who enter into relationships with providers are protected by a set of norms that outline, at least in part, how the roles of provider and patients are to be enacted and exactly what privileges and responsibilities it is that these roles entail. The reality of practicing as a healthcare provider includes risks as well as rewards. In this era of malpractice controversies and the emerging legal considerations of managed care, these risks become more than just hypothetical circumstances or philosophical debates. The rights and privileges of patients regarding their care and communications with providers should be taken very seriously.

Many kinds of legal and ethical issues confront healthcare providers. These vary from what seem to be straightforward issues of informing patients of their diagnosis to more complex issues related to extending patients' lives. From a legal and ethical standpoint, we are concerned with patient safety, liability, incident reports, and malpractice litigation. From a communication perspective, we are concerned with the basic challenge of effectively communicating with patients to maximize their privileges of choice and execute our responsibilities. There are several sources of pressure that influence our actions. Licensure and accreditation of healthcare facilities support practices that are respectful of patients' rights and sanction those that are not. These sanctions range from very severe to merely warnings. Providers' own professional licensure requirements, however, strongly enforce adherence to basic fundamental patients' rights.

Additionally, legal systems have evolved in elaborate ways to address the complexity of provider–patient encounters. Federal and state laws regulate practice through professional practice acts. Each state must assume the responsibility for developing these guidelines and for providing regulatory measures to ensure that professional standards are upheld. This legislative authority is both ethically and legally binding. It is important to note that providers are expected not only to practice within standards, but they are also expected to protect patients from abuses within the healthcare system. It is this latter area that can create dilemmas that are not easily resolved. Many providers are clear about their own level of practice; however, when the system and/or other providers are involved and place the patient at risk, indirectly or directly, the fundamentals of practice and of protecting healthcare systems becomes complex. These conflicts raise a number of professional consequences that create stress in providers. Thus, the role of providers in protecting patient rights is influenced by many factors. The communication and interpersonal competencies of providers are intimately connected to safeguarding patients' rights.

ISSUES OF PROVIDER–PATIENT PRIVILEGE

Perhaps the most noteworthy examples of provider–patient privilege are embedded in the concepts of informed choice and informed consent. The underlying assumption behind the issues of informed choice and informed consent is that in healthcare arenas, the balance of power rests with providers. After all, the patient is ill or otherwise incapacitated and is at the mercy of the system's definition of when, where, what, and how actions will be taken. By virtue of this inequitable power distribution, patients' rights for self-determination must be protected. Inherent in this objective is the standard to act and communicate in ways that respect the dignity and worth of every patient. We, as healthcare providers, are morally obligated to respect human existence and the individuality of all patients who are recipients of our care, but our values may run counter to traditional treatment measures. Resolving these conflicts is not easy; an entire science of bioethical decision making has emerged in the past two decades to assist us with these complexities.

Informed Choice

In each and every healthcare situation, providers have a duty to offer patients choices and participation in decisions that are germane to their case. These choices are always reflective of the medical technology and resources available. A provider cannot offer an alternative surgical procedure if that procedure is contrary to hospital policy or is not available due to lack of medical and professional resources. Providers are, however, obligated to describe the alternatives that are available. Informed choice requires providers to clearly communicate about the treatment of choice, but also about other less-favored approaches. Sometimes, providers perform this task ineffectively and options are not fully and adequately discussed.

Haas et al. (1993) reported on the barriers that providers had in discussing resuscitation with AIDS patients. In this study, the majority of persons with AIDS had not discussed their preferences for life-sustaining care with their physician, despite their desire to do so. Healthcare providers need to be well-informed about advance directives for medical care in the event that a patient becomes incapacitated. The Patient Self-Determination Act (PSDA) was a step in this direction. On November 5, 1990, Congress passed this measure as an amendment to the Omnibus Budget Reconciliation Act of 1990. It requires providers to give adult individuals, at the time of inpatient admission or enrollment, certain information about their rights under state laws governing advance directives, including (1) the right to participate in and direct their own healthcare decisions, (2) the right to accept or refuse medical or surgical treatment, (3) the right to prepare an advance directive, and (4) information on the provider's policies that govern the utilization of these rights. The act also prohibits institutions from discriminating against a patient who does not have an advance directive. The PSDA further requires institutions to document patient information and provide ongoing community education on advance directives. Whereas attitudes toward advance directives are positive, many providers have little knowledge of the Durable Power of Attorney for Health Care Act and are poorly equipped to discuss it with patients, not only out of ignorance, but because of their own personal discomforts.

In cases where providers must offer informed choice, a number of factors influence the process, including the historical and technological treatment patterns as well as the philosophical and even religious background of providers. These factors often explain why providers may hold different attitudes about the same issue and why some providers are more comfortable in their communication than others.

Some providers come from cultural backgrounds that do not place much value on principles of autonomy and self-determination. We might expect these providers to understand and practice informed-choice procedures somewhat differently. Without accusing or critically evaluating these providers, we can say that their approach to informing patients of treatment choices may be influenced by their underlying belief system. For example, they may fail to address all potential treatment choices, or they may overemphasize their authority in directing patients' choices. On a more subtle level, they may verbally present choices but nonverbally suggest that their opinions should be followed. Their encounters with patients and families may also suggest that if their advice is not followed, there may be negative repercussions. This type of response from a provider is unacceptable and unethical. Patients' fear of abandonment or retaliation, real or imagined, can influence whether they will exercise their autonomy. Fears could include concerns that the treatment they receive will be withdrawn or will be of lesser quality or that they will suffer unnecessary pain or discomfort. For these reasons, patients may be very sensitive to any variances in the context of discussions of choices. They may react to perceptions of the providers' bias or preference, or even imagine what those biases might be.

Despite this subtle, and not so subtle, interplay between providers' preferences and patients' choices, one thing must be generally clear: the patient is the primary decision maker. With the advancement of the science of bioethical decision making, there has been a renewed concern for patients' roles in their care and their personal freedom to direct this care. It is generally maintained that patients are critical participants and should retain significant control over healthcare decisions that affect their welfare, and they can only do this if the communications between the provider and patient are open and fluid.

In 1983, the President's Commission for the Study of Ethical Problems in Medicine and Biomedical and Behavioral Research issued a recommendation with regard to patients' roles in healthcare decisions (Thompson & Thompson, 1985). This document supported the important concept that patients with the capacity to make decisions be permitted to do so. The Commission, however, indicated that the process is based on mutual respect and shared information, although this choice is not absolute. For example, patients cannot expect healthcare providers to render services that violate standards of practice or the providers' moral beliefs. This deliberation also touched on the issue of reasonable rights; that is, the patient cannot insist on services that draw on limited resources to which the patient has no binding claim.

We could say, for example, that expensive one-to-one nursing care, although desired by a patient as a routine aspect of his or her care, is outside the realm of possibility—the patient has no binding contract with the facility to receive this type of care. This clarification of the limits of patients' choice in health care is made on a case-by-case basis. The institution's rights may predominate, but this is not just an issue of providers' maintaining power over patients. Rather, it provides some protection to the healthcare facility and provider groups as they attempt to balance patient autonomy with instances in which it is inappropriate to let patients make the final choice.

What remains critical here is that regardless of the request, respectful discussions, in which information is provided in ways the patient can comprehend, must be ensured.

Informed Consent

That physicians and nurses are competent in ethical decision making is no longer a given (Thompson & Thompson, 1985). One reason for this is that clinical and technical skill and expertise cannot be easily generalized to ethical decision making. Rees (1993) suggests that political, legal, ethical, social, economic, and technological changes in the 20th century have profoundly changed the way in which providers and clients communicate. As patients now assume two identities—health consumers and active participants in medical decision making—they are more and more concerned not only about symptoms, disease, and treatment, but are also equally preoccupied with issues about cost of, quality of, and access to health care.

There are many more decisions to be made in healthcare practice than there were a century ago; even within the last decade, technological advances have made bio-behavioral medical decision making exceedingly complex. This advancement in technology has created choices and options in patient care that did not previously exist.

In its landmark 2001 report on *Crossing the Quality Chasm*, the Institute of Medicine (IOM) listed "patient-centered care" as one of the six fundamental aims of the U.S. health care system. The IOM defines patient-centered care as:

> *Health care that establishes a partnership among practitioners, patients, and their families (when appropriate) to ensure that decisions respect patients' wants, needs, and preferences and that patients have the education and support they need to make decisions and participate in their own care.*

To fulfill participatory expectations, patients must have access to information and be offered the opportunity to make decisions. The issue of informed consent is derived from the value of self-determination, wherein information is the prelude to informed choice. That is, under normal circumstances, informed patients are capable of making decisions about their care. Exceptional circumstances are those in which families make decisions, and many times providers fail to communicate effectively with the family.

There are many difficulties in achieving patient-informed consent; these difficulties cause us to consider whether informed consent can, in actuality, be met. First, patients, families, and providers frequently come to decisions with dissimilar values and beliefs. Even if these values and beliefs appear compatible, their translations may be quite different. For example, both patient and provider may want the best possible surgical intervention and on the outside, their views seem compatible. When these views are translated to specific steps and "surgical cuts," however, we find that the provider's views are more radical than the patient's. Because values and beliefs are always subject to individual interpretation, they are best presented explicitly by the patient and not simply inferred from what the patient has said. If the patient is unable to verbalize the specifics, then the provider can address gaps or problems in understanding by qualifying, clarifying, or offering the patient multiple-choice options.

Knowing the views of the patient requires time, and this time is not vacuous—it is time within the context of a therapeutic relationship. Does the provider have the time that is required to learn the views of the patient? Some providers feel that too much time spent in extracting patients' views may inhibit decision making rather than facilitate it. They are concerned that the process can get bogged down. In extended communications of this sort, it is common that many options are raised. Sometimes these options are impractical or have never been tried before. Too many options can contribute to the confusion of what decision to make. The patient, family, and provider may have already had difficulty with only two options for action; now the situation is complicated with still additional choices.

On the whole, providers would agree that the time spent in learning to understand the patient's concerns, personal, and cultural beliefs is worthwhile. There are many of us who would say that this process is not only valuable, it is an imperative. That is, providing the best care possible rests on our knowing our patients well.

Patients' rights for self-determination include their protection from deception. Deception in health care is a type of manipulation that subverts patients' capacities to exercise rational and deliberate choice. Kirlin (2007) explains that when a physician fails to tell the patient the truth, about diagnosis, prognosis, or even risks and benefits of alternative treatments, it has the effect of making a unilateral decision to deny the patient his or her right to participate autonomously in care decisions.

Deception, when translated into specific acts, includes withholding information, deliberately making the information unclear or difficult to understand, minimizing important aspects, and presenting an unbalanced picture. Historically, providers have considered that less information leads to greater satisfaction, at least in the short run. This point of view is highly inconsistent with today's thinking. It is currently held that with each act of deception, however minor, there is a corrosive effect on the patient–provider relationship. The trust that is necessary in patient–provider relationships suffers with even the most minor instances of deception.

Given the importance of truthfulness in the professional provider–patient relationship, it may come as a surprise to realize that the codes of professional ethics have not always presented a strong case for truthfulness. Bok (1978), cited in Benjamin and Curtis (1992), points out that professional oaths and codes as well as the writings of physicians have made little to no mention of the need to be truthful.

For whatever reasons the issue of truthfulness has not been stressed early on, the current shift away from paternal dominance to individual rights through knowing is both a serious and important shift. The Patient's Bill of Rights, endorsed by the American Hospital Association in 1992, clearly recognized the importance of a high level of honesty in patient–provider communications (see Exhibit 20–1).

Exhibit 20–1 Patient's Bill of Rights, American Hospital Association (October 21, 1992)

1. The patient has the right to considerate and respectful care.
2. The patient has the right to and is encouraged to obtain from physicians and other direct caregivers relevant, current, and understandable information concerning diagnosis, treatment, and prognosis. Except in emergencies when the patient lacks decision-making capacity and the need for treatment is urgent, the patient is entitled to the opportunity to discuss and request information related to the specific procedures and/or treatments, the risks involved, the possible length of recuperation, and the medically reasonable alternatives and their accompanying risks and benefits. Patients have the right to know the identity of physicians, nurses, and others involved in their care, as well as when those involved are students, residents, or other trainees. The patient also has the right to know the immediate and long-term financial implications of treatment choices, insofar as they are known.
3. The patient has the right to make decisions about the plan of care prior to and during the course of treatment and to refuse a recommended treatment or

continues

plan of care to the extent permitted by law and hospital policy and to be informed of the medical consequences of this action. In case of such refusal, the patient is entitled to other appropriate care and services that the hospital provides or transfer to another hospital. The hospital should notify patients of any policy that might affect patient choice within the institution.

4. The patient has the right to have an advance directive (such as a living will, healthcare proxy, or durable power of attorney for health care) concerning treatment or designating a surrogate decision-maker with the expectation that the hospital will honor the intent of that directive to the extent permitted by law and hospital policy. Healthcare institutions must advise patients of their rights under state law and hospital policy to make informed medical choices, ask if the patient has an advance directive, and include that information in patient records. The patient has the right to timely information about hospital policy that may limit its ability to implement fully a legally valid advance directive.

5. The patient has the right to every consideration of his/her privacy. Case discussion, consultation, examination, and treatment should be conducted so as to protect each patient's privacy.

6. The patient has the right to expect that all communications and records pertaining to his/her care will be treated as confidential by the hospital, except in cases such as suspected abuse and public health hazards when reporting is permitted or required by law. The patient has the right to expect that the hospital will emphasize the confidentiality of this information when it releases it to any other parties entitled to review information in these records.

7. The patient has the right to review the records pertaining to his/her medical care and to have the information explained or interpreted as necessary, except when restricted by law.

8. The patient has the right to expect that, within its capacity and policies, a hospital will make reasonable response to the request of a patient for appropriate and medically indicated care and services. The hospital must provide evaluation, service, and/or referral as indicated by the urgency of the case. When medically appropriate and legally permissible, or when a patient has so requested, a patient may be transferred to another facility. The institution to which the patient is to be transferred must first have accepted the patient for transfer. The patient must also have the benefit of complete information and explanation concerning the need for risks, benefits, and alternatives to such a transfer.

9. The patient has the right to ask and be informed of the existence of business relationships among the hospital, educational institutions, other healthcare providers, or payers that may influence the patient's treatment and care.

10. The patient has the right to consent to or decline to participate in proposed research studies or human experimentation affecting care and treatment or requiring direct patient involvement, and to have those studies fully explained prior to consent. A patient who declines to participate in research or experimentation is entitled to the most effective care that the hospital can otherwise provide.

continues

11. The patient has the right to expect reasonable continuity of care when appropriate and to be informed by physicians and other caregivers of available and realistic patient care options when hospital care is no longer appropriate.

12. The patient has the right to be informed of hospital policies and practices that relate to patient care, treatment, and responsibilities. The patient has the right to be informed of available resources for resolving disputes, grievances, and conflicts, such as ethics committees, patient representatives, or other mechanisms available in the institution. The patient has the right to be informed of the hospital's charges for services and available payment methods.

Source: Reprinted with permission from the American Hospital Association, Chicago, Illinois, © 1992.

This bill of rights recognized the patient's right to complete, current information concerning his or her diagnosis, treatment, and prognosis in terms that the patient can be reasonably expected to understand. Except in emergencies when the patient lacks decision-making capacity and the need for treatment is urgent, the patient is entitled to the opportunity to discuss and request information related to the specific procedures and/or treatments, the risks involved, the possible length of recuperation, and the medically reasonable alternatives and their accompanying risks and benefits.

Perhaps the most dramatic example of the shift to provide patients with information is seen in the following example. Not more than two decades ago it was unthinkable for a patient to exercise his rights to the extent of requesting copies of everything in his medical record, including notes, lab test results, doctors' orders, and so forth. Today, this is a patient right. This request occurs, albeit infrequently, and while the entire chart is not usually provided, excerpts of the contents of the record are summarized for the patient. This request is not only for the purpose of completing referrals, it is in response to a direct request of the patient to have access to and therefore to be able to pursue and deliberate, for himself and under conditions he chooses, aspects of his illness and treatment.

The process of informed consent becomes even more deliberate when the patient is involved in research studies. Research studies are usually of two kinds: (1) those focused on specific medical experiments (e.g., studies involving experimental drugs or devices) and (2) those focused on nonmedical research (e.g., studies in the social and behavioral sciences that study attitudes, beliefs, and behaviors through the use of surveys and interviews).

Research studies involve several issues around patient's rights and, therefore, undergo a great deal of scrutiny in institutional review boards (IRBs) and human subject protection committees (HSPCs). Issues of concern to review committees include (1) risk (minimal and major) of physical and/or emotional injury; (2) freedom to withdraw without consequences to care and treatment; (3) physical and/or emotional (mental) discomfort or pain related to the research process; (4) loss or invasion of privacy, dignity, and/or autonomy by consenting to participate; and (5) the time and energy required to participate.

In any research study, these issues must be addressed clearly and truthfully by researchers. Under review, these issues are extensively examined, including the clarity of the investigators' descriptions. An approval issued by an IRB or HSPC always means that the risks of the study outweigh the benefits and that any conditions placing the patient at risk are explained and provided for and that all this information has been adequately communicated by the investigator.

Additionally, IRBs will expect to be assured that specific issues related to subject recruitment, procedures for obtaining informed consent, and protecting confidentiality are addressed. They are concerned with how subjects will be selected and contacted as well as what subjects will be told on the first contact. IRBs are concerned about whether subjects and data about subjects will be identifiable by name and, if patients are identified by name, what procedures will be used to collect, process, and store data that will protect patient identity. Review boards expect patients to be informed of the purpose of the study; the expected duration of their participation; and the reasonably foreseeable immediate and long-term discomforts, hazards, risks, and potential consequences. Every consent must include certain guarantees; these vary from institution to institution but generally include stated reassurances that (1) the patient may refuse to participate or may withdraw from participation at any time without any negative consequences; (2) no information that identifies the patient will be released without the patient's separate consent (except as specifically required by law); and (3) if the study, design, or use of data is changed, patients will be informed and their consent re-obtained. The informed-consent forms (ICFs) tell the patient who to contact with concerns or questions about the study and how to proceed if this avenue does not satisfy the patient. A copy of the written consent along with a statement of the Patient's Bill of Rights is provided to each subject. In the case that a subject is unable to sign (e.g., in the case of minors), a signature (and date) is obtained from a parent or guardian. If the patient cannot sign because of physical disability or illiteracy but is otherwise capable of being informed and of giving verbal consent, a third party not connected with the study (a next-of-kin or guardian), would be asked to witness the discussion, sign, and state the reason for standing in for the patient. When a subject's native language is one other than English (or the person is poorly versed in English) an accurate translation must be used.

Studies of a medical nature involving treatment of disease or illness (e.g., those involving experimental drugs or medical devices) must provide additional information to patients. Studies of this kind must include a statement that describes any appropriate alternative procedures or treatment that might be advantageous, including both risks and benefits.

THE LEGAL STATUS OF THE PATIENT–PROVIDER RELATIONSHIP

Healthcare providers are confronted with many legal and ethical issues, but advancing medical technology is not the sole reason for this circumstance. Healthcare delivery has become exceedingly complex. The emerging system of managed care brings myriad important issues to the surface that include who decides, who gives care, and who, ultimately, is accountable for outcomes. A good deal of this complexity is played out in one-to-one encounters with providers.

Accountability, responsibility, and, subsequently, liability, is understood or misunderstood in the specific context of patient–provider relationships.

Just about every ethical and/or legal issue reflects the inadequacy of patient–provider communication and the trustworthiness of the relationship. Refusal or withdrawal of treatment, for example, occurs in the context of patients' and providers' understanding of one another's roles and beliefs. When "push comes to shove," patient dissatisfaction and/or the decision to pursue litigation reflects, in large part, the poor quality of communication within the patient–provider relationship.

Legal Duty to Provide Care

Duty to the patient, including a breach of duty, underlies standards of practice for all healthcare professionals. When healthcare professionals enter into a relationship with a patient, a duty or obligation that is recognized as a legal relationship ensues. This legal relationship holds the professional accountable for practicing within established standards of care. When this duty includes providing care as well as protecting patients from harm, the legal relationship becomes even more complex. Clearly, we can comprehend the circumstances of a particular provider neglecting the patient and performing below standards, which is grounds for malpractice.

Providers, however, are also commonly confronted with situations that impinge on, or have the potential to impinge on, patients' rights. The four basic consumer rights outlined by the American Hospital Association (AHA) are (1) the right to safety, (2) the right to be informed, (3) the right to choose, and (4) the right to be heard. What happens if the provider witnesses infractions of these rights by others in the healthcare system?

Most clearly, our legal duty includes protecting patients from harm and from violations of their rights. Consider, for example, a particular patient who is not warned of the consequences of research protocol or of a drug trial. Let us also say that another provider, or even a group of providers, is aware of this problem. It is obvious that the provider who is prescribing the treatment is at risk for malpractice through negligence. Still, are the providers who are aware of the problem and who do not intercede also negligent? We could argue convincingly that this is the case; in truth, however, malpractice claims are usually levied against the institution as well as the individual practitioner. Is this because the attorney understands that the institution has more money than does the individual provider? Maybe. But, the real issue here is that other professionals were aware of the situation and did not correct it. As providers, we have a moral, ethical, and legal duty to intervene.

Providers Who Refuse to Provide Care

Essentially, providers have the right to refuse to provide care if the interventions to be used stand in opposition to the provider's ethics or values. Additionally, if the provider feels incompetent to care for a patient, this refusal is supportable. If providers assume care that they are not competent to perform, they may be disciplined for incompetence or negligence.

There are other circumstances that may also surround providers' refusals to provide care: (1) physical risk (when there is strong evidence to suggest more than minimal risk to self), (2) rendered care that violates patient autonomy and rights to self-determinations, and (3) religious and/or moral issues that cause the provider to object. Most institutions will support a provider's personal objections, provided that these are stated well in advance and result in no harm or negative consequences for patients.

> A physician shall, in the provision of appropriate patient care, except in emergencies, be free to choose whom to serve, with whom to associate, and the environment in which to provide medical care. (Adopted by the AMA's House of Delegates, June 17, 2001)

While the duty to provide care is quite clear, providers' refusals to provide care are not infrequent occurrences. Early on in the AIDS epidemic, many providers expressed their fears, and even distaste, about caring for patients with AIDS. These fears, expressed as fear of AIDS contagion, were questioned because the chance of a provider contracting HIV infection was extremely small. These fears were often worsened by conflicting values and underlying prejudice against persons or groups who practiced risky behavior. As the epidemic spread into the heterosexual population, attitudes shifted somewhat; still, the ways in which the majority of people contract HIV in the United States (through intravenous drug use, unprotected sex with an intravenous drug user, or male homosexual sexual encounters) fuel a great deal of negative reaction in providers who cannot accept those lifestyles. In a recent study regarding stigma among healthcare providers (Kinsler, Wong, Sayles, Davis, and Cunningham, 2007) the concern that provider bias could result in serious consequences was raised. Essentially, stigma can affect healthcare utilization, and lack of access or delayed access to care may result in clinical presentation at more advanced stages of HIV disease. These authors called for interventions to reduce perceived stigma in the healthcare settings, which might include teaching by modeling nonstigmatizing behavior.

A provider's reluctance to care and refusal to care are frequently communicated to patients. This reluctance may be blatantly disloyal and may take the form of refusal to enter a patient's room, exaggerated protective measures, and even direct comments to patients, implying that they have some form of character weakness. It may also be covert (e.g., in little time spent with the patient and minimal communication responsiveness). Historically, provider refusal to provide care was viewed as unethical. Ethical codes focused on patients' rights, ignoring providers' values and beliefs, but times have changed. The shift toward recognizing providers' limits to providing care have largely been regarded positively, because forcing them to provide care would be detrimental to both patient and provider.

Limitations on Patients' Personal Choices

The doctrines of personal choice and informed consent originated largely from malpractice litigation. Historically, patients' rights to informed consent were blatantly violated; patients knew little of the nature of their treatment, outcomes, or alternative procedures (and/or the outcomes of no intervention).

There was no conceivable way in which they could enter into a personal cost–benefit analysis. To correct this situation, numerous changes occurred, but the outcomes of these changes did not respect the limitations of patient decision making. The President's Commission for the Study of Ethical Problems in Medicine and Biomedical and Behavioral Research (1983) recognized that patients' choices were not absolute. This limitation was described as irregularities in patients' requests such that they violated standards of practice or overtaxed clinical resources.

There are specific circumstances wherein providers' recommendations clearly need to be heeded in spite of contrary beliefs of patients. In these cases, it is appropriate for providers to make the final decision for action. Perhaps the most obvious situation is when the patient clearly and directly requests the provider to make the decision. In this case, it is important for providers to understand why the patient or patient's family has requested that the provider decide. There is at least one problem area in respect to the traditional deference given to providers. Some cultural groups are more likely to defer to authority figures. When their request is an unnecessarily dependent one, the provider has an obligation to engage the patient or patient's family more actively in the decision-making process. In any case, providers should not take the relinquishing of decision making by the patient lightly.

THE PROBLEMS WITH INFORMED CONSENT AND INFORMED CHOICE

Assumptions about Patients

The concept of informed choice and informed consent is based on the important assumption that the patient (and/or family) is adequately informed. Prerequisites are that the patient is willing, capable, and competent to receive the information. Questions that must be satisfied include:

- Does the patient have the ability to hear or read?
- Is the language used appropriately for his or her understanding?
- Is the method used to present the information respectful of the patient's age and educational level?
- Is the patient's attention span and memory sufficient enough to allow him or her to process the information?
- Will the patient clarify the information he or she cannot fully comprehend?
- Does he or she understand his or her rights to decide even if his or her decisions run counter to those of the provider?
- Does he or she have the ability to communicate his decisions and preferences?

Special Problems with Certain Patient Groups

It is important to recognize that all patients have handicaps in one or more of these areas. Patients' willingness to be informed, their abilities to receive and to process data, and their abilities to express themselves are due to many factors. These factors include illness; the effects of treatment; the psychological responses to illness and injury; trauma and crisis states generated by the awareness of a guarded prognosis; recency of diagnosis; and other personal demographic factors, including age, education, and sociocultural background. Historically, certain groups have been recognized because of their special limitations. These groups include the mentally impaired and developmentally delayed, the mentally ill, children, and the elderly. These groups are known to have limitations in one or more areas of communication (reception, processing, and/or expression of thoughts and feelings). A group that is particularly vulnerable to infringement of personal choice are those individuals who are institutionalized or imprisoned. In these cases, the freedom that patients can exercise in making choices, even if they are fully informed and communicated competently, may be severely restricted. Coercion, in the form of implied or expressed threat, is considered to be a factor in restricting choices, and, therefore, is an actual or potential threat to individual rights.

The problem that engages any patient groups who have known impairment is complicated further by instances in which patients belong to more than one group. For example, the elderly, mentally ill, and children with mental impairments may not be able to participate in the informed-consent, informed-choice process. Usually, family or court-appointed guardians represent patients in instances wherein healthcare decisions must be made.

Some providers, even when they attempt to fully inform patients, observe that patients do not want to know everything, and they prefer to defer to the provider. Although this may, in fact, be the case, it is not adequate justification for short-circuiting the process of informed consent. In many situations, short-circuiting can occur despite full and appropriate procedures to engage patients in the informed-consent process because informed consent forms can be prohibitive. They may be very long (three to eight pages), and they may express ideas in legal jargon unfamiliar to the patient. These elements add to a patient's resistance to hear and/or read in a comprehensive manner all of the information contained in the consent. For this reason, patients are always provided with their own copies of both the signed consent form and a copy of the Patient's Bill of Rights.

CONCLUSION

A lack of effective communication between providers and patients is at the root of the violations of patients' rights. Whether the problem is one of informed choice or informed consent, a lack of effective communication can lead providers into serious ethical, moral, and legal problems. Providers have an obligation to care and also to protect patients from harm. When the problems in communication are not a result of their interactions but involve encounters with other providers, there remains the obligation to intervene and change existing circumstances. If a patient does not know about treatment options, is not aware of the consequences of a chosen treatment, or feels that the choice provided is not a "real choice," patients' rights are in jeopardy.

Issues of standard communications are increasingly important in cases of informed choice and informed consent because of the medical and legal implications (Sharpe, 1994). Providers have not always been convinced of the patient's need for or desire to be told the details of their diagnosis, prognosis, or even alternatives for treatment. However, current Western medical practices place a high value on providing adequate and accurate truthful information to patients, which is indicative of the commitment to patient autonomy and participation in decision making (Gold, 2004).

Above all else, professionals are members of a moral community. This community is made stronger by the support of and adherence to standards of practice that protect patients' rights. The privileged nature of patient and provider relationships derives meaning from the morality of the health professions and healthcare system.

CHAPTER 21

The Privileged Nature of Patient and Provider Communications: Issues of Confidentiality, Anonymity, and Privacy

In the area of the confidentiality of patient's communications, what may be "right" in most instances, may be terribly wrong in others.
—Gwen van Servellen

CHAPTER OBJECTIVES

- Discuss the regulations surrounding the principle of protecting patient–provider confidentiality.
- Describe ways in which provider–patient communications are privileged.
- Discuss the strengths and limitations imposed by the principle of confidentiality.
- Discuss how anonymity and privacy can be maintained.
- Discuss the inability to provide absolute protection for confidentiality of patient–provider communications.
- Discuss alternatives to absolute confidentiality.

In the past 30 years, a great deal of attention has been given to the issues of privileged communications in relationships between patients and providers. The majority of this discussion has been sparked by two important and related issues: the confidentiality of the clinical and research process and infractions of patients' rights that reached the level of litigation. The issue of privileged communications in health care is extremely important in regard to patient–provider relationships. Many states have granted statutes that guarantee privileged communication for healthcare professionals. Still, these statutes have been challenged by arguments against privileged communication. A case in point centers around the threat of societal exposure to HIV. The argument addresses the issue of social good versus individual rights. That is, it is deemed essential to reveal certain health information that would otherwise be held confidential because reporting it is essential to protect society. A most notable example, where the rights to confidentiality were challenged, was in a landmark case in California (*Tarasoff v. Regents of the University of California*, 1974). This case set an important precedent in the United States and many other parts of the world. The critical incident involved a therapist who knew that a patient had homicidal thoughts toward a specific person but who did not warn the person who was in danger. The situation resulted in the stabbing to death of the targeted person. The patient (Mr. Poddar), seen at the college student health services, had confided to his psychiatrist, Dr. Moore, that he was going to kill Ms. Tarasoff when she returned from summer break.

Dr. Moore subsequently informed the campus police that he felt Poddar was dangerous and that he should be hospitalized involuntarily. The police picked up Poddar, but after questioning felt he had "changed his attitude" and released him after he promised to stay away from Tarasoff. He did not, and Ms. Tarasoff was not informed of the threat. It was also argued that the patient (Poddar) should have received involuntary hospitalization because of his threat to others. This landmark case established that despite the preservation of patient–provider communications, it was a therapist's duty to warn endangered parties if the patient intended to harm them. Thus, providers can be held liable for failing to inform appropriate people if their patient reveals a risk to self or against a specific named person.

In truth, the issue to disclose or not and protection of individual versus societal rights is not as straightforward as we could hope it to be. Each individual case must be evaluated with respect to the particular facts and consequences that surround the case. Absolute confidentiality, anonymity, and privacy cannot be guaranteed; however, protection of patient information must be respected and provided. Practices that do not reflect a conscious effort to provide for these rights are subject to severe ethical and moral scrutiny.

THE SACROSANCTITY OF PROVIDER–PATIENT COMMUNICATIONS

When patients seek medical intervention, they reveal very intimate details about themselves and their families. In fact, effective patient–provider relationships rely on the patient's willingness and ability to talk frankly and openly about their situations. The information may be denunciatory or incriminating. For many patients, this information has rested in the realm of secrecy. It is data that may not have been shared with any other individual. A great deal of the time, the information that patients divulge, because it is related to problems, causes them distress. It is generally recognized that professional healthcare providers have an explicit obligation to hold all information in confidence with the understanding that the patient's welfare and trust could be jeopardized by the disclosure of this confidential information (Stern, 1990).

Confidentiality

Confidentiality as it relates to professional patient–provider communications has the sole purpose of protecting the patient from unauthorized disclosures (Taylor and Adelman, 1989). Regulations and laws (both state and federal) surrounding the right for confidentiality have existed long before the Internet system was in place. Unfortunately, even before the Internet, not all providers took these regulations seriously. It is the patient's basic right to have his or her privacy respected. This privacy cannot be breached. Only the patient has the authority to release information in his or her medical record. Any breach in confidentiality, no matter how minor, can be construed as a grounds for mistrust and potential litigation and disciplinary action (American Medical Association [AMA], May 7, 2007).

This ethical principle is concerned with privacy, with secret knowledge, and with knowledge known only to a select few. *Confidential communication* refers to personal or private matters that are revealed to a provider, who cannot be compelled by law to repeat this communication or be a witness against the patient. Codes of professional ethics address the issue of confidentiality explicitly. Essentially, patients should be able to assume or be explicitly assured that their private communications with the professional will not be passed on to others, except in a few specific situations. Exceptions include the need for professionals to seek other professional opinions about the patient in consultation.

A field of practice that has addressed the issue of privileged communication in detail is that of mental health. There are precise stipulations governing conditions under which information can be disclosed. As previously explained in the discussion of *Tarasoff v. Regents of the University of California* (1974), in specific situations (e.g., psychiatric–patient encounters), the provider must disclose any threats that the patient has made to him- or herself, or to others. Generally, however, the guideline is that providers should disclose that which is needed and specifically requested. That is, the provider should and is allowed to keep in confidence those disclosures that are immaterial or irrelevant (Stern, 1990). Thus, unless otherwise specified, information about the patient's sexual preferences or fetishes would not be disclosed if deemed irrelevant.

On the issue of confidential written records, the provider has the obligation and duty to maintain patient records in a manner in which there is no reasonable chance of their getting lost, stolen, or falling into the hands of unauthorized persons. With the advent of e-records and e-mails between provider and patient, interpretations and guidelines are not so straightforward. However, it is just a matter of time before explicit restrictions and guidelines will specifically address this avenue of communication and disclosure.

Confidentiality, it would seem, is like anonymity, privacy, and other such phenomena. There are specific differences, however, and these differences have been addressed (Shah, 1970a). Essentially, confidentiality protects the patient from unauthorized disclosures of any sort by the professional without the informed consent of the patient.

Examples in which providers are or are not at liberty to reveal details to family members are cases of interest. Consider, for example, a terminally ill patient who expresses a desire to commit suicide; or a woman who, unbeknown to her husband, admits that she has had two therapeutic abortions; or a cancer patient who pulled her nasal-gastric tube out. What is the provider's obligation to keep this information confidential? And, confidential to whom and for what purposes? The ethical codes of professional organizations aim to safeguard the patient's right to confidentiality, even though it could be argued that the patient's significant other(s) may have an equal right to know this information. Professional ethics would support the sanctioning of any healthcare provider who violated the patient's rights to confidentiality in these instances, even if this meant only sharing this information with family members.

Other specific instances in which rules of confidentiality are taken extremely seriously include cases in which patients are the research human subjects. In research studies, the issues of confidentiality are clearly stated. Research subjects should not be identifiable (e.g., by name, Social Security number, medical record number); rather, another procedure (e.g., a code number or other method) should be used that is impossible to link with the subject.

On the chance that identifiable data (name, Social Security number, address, phone number) are obtained, the researcher must explain the specific procedures that will be used for collecting, processing, and storing data, including who will have access to the data and what will be done with the data when the study is completed.

The Health Insurance Portability and Accountability Act (HIPAA) privacy rule sets the standards for protecting individuals' medical records and other personal health information. It gives patients more control over their health information and sets boundaries on the use and release of health records, holding violators accountable with civil and criminal penalties that can be imposed if providers violate the patient's right to privacy. HIPAA requires that patients be notified of their privacy rights and of how their information may or may not be used. It was created to facilitate communication between healthcare organizations; however, the fears and misinterpretations of this act have also led to negative consequences. Despite the importance of this regulation in protection of patient confidentiality, concern has been raised that it may delay important information transmission to healthcare providers and may place the patient at risk. What might result is that misconceptions and misinterpretations of HIPAA are hampering communication among those who need to know, and patients may not be receiving the best treatment because vital information is not being shared. For more information on HIPAA see: http://www.hhs.gov/hipaafaq/about/187.html.

Privileged Communication

Historically, the doctrine of *privileged communication* simply meant that patients have a legal right by law to have their communications protected. This protection was very specific. That is, the patient has the legal right where that right exists, to not have his or her confidences revealed publicly from a witness stand during legal proceedings without his or her expressed permission. Through judicial interpretation, this protection can be extended to legislative and administrative proceedings as well. Privileged communication statutes exist to govern patient–provider communications in many, but not all, states. Currently, the physician–patient privilege is a recognized statute in 33 states and the District of Columbia. In states without such statutes, the right to privileged communication can be affirmed by common law on a case-by-case basis.

What is meant by patient–provider privilege is that the privilege is assigned only to the patient. They alone have the right to employ it. The privilege does not extend to a family member or provider. For example, providers must withhold information and cannot relinquish the information to protect themselves. It cannot be used in any way to enhance the well-being of another. For example, if the physician was engaged in litigation about a certain surgical procedure and her abilities to perform this procedure, she could not provide the attorney with information on other cases she attended because this would be an unauthorized use of the data in which the provider would be in a position to gain from the disclosure. When a patient dies, it is usually the case that the person that represents the patient (e.g., in a wrongful death case) usually has the power to waive the physician–patient privilege.

The history of privileged communication dates back to early English law, where the responsibility to testify in a court of law was the issue. Despite the stated duty to provide witnessed data, it was argued that some relationships were of sufficient importance that communications originating in these relationships should be privileged. Recent cases, such as those related to the AIDS epidemic, have reaffirmed the need for strict statutes pertaining to privileged communication. Arguments in favor of privileged communication include the need to promote patient disclosure, not only to adequately care for the patient but to ultimately reduce threat to others. It is logical, taking this argument into account, that the provider–patient interaction be protected to inspire trust and confidence both for the good of the individual and society at large. Under these conditions, confidence in providers is nurtured and a full account of symptoms is made available to the providers.

As has always been the case, the issue of privileged communication involves striking a balance between two important social values: (1) society's right to access information critical to fact finding and (2) the individual's right to privacy. But (as has been previously discussed) these principles are far from simple to apply in selected instances.

Anonymity and Privacy

Shah (1970b) states that the U.S. Supreme Court first recognized the "right to privacy" as an independent constitutional right in the case of *Griswold v. Connecticut* in 1965. This case concerned the unsuccessful attempt by the state of Connecticut to prevent by statute anyone, including married couples, from using contraceptive devices. In their decision against Connecticut, some of the Supreme Court justices claimed that the right to privacy was not to be found in any specific constitutional amendment but in the implications cast by several amendments (First, Third, Fourth, Fifth, and Ninth amendments). But how many times have healthcare providers themselves witnessed infractions of the principle of patients' rights to anonymity and privacy? The infractions occur so frequently that providers sometimes become insensitive and oblivious to them. *Anonymity* refers to the right of patients to have their identity protected from its being known to others. *Privacy* more generally refers to the right of the patient to limit any knowledge about himself or herself known to others.

Consider, for example, the pharmacist who speaks loudly to a person in the presence of several other people standing in line to pick up medications: "Mr. Smith, your Trizivir is not ready for pick up, can you come back in 20 minutes?" Trizivir is an anti-HIV medication in a category called nucleoside reverse transcriptase inhibitors (NRTIs) that prevents the development of new virus and decreases the amount of virus in the body as a whole. This specific information is about medications, but it could also include his diagnosis, explicitly or implicitly revealed; the patient's Social Security number; and the spelling of his first and last name. This would be a violation of patient rights, even though no one in line might recognize that it is prescribed because the patient has HIV/AIDS.

Consider also the medical resident or student nurse who discusses the details of a patient's case (revealing the patient's name) in a clinic or hospital elevator. If you watch such events you will notice that onlookers waiting nearby will turn their heads and look down or look away. People are aware that such data about another person are privileged and that they are not really entitled to know this information. The provider, however, appears oblivious to the situation. When this occurs, most people feel anger and concern but do not know how to deal with the situation. People waiting in line for their medications worry that this will happen to them and they may speak softly or withhold verbalizing information in hopes of decreasing the likelihood that their rights to privacy and confidentiality will be preserved. Assertive providers, such as the bystanders in the elevator scenario, may pull the violators aside and reprimand them for their misconduct. In either case, the patient could file a case against these providers, and it would be upheld in a court of law. Every patient who experiences a violation has the opportunity to file a health information privacy complaint with the Office for Civil Rights (OCR). There are many examples of this same infraction. Consider the patient in an outpatient clinic who is awaiting diagnostic-testing procedures. The receptionist broadcasts the name of the patient to the room of six to seven patients and family members. Having not obtained all the information initially, she requests the patient to call back to her (behind the desk) the reason for the diagnostic test, where the patient lives, and home and work phone numbers. Can we say that the information that is revealed publicly in these situations does not have to be confidential? Not so, given the rights of patients for anonymity and privacy. These infractions are serious ethical errors. Again, could the patient sue the provider, assistant, and/or healthcare facility? The answer is yes.

In general terms, the concept of privacy acknowledges the freedom of patients to pick and choose for themselves the time, circumstances, and, particularly, the extent to which they wish to share or withhold their identity, attitudes, opinions, beliefs, and current, past, or future behaviors. The right to privacy is not just the entitlement to have the curtain pulled during a physical exam or medical procedure, it is an affirmation of the importance of the uniqueness and individuality of patients and their desired freedom from unreasonable intrusion by others.

COMMON DILEMMAS AND ALTERNATIVE RESPONSES

Responsible actions by providers need to reflect the fact that with issues of privacy, confidentiality, and the privileged nature of patient–provider communications, dilemmas will always arise. In fact, as stated earlier, these issues are not translated into absolute terms. The particular facts and consequences of each individual case must be considered. Additionally, patients' bills of rights, professional codes of ethics, and the legal statutes of a specific state will influence the resolution of the dilemmas. However, the HIPAA regulations trump any state codes; they are national standards.

CONCLUSION

Patients who seek treatment reveal important intimate information that is known to very few or, often, to no one else. Some of this information or the meaning of the information may be out of the patient's immediate awareness. Thus, patients could be revealing not only data no one else knows but also data previously unknown to them. Because the provider uses techniques to promote patient self-disclosure, the chances of the patient revealing personal and private information are very high. Many times, the contents of this private and personal communication can be distressing or even self-incriminating. Therapeutic relationships with providers rely on both the patient's willingness to self-disclose as well as on the provider's skill in promoting patient self-disclosures. HIPAA, the first-ever federal privacy standard, regulates the disclosure of medical record information and other health information.

There are inherent professional obligations in patient–provider encounters to hold patients' communications, both written and verbal, in confidence. Although not absolute, these principles of confidentiality, anonymity, and privacy characterize professional–patient relationships. The patient's welfare and trust may be severely compromised by the disclosure of information provided in confidence or by the disclosure of identifying information to others outside the immediate circle of healthcare providers responsible for the patients' care. Exceptions do occur, particularly when the welfare of others is in question (e.g., when the patient is an immediate threat to himself or a specific other).

A full and detailed discussion of the principles and skills of therapeutic communications is appropriately closed by the affirmation of the special professional obligation that underlies the treatment of patient self-disclosures once they are effectively elicited.

PART VI

Transforming the Role of Communications in Health Care

Successful professional role development depends on our grasp of advanced issues in the use of healthcare communications. Theories of behavior change explain the use of communication principles in the context of a theoretical or conceptual framework. Knowledge of behavior change theories puts us at an advantage in understanding how communication skills and concepts fit within paradigms of knowledge. Healthcare communications are undergoing significant changes in the way in which they occur, the use of Internet communications being the most significant change in the last decade. There are important issues with Internet communications between patient and provider, and these are addressed in this section of the text. Finally, providers and patients alike are in positions to make changes to improve healthcare communications.

The role of healthcare systems in shaping health communications is clearly outlined. The structure of the healthcare system is less studied for its impact on the nature of communications between patients and providers and providers with one another; however, the structure of systems of care clearly influences communication and, subsequently, quality of care. The content and issues presented in this section of the text are compelling and will encourage the reader to further examine possibilities for change in the communications they observe in a variety of healthcare arenas.

Chapter 22, Health Communications to Enhance Behavioral Change, describes the role of communication in supporting behavior change in patients. The chapter describes and discusses specific theories guiding health promotion and disease prevention in groups of clients. These theories include Social Learning Theory, the Theory of Reasoned Action (TRA) and Theory of Planned Behavior (TPB), the Health Belief Model (HBM), the Transtheoretical Model of Change™, and the Social Ecological Model. With each framework, the provider, through relationships and communications, creates situations for change. Providers, friends, and family are sources of interpersonal influence that can encourage health promotion behaviors. When these influences are in agreement and are coupled with patients' sense of self-efficacy (believing they can make the change), patients are more likely to change their behavior in positive ways. When these sources of interpersonal influence offer conflicting views, even if the patient feels he or she can make a change, the change may not occur, or, if it does, it might not be sustained.

Chapter 23, Internet Use and Communications of Patients and Providers, addresses the newest intervention to alter the nature of patient–provider communications. Patients and their families will frequently turn to other sources for health information. They might seek out lay providers, advice from family or friends, or Internet sites (e.g., search engines, including chat rooms). This chapter reviews the various uses of Internet communications that have implications for information exchange and support to patients and their families. The discussion includes the advantages of Internet sources to build credible information and serve to expand patients' readiness to participate interactively in making healthcare decisions. It also addresses the downside, which is the potential for inaccurate information or exchanges that may be counter to the productive communication between patient and the healthcare provider. A critical issue surrounding patients' use of the Internet is that communication that should occur in a specific encounter with the provider may be heard in an inappropriate venue. It is clear that delivery channels affecting the way providers communicate and what information patients receive will have a growing impact on future communications between providers and patients.

Chapter 24, Altering Systems of Care to Enhance Health Care Communications, examines the many ways systems of care influence and shape communications with healthcare providers. Providers and communities alike, independently or collectively, are in a position to make at least minor changes in the organization of care delivery to enhance therapeutic communication. This chapter discusses various system-level factors that promote therapeutic communication (e.g., the impact of continuity in building therapeutic alliances). A report of findings from selected research studies and a description of the program of change are described. Examples such as transitional care, telephone-based continuing care, and systematic care are discussed, and the methods of communication between provider and patients/families are detailed.

CHAPTER 22

Health Communications to Enhance Behavioral Change

Drugs don't work in patients who don't take them.
—U.S. Surgeon General C. Everett Koop

CHAPTER OBJECTIVES

- Identify key theoretical models that explain behavior change.
- Discuss key principles of the humanistic movement.
- Discuss key principles underlying the social learning model.
- Discuss key principles of the Transtheoretical Model of Change.
- Discuss key principles of the Theory of Reasoned Action and the Theory of Planned Behavior.
- Discuss key principles of the Health Belief Model.
- Discuss key principles of the Social Ecological Model.
- Consider obesity as a health problem, and differentiate the approaches each theory might recommend to support behavioral change.
- Identify concepts common in each model.

A good deal of what health providers do is to communicate in ways that promote behavioral change. Helping patients change behaviors is an important aspect of the role, yet few providers have an understanding of the dynamics of patient behavior change. Historically, patient–provider communication has been viewed as an art unique to the particular patient in response to the approach to the provider. Over the past 50 years or more, there have been a number of theories or analytical models put forth to enable us to better understand how providers can communicate to derive the most effective outcomes of behavior change. These theories are not altogether different from one another, but there are usually a number of assumptions or principles that set them apart.

In this chapter, several models of communication to elicit behavioral change are described and illustrated. Of particular concern are communications that promote lifestyle changes to encourage health promotion and disease prevention. The social behavioral models that will be discussed in this chapter include, but are not limited to: social learning theory, the Theory of Reasoned Action (TRA) and the Theory of Planned Behavior (TPB), the Health Belief Model (HBM), the Transtheoretical Model of Change™, and the Social Ecological Model. Within each paradigm are certain skills and knowledge that help the provider focus communications toward a spirit of changing behavior. Providers and researchers have developed an array of interventions that spring from theories of behavior change and target social support, provider–patient interaction, self-efficacy, and coping. These interventions have a basis in a wide variety of behavioral change theories, some of which clearly overlap. The following is a description of the frameworks and models and specific advances that have affected the way providers interact with patients.

THEORETICAL FRAMEWORKS AND MODELS OF BEHAVIOR CHANGE

We know what we have to do: *eat healthy, stop smoking, don't use drugs, and exercise*. But, how is this done? Theoretical or conceptual models provide answers that can guide providers' responses to patients. Of late, there has been a considerable amount of interest in how to create change in behavior: such as with smoking cessation, alcohol abuse, healthy eating, and increasing physical activity. *Healthy People 2010* (http://www.healthypeople.gov/About/goals.htm) proposed two overarching goals: to increase quality and years of healthy life and to eliminate health disparities among different segments of the population. The first goal—to help individuals of all ages improve their life expectancy and quality of life—has direct implications for providers to implement and evaluate their approach to helping individuals and families changing unhealthy behaviors.

Integral to understanding theories of behavioral change are specific principles of change theory:

1. Change happens incrementally. Change is rarely a single event or something accomplished over a specific period of time. Change is ongoing; therefore, it is of particular importance to consider that you are interacting with individuals at a specific point in an ongoing process.
2. Permanent change is not likely to occur if the motivation to change is not internalized. Thus, simply telling the patient that they must or should change is not likely to create the change that is needed.
3. Reinforcement motivates individuals either to continue or discontinue behavior and behavior change. Reinforcement can be negative or positive. For example, voicing to patients that they did a good job in starting to make changes is likely to motivate them to continue.
4. Individuals' motivation to change is integrally bound to their perceptions of the need to change. Providers, in part, are agents for cues to action. When voicing the need to change, the provider brings patients' needs to the forefront.
5. Social environment (social network and social support system) has a direct effect on the individual's desire to change and maintenance of the behavioral change. Patient changes are reinforced not only by the provider but the social environment. If the provider and social network agree in the need to change, the patient is more likely to attempt a change. Dissonance between the provider and environment is likely to yield confusion.
6. Persons must believe in their ability to execute the behavior change if they are to approach change (intention to change). Self-efficacy (belief in one's capacities to change) motivates patients to try or continue a

behavior change. Expressed support and confidence in the patient to change will also enhance behavior change.

As each of the theoretical models is discussed, it will become clear that there is a good deal of similarity in the models of understanding and motivating behavioral change. A background description of the field of human psychology helps lay the foundation for understanding current models.

The study of behavioral change and how to enhance change has a long history dating back to early thoughts of behavior and what to do to eradicate undesirable expressions. Psychology and psychiatry, particularly those models of personality theory, are most credited for change theory. Among these theorists is Carl Rogers (1902–1987) from the field of humanistic psychology. The principles of Rogers's personality change theory (1959, 1961, 1977, 1994 [posthumously, with Freiberg]) have affected providers' approaches to patients and can still be observed in providers' responses to patients. Rogers's view of change evolved from his overriding belief that humans have an underlying *actualizing tendency* and will approach change as a natural result of this tendency. Several theorists in this category of creating change would agree that self-acceptance is key to growth, and unconditional positive regard nurtures change. Rogers's person-centered approach is most obvious today in the belief that motivation to change requires an individual approach to the patient. In 1982, *American Psychologist* ranked Rogers number 1 out of the 10 most influential psychotherapists.

Rogers put considerable faith in the individual's experiential learning, which he thought could be facilitated by the provider's approach. Rather than thinking he could solve the problems for the client, he believed that clients could solve their own problems and that doing this creates the change to make the client better. The role of provider as facilitator (or teacher as Rogers described) would include (1) setting a positive environment for learning, (2) clarifying the purpose of the learning with the client, (3) organizing and making available learning resources, (4) balancing both intellectual and emotional aspects of learning, and (5) sharing thoughts and feelings with clients without dominating the conversation (Retrieved from http://www.tip.psychology.org/rogers.html).

One of Rogers's most well-known techniques is *rephrasing* (the belief that knowledge comes from within). Otherwise, instead of answering a patient's question directly, he would rephrase the question and ask the patient what he thought. (*Note:* A fuller description of the technique of rephrasing or restatement is provided in Chapter 11.) Not only would he ask the patient the question, he would then ask the client how he felt about the answer. (Retrieved from http://www.enotes.com/psychology-theories/rogers-carl-ransom.) Rogers devoted his time to improving communications between clients and health care providers.

I. Focus on the actualizing tendency:

Instead of:

"Well I don't seem to convince you that if you don't control your diet, things are going to get worse." *Consequence:* Patient feels hopeless and shameful that they are unable to satisfy the provider's expectation.

Use:
"I know you are moving toward changing your diet . . . it's what you want to do . . . but, it is taking time. . . . I believe you will find a way." *Consequence:* Patient may ask for resources and explore small steps which are more realistic.

II. Rephrasing
Instead of:
"What do you mean you can't change your diet?" *Consequence:* Patient is unconvinced that they can change their diet.
Use:
"You are saying you can't change your diet." *Consequence:* Patient takes ownership of the problem and is encouraged to explore the reasons.

While Rogers's work influenced the early foundations of humanistic psychology, the literature addressing his theory and the empirical evidence is limited. Most often researchers will use a qualitative design using his general principles. Much progress has been made in both the development of behavior change theories and evidence supporting or showing mixed results using these theoretical frameworks. Current theories of planned behavioral change explore the importance of internal motivation and the potential of individuals to make changes in light of internal and external barriers and facilitators. We begin with a description of social learning theory.

SOCIAL LEARNING AND SOCIAL COGNITIVE THEORY

Social learning theory maintains that change occurs in the context of a cost–benefit analysis, where the consequences of changing offset any negative consequences that the change may produce. Environmental factors, personal factors, and attributes of the behavior itself all affect the process of behavior change. These factors act both independently and interdependently on the change process (e.g., patients' environments, which include social resources, have a direct impact on patient behavior change, social resources, patients' personal skills and knowledge in turn affect behavior change). Social cognitive theories combine social learning theory and cognitive behavioral approaches. Social cognitive theories emphasize the importance of considering the individuals' subjective perceptions of situations and interpretations of the meaning of events. All groups of individuals are influenced by the norms, beliefs, and ways of behaving consistent with their social reality. Behavior change can be approached or avoided, depending on the support of the groups with which the individual affiliates. Lack of support and encouragement may cause individuals to be uninterested in change.

A critical principle of social learning theory is the concept of self-efficacy. *Self-efficacy* refers to the belief individuals have that they can actually perform a certain behavior or behavior change. Self-efficacy—a sense that one has control over one's environment and behavior—is said to predict intention to change and maintenance of change after it is implemented. In Bandura's vision, "self-efficacy is the belief in one's capabilities to organize and execute the sources of action required to manage prospective situations" (Bandura, 1986). According to Bandura (1997), a personal sense of control enhances behavioral change. Self-efficacy also affects how goals will be set, with persons having a low sense of self-efficacy expressing goals in hopeless ways. Individuals with high levels of self-efficacy may create more challenging goals.

While Bandura did not conceive a general overall sense of self-efficacy (it was conceived in the context of a specific situation), it is possible to think about self-efficacy in a more global context. To measure general self-efficacy, a provider would ask how confident a person feels—"I am certain that I can do most things"—and the required response could range from "definitely not" to "exactly true." An example from the general self-efficacy (GSE) scale (Schwarzer and Jerusalem, 1995) would be: "When I am confronted with a problem, I can usually find several solutions." However, to make the measurement more situation specific, you would ask the patient to respond to such items as "I am certain that I can lose weight, even if I have periods where I eat unhealthy things" or "I can manage to stick with healthful foods, even if I have to try several times until it works" (the nutrition self-efficacy scale; Bagozzi and Edwards, 1998). In the literature there are numerous specific self-efficacy measures: smoking cessation self-efficacy, condom use self-efficacy scale (Brafford and Beck, 1991), physical exercise self-efficacy measures (Fuchs, 1996), and an alcohol resistance self-efficacy scale.

For social cognitive theorists, two essential aspects of the behavior change must be tracked over time: (1) the intention to change a behavior and (2) the actual behavior. These are not always congruent in that someone may have high intentions to change but the behavior suggests the intention is very low. Self-efficacy is important to both because self-efficacy is said to influence intentions to change as well as resultant behavior.

According to Bandura (2000), the paths of influence through which perceived self-efficacy affect other social cognitive factors is complex. For example, self-efficacy might have a direct impact on behavior but factors such as *outcome expectations*, goals, and sociostructural factors (facilitators or impediments) would mediate the relationship of self-efficacy and goal setting. For example, perceived impediments might predominate in the patient's view of behavior change. This would influence the patient's goal setting toward choosing weak goals or no goals at all.

The role of the provider in influencing how patients perceive the need to change, the goals they set, and their attitudes toward impediments to change is critical. Communications with providers can be relatively perceptive to the patient's views and considerations, and when there is just the right amount of empathy and understanding, providers can help patients navigate the change process. Perceived self-efficacy plays a role in the beginning, when the patient is developing goals for behavior change, and in the maintenance stage, when self-efficacy to maintain the change is in question.

Using principles of social and cognitive-behavioral learning, providers might select from a number of communication strategies that would build on patient self-efficacy and assess how feelings of self-efficacy might fluctuate over time.

For example, an area of assessment would be the patient's beliefs about being able to change an unhealthy behavior, how the unhealthy behavior plays a role in everyday life, what the *impediments* and *facilitators* are:

> *"Tell me about your overeating: when, how often, what seems to work and not work."*
> *"How much do you want to stop overeating?"*
> *"How much do you believe you can control overeating?"*
> *"What might stand in the way of being able to control overeating?"*
> *"What can help you to keep on track?"*

This line of inquiry demonstrates empathy and understanding and can help patients feel they have support in the change process and that, with the provider's continued interest, they may reduce the barriers they face.

A number of studies have examined the use of social cognitive behavioral learning and prediction of behaviors. Among these is the important work of Christiansen and colleagues (2002), who examined the impact of positive and negative outcome expectancies on heavy alcohol use, which indicated that positive outcome expectancies were significantly related to heavy alcohol use among college students. Others expanded this work and were able to show positive expectancy and drinking refusal self-efficacy were strongly related to college student drinking (Young et al., 2006). Using social cognitive theory, Rovniak and colleagues (2002) studied the potential predictors of physical activity among university students. They examined the impact of social support, self-efficacy, outcome expectancies, and perceived self-regulation on engagement in physical activity. Perceived self-efficacy had the largest effect on self-reported physical activity, mediated by self-regulation, which directed predicted activity. Also, social support affected activity through its relationship to self-efficacy. In sum, social support, self-regulation, and self-efficacy were important factors in explaining whether university students would participate in physical activity. Dilorio and colleagues (2000) studied condom use behaviors among college students, testing the predictive value of several social cognitive variables (self-efficacy and outcome expectancies, in addition to anxiety). Self-efficacy (belief that one could use condoms) was directly related to condom use behaviors and indirectly through its impact to lower anxiety. However, anxiety was not directly related to condom use behaviors. For the most part, these studies provided support for the social cognitive behavioral model.

THEORY OF REASONED ACTION AND THEORY OF PLANNED BEHAVIOR

A major concern of all behavioral change theorists is *why do people behave the way they do and how do we influence them to change.* The Theory of Reasoned Action (TRA) was first developed in 1967 by Martin Fishbein and then revised and expanded by Azjen and Fishbein in 1975, 1977, and 1980. The roots of this theory are from social psychology with an emphasis on how individuals' attitudes affect behavior. The major premise is that attitude and behavior are positively correlated. An individual's belief that a behavior leads to certain outcomes and positive attitudes about these outcomes influence attitudes toward the behavior, which in turn influence performance of behavior. Only some attitudes are influential in this way, and these are referred to as *salient attitudes* formed from salient beliefs toward an outcome. Attitudes, subjective norms, intentions, and behavior are the primary concepts of TRA.

Attitudes are influenced by the opinions of others, and *intentions* shape behavior. Intention is the probability that the individual will perform a behavior, which is influenced by both attitudes and subjective norms. *Subjective norms* are what the individual perceives others will think of the behavior. For example, subjective norms about illicit drug use among substance abusers is that drug use is OK. Other substance abusers form the normative beliefs of the individual and the degree to which the behavior change will occur. Otherwise, if the norms are to *use*, then drug-using behavior is in concert with the individual's norms. Intentions are the individual's reported statement of the likelihood that he or she will perform the behavior.

Although Fishbein recognized that other factors may influence behavior (e.g., demographic characteristics), he believed that those factors would not be important in the context of things unless they had affected the individual's attitudes or normative beliefs. Any given behavior is a product of intention to action influenced by the individual's attitude toward the behavior and anticipated outcome of performing the behavior. That is, the person with an intention is likely to perform the behavior provided that the attitude about the behavior and subjective norms support the behavior. The following is an example of how this theory is operationalized:

Attitude: *"I think eating and not exercising is bad for me."*
Subjective norm: *"Other people I know tell me I need to lose weight."*
Intention: *"I want to do things to lose weight."*
Behavior: *"I am going to start an eating and exercise program to help me lose weight. And, if that doesn't work, I will ask my doctor for advice."*

Perhaps the most noteworthy strength of this model is that it is simplistic and has been shown to support interventions for behavior change in a number of populations (e.g., weight loss, condom use, and preventing sun exposure). A major weakness of this theory is the presumption that behavior is under volitional control and that there is a reasoning process that occurs that is systematic and always follows a particular route. Behaviors that are spontaneous and not thought out are not explained by this framework. Also, the pattern of variance in behavior is not fully addressed in this framework. To correct for these limitations, Ajzen revised the model to incorporate other variables (e.g., how difficult the behavior change is and whether the individual perceives that he or she will be successful in changing). The revision of the original TRA model is described as the Theory of Planned Behavior (Schifter and Ajzen, 1985). Thus, TPB which appeared in the 1980s, is an extension of TRA. TPB views behavior change as a result of the interaction of three constructs: attitude, subjective norms, and perceived behavioral control (self-efficacy as interpreted here). Subjective norms are the perceived social expectations about what is valued or accepted in the individual's social network.

Studies by Quo and colleagues (2007), Sable and colleagues (2006), and Onibokun (2002), using different populations and different target behaviors, illustrate the application of the TRA model. In Quo and colleagues' study of smoking behavior in Chinese adolescents, the applicability of TRA and TPB were tested. Although they thought TPB was superior to TRA, they also found that TRA can better predict smoking among students with lower (rather than higher) perceived behavior control. The independent effects of attitudes about smoking and perceived norms on smoking behavior were partially mediated by intention, pointing to the utility of TRA factors in predicting behavior. Sable and colleagues examined physician behavior in prescribing contraceptives to a largely female population seen in emergency room settings. They found that high intentions to prescribe contraceptives were positively associated with attitudes toward doing so and with the perception that their colleagues and professional groups support prescribing condoms. Onibokun studied the risk behaviors of female commercial sex workers in Nigeria and found support for the utility of TRA. Results of the multiple regression analysis revealed that those who perceived subjective norms to be more supportive of condom use (others they respected supported using condoms) and had favorable attitudes toward their use were more likely to report firm intentions to use condoms in the next three months. Key normative influences in this case referred to their sexual partners and peers.

THE HEALTH BELIEF MODEL

The Health Belief Model (HBM) originated from the work of Rosenstock, Strecher, and Becker (1988) and at the time was considered a social learning model that contributed an expanded view of motivation to change incorporating beliefs and perceptions of individuals that speaks to motivation as an underlying propelling element affected by a logical examination of the need for change. The HBM rests on general principles of behavior change in response to perceptions of the likelihood of illness. There are four critical areas: (1) perception of the severity of a potential illness or disease, (2) individual's perceived susceptibility to a given illness, (3) the benefits of taking action, and (4) the barriers to taking action. The model also includes a concept—*cues to action*—that is an important element in eliciting and maintaining behavior change. Cues to action may be as simple as a note posted on the refrigerator to remind a person about eating vegetables and fruit or more complex such as the cues subtly played out in a social situation in which everyone is slim and is avoiding the unhealthy foods attractively set at the table. Perceived threat is activated by cues to action. The concept of self-efficacy, discussed earlier for social learning theory, has been added to the Health Belief Model. Self-efficacy beliefs in this model help explain why, when severity and susceptibility are believed to be high, benefits are clear and barriers are minimal but an individual has little hope in their being able to successfully accomplish the behavioral change.

The distinct approach of the HBM is that behavior is seen as a result of rational appraisal of needs, benefits, and barriers. It presumes that individuals do not act but through the logical analysis of disease and illness using an empirical process. High perceived threat, low barriers, and high perceived benefits will increase the likelihood of participation in the recommended behavior change. There is some disagreement about whether susceptibility is more important than perceived threat because perceived severity has a weaker association with taking action than the perception that one is at risk. The essence of this model is that all elements interact to result in action or no action. Consideration of other important mediating factors (e.g., age, socioeconomic status, and other socio-psychological variables) does not have an active place in this theory.

Using the HBM, Lin and colleagues (2005) wanted to examine its utility in predicting sexual behaviors in Taiwanese immigrants. Students completed an online survey which asked them about several health belief factors and their sexual behaviors. HBM variables, as a set, predicted participants' sexual behavior (number of partners and frequency of intercourse). Although the study had several limitations in measurement, the authors suggested that self-efficacy be targeted in this group and that both measures and interventions be culturally sensitive. An interesting application of the HBM was applied to clinic appointment keeping among persons with chronic illness. Mirotznik and colleagues (1998) explained that although there has not been major support for the use of HBM, they thought it useful to examine the framework as it applies to keeping appointments for systemic lupus erythematosus (SLE), which, unlike some chronic illnesses, is potentially fatal. As expected with the use of this model, they found that perceived severity of this condition and general health motivation were uniquely associated with intent to keep appointments as well as the number of scheduled appointments kept (using medical record data during a 12-month retrospective period). The authors noted the limitation of modest effect sizes and recommended future studies. A third study applied the HBM to prevention of osteoporosis in Iranian middle school girls. Hazavehei and colleagues (2007) reported that mean scores for those in their health education program, modeled after HBM, showed increased knowledge about osteoporosis, perceived susceptibility, perceived severity of the condition, perceived benefits of reducing risk factors, and perceived benefits of taking health action. Mean scores in the education group not modeled after HBM showed improvement in knowledge and perceived susceptibility. And those in the third group without a specific education program in osteoporosis showed no significant changes on the HBM components. The authors were optimistic about the use of a theory-based educational program to induce behavior change for disease prevention in this group.

TRANSTHEORETICAL MODEL OF CHANGE

The Transtheoretical Model (TTM) of Change, first described by Prochaska and colleagues (1983, 1985, 1992, 1993, 1997), is also known as the Stages of Change Model (Zimmerman, Olsen, and Bosworth, 2000). Like many of the behavioral change models, this model can be used to both describe and change behavior. There are two major constructs in this model: stages of change and processes of change.

Essentially, the TTM theory proposes that change occurs as spiral processes of change. These are called stages and include:

1. Pre-contemplation.
2. Contemplation.
3. Preparation (for action).
4. Action.
5. Maintenance.

The TTM has been widely used in the literature to describe and track patients' readiness to change. In keeping with this model, providers need to use stage-specific approaches. That is, if someone is in the pre-contemplation stage, they are not just beginning to be exposed to information about the need to change, but they have not yet considered that this information really applies in their situation. It is the task of the provider to point out how this information does apply to them. Likewise, when a patient is taking action to change unhealthy eating behaviors, it would be inappropriate to focus solely on bringing the patient to considering making a change. The more appropriate approach would be to acknowledge that the patient is taking action and that there may be unanticipated barriers that are interfering with his or her progress. Thus, the communication between the patient and provider is stage specific. Teaching skills and providing knowledge is important in every stage of change, but the actual content can also be stage specific. Once the patient has taken action to change a behavior, then appropriate knowledge and skill would be controlling triggers that bring on negative behaviors.

This model is most useful in exploring the underlying components of long-term changes and thus changes related to the prevention and management of chronic illness. It may be difficult for providers to engage in long-term changes for two reasons: (1) they may not see themselves as the only or only ongoing provider that will make the difference, and (2) the prospect of long-term change may appear overwhelming to them, and they might overestimate the steps that need to occur to cause even the most minor change.

An offshoot of the Transtheoretical Model is an interviewing process called *motivational interviewing*. Rather than a distinct theory, motivational interviewing describes an approach based on theories of change stages (Miller and Rollnick, 1991). Like the Transtheoretical Model, motivational interviewing looks at changing behavior in stages. It is an approach to facilitating patient change with the understanding that providers are interacting with patients on some level of the continuum. It is critical for providers and patients to understand that change is contingent on motivation but motivation is not sufficient to create change.

Miller and Rollnick (1991, 2002) developed a template for appropriate interactions with patients based on change stages, and it is perhaps most useful in the early stage of change when motivation is critical. Motivational interviewing is most important in promoting motivation for change and relies on specific approaches to achieve changes in a wide variety of life issues beyond the specific targeted change. Three specific concepts are inherent in providing motivation for change: expression of empathy, developing discrepancy, and rolling with resistance. Like many behavioral theories, this model was developed out of dissatisfaction with current alternative models. The idea that the health provider should confront the patient with the worst possible scenario to cause change is alien to this approach.

In keeping with TTM of *change*, rather than confrontation or persuasion, providers need to foster an environment in which individuals are encouraged to engage in self-exploration and contemplation of change. The outcome is improved motivation to change because the perception of the need to change comes directly from the patient rather than the health provider. The idea is that together, the patient and provider are examining the need for change and that without bringing the patient along in decisions about change, there can be no effective long-standing approach to the targeted behavior change. The application of motivational interviewing is problematic in that a single expression from the patient of a desire to change may not mean that the provider and patient are ready to move on. Take for example, the individual addicted to prescription pain medication who approaches the provider with the intention to change. Perhaps he or she has been confronted by a family member or has been arrested for possession of drugs and is feeling both panic and motivation to change. Taken simply, the provider using motivational interviewing would view this state as positive because the patient is motivated to make a change. However, the provider may come to learn that the readiness to change is not fully integrated, and this momentary motivation to change is short-lived.

As with other behavioral change models, TTM has been used to predict and substantiate the usefulness of intervention programs based on the theory. Di Noia and colleagues (2006) studied the fruit and vegetable consumption behaviors among economically disadvantaged African American adolescents. The results of this study gave support to the fact that the stages of *action* and *maintenance* were different from beginning stages. Participants found to be in the action–maintenance stages reported higher levels of pros and lower cons as well as higher self-efficacy and greater consumption of fruits and vegetables than participants said to be in the pre-contemplation and contemplation–preparation stages, suggesting movement toward better behaviors in the later stages of the change process. This investigator suggested that with replication, the TTM could be appropriate in designing interventions to increase fruit and vegetable consumption among these youth. Johnson and colleagues (2006) examined the usefulness of an intervention built on TTM to improve adherence and increase exercise and diet in an adult population receiving treatment. They substantiated the effectiveness of the program in moving intervention subjects from the pre-action stage to the action and maintenance stages for adherence at the end of the 18-month randomized clinical trial. Further, those who were in the treatment group were more likely to progress to the action and maintenance stages for exercise and dietary fat reduction.

BEHAVIORAL OR SOCIAL ECOLOGICAL MODEL

The evolution of behavior change theory has been heavily influenced by a concentration on the individual (perceptions, attitudes, beliefs, intentions, personal norms, and self-actualizing capacities). The Behavioral Ecological Model was articulated early on by McLeroy and colleagues (1988), who hypothesized that multiple levels have to be considered in the change process. Emphasizing behavior change at the individual level can create bias and blinding to factors that are also critical in considering behavioral change and program intervention (e.g., sociocultural and physical environmental factors that also influence behavior change). The Social Ecological Model, sometimes referred to as the Behavioral Ecological Model, places these factors on a scale equal to individual skills and knowledge and intentions to change. Otherwise, physical and sociocultural supports have much to do with producing change in individuals' behaviors. Exercising is more likely if there are places to exercise (free gyms, parks, bicycle paths, etc.). Environmental conditions can significantly influence exercise behavior.

The basic premise behind the Social Ecological Model is that change is more likely if the approach is at both a macro and micro level, where attention is placed simultaneously on the physical and cultural environment. Such an approach would include intrapersonal, interpersonal, group, institutional, community and public policy factors. Effective intervention would include consideration of multiple levels of intervention (e.g., transportation, accessibility of program, motivation to enroll, family support to enroll, and racial and cultural factors).

The studies selected to illustrate the application of the Social Ecological Model address communications about cancer, influencing women to join WIC programs (Supplemental Nutrition Program for Women, Infants, and Children), and suggesting a pathway to target the obesity pandemic. These articles include either databased research or policy implications. Patrick, Intille, and Zabinski (2005) provide a compelling exposé about the impact of computer-supported interactive media on etiology, prevention, early detection, treatment, and post-treatment survival. Recent technology directs us to examine other influences that rely only on psychosocial and cognitive theories. These latter approaches may lack meaningful evaluation of the potential effect of a wide range of environmental factors, which is unfortunate in an era of increasing understanding of the complex relationships of genetic, behavioral, and environmental factors in the cause of cancer. The Social Ecological Model's multiple levels and interactions are key, and it is this theory that is more inclusive of many elements of the environment both at the micro and macro levels. Patrick and colleagues cite the example of tobacco use and the many important elements that need to be addressed to target this problem. Recognition of the limitations of intrapersonal and interpersonal factors alone for health behavior change—as in alcohol use, obesity, and physical activity—are leading the movement in the application of social ecological frameworks to research, practice, and policy.

Debate and Pyle (2003) used the Behavioral Ecological Model to assess what predicted women's early use of the WIC. Their findings indicated that cultural, intrapersonal, and interpersonal contingencies and perceived systemic barriers influenced WIC enrollment. They urged that in building programs of this kind, attention should be given to personal, cultural, but also environmental influences.

In an analysis of approaches to effectively examine the obesity pandemic, Egger and Swinburn (1997) discuss the environment as a co-conspirator in the obesity epidemic. They claim that previous views that regarded obesity as a personal disorder that required treatment must be reconsidered as a normal response to an abnormal environment, stating that understanding and altering the "obesogenic" environment must be attended to. The model presented in this article is a classic approach to examination of factors outside the individual's domain of control.

Interventions that simultaneously influence these multiple levels and multiple settings may be expected to lead to greater and longer-lasting changes and maintenance of existing health-promoting habits. The Social Ecology Model has significant implications for future interventions. Using this model, communications at a much larger level (governmental, community-level, widescale broadcasting) would be an important influence on patients' desires, intentions, and actions to modify unhealthy behaviors. Providers need only to examine recent nationwide weight loss and exercise campaigns to understand the importance of this level of communication and behavior change.

CONCLUSION

Theories of behavior change may be useful to clinicians, provided they know of them and can apply them to their particular patient population. Many theoretical frameworks overlap. For example, the concept of self-efficacy is addressed in the Social Cognitive Theory but again in the Theory of Planned Behavior (TPB), the Transtheoretical Model (TTM), and the Theory of Reasoned Action (TRA). In each theory, the role of self-efficacy may play a more or less prominent role. The fact that self-efficacy appears in multiple cases should not be a criticism. It may be indicative of the importance of the phenomena across several domains.

Despite their importance to an understanding of the behavioral change process, there may be a number of reasons that theories or conceptual frameworks are not applied. First, there is some support for these theories, but in several instances the findings are mixed. Second, because behavioral theories overlap, providers may think that there are no unique theories, just a few major principles that seem to reappear. Third, providers may have difficulty using the theories because they do not capture the full significance of behavior change as they see it. There have been criticisms that behavioral theories have heretofore neglected consideration of situational variables, physical, social, and economic factors (e.g., poverty and poor access to care). A framework that has emerged from this criticism is the Social Ecological Model that maintains that many factors influence behavioral change, not just psychosocial phenomena, which are somewhat difficult to observe and measure. In certain populations, environmental factors may have as much or more influence than behavioral science variables. Of particular concern is that theories may limit our vision to the extent that we ignore problems that do not fit the theory in question.

There is a movement nationwide to construct theories of change that will be useful in an analysis of change over time, not just in isolated short-term increments. Management of chronic illness, for example, requires a long-term perspective on multiple behavioral changes, and concerns about the use of current theories are that these theories have been found to be insufficient in predicting and guiding behavior change over time. Many of these theories stop

Table 22–1 Social and Behavioral Theories of Behavioral Change

Theoretical/ Conceptual Framework	*Key Concepts and Principles*	*Patient Behavior Change Targets*	*Studies Using Framework*
Social and Cognitive Behavioral Model	Perceived self-efficacy	Physical activity	Rovniak et al. (2002). Determining predictors of physical activity in university students.
	Behavioral intentions	Alcohol use	Christiansen et al. (2002). Alter college students' heavy alcohol use.
	Outcome expectancies	Condom use	Dilorio et al. (2000). Understanding condom use among college students.
Theory of Reasoned Action (TRA) and Theory of Planned Behavior (TPB)	Attitude toward behavior	Smoking behavior	Quo et al. (2007). Smoking behavior in Chinese adolescents.
	Behavioral intention	Physician contraception prescription practices	Sable et al. (2006). Physician intention to prescribe emergency contraceptives.
	Subjective norms Control beliefs	Risk for transmitting sexual diseases among sex workers	Onibokun (2002). Risks for transmitting sexual diseases and HIV among sex workers in Nigeria.
Health Belief Model (HBM)	Perceived susceptibility Perceived seriousness of disease	Building osteoporosis prevention programs	Hazavehei et al. (2007). Osteoporosis prevention education among Iranian middle school girls.
	Perceived benefits of behavior change	Clinic appointment-keeping in those with chronic illness	Mirotznik et al. (1998). Using the Health Belief Model to explain clinic appointment keeping in chronic disease management.
	Perceived barriers to change Cues to action	HIV risk behaviors	Lin et al. (2005). Predicting HIV risk behaviors among Taiwanese immigrants to the United States.
Transtheoretical Model (TTM) of Change	Five stages of change Linear stages of change occur in linear fashion	Unhealthy eating	Di Noia et al. (2006). Changing fruit and vegetable consumption among economically disadvantaged adolescents.
	Specific patient behaviors evidenced in each stage Stage-specific interventions	Lipid lowering	Johnson et al. (2006). Lipid lowering through intervention to increase exercise and diet and improve treatment adherence among adults.

continues

Table 22–1 Continued

Theoretical/ Conceptual Framework	*Key Concepts and Principles*	*Patient Behavior Change Targets*	*Studies Using Framework*
		Drug use in treatment-seeking adults	Gossop et al. (2007). Decreasing drug use among treatment-seeking adults.
Ecological Model	Interaction of physical and social contingencies	Communicating about cancer	Patrick et al. (2005). Implications for communicating about cancer and the ecological framework.
	Intrapersonal factors Interpersonal processes and primary groups	Entry into pregnancy programs	Debate and Pyle (2004). Understanding women in their first trimester and entry into WIC.
	Institutional factors Community factors Public policy	Understanding and intervening in obesity pandemic	Egger and Swinburn (1997). Understanding and treating the obesity pandemic through public policy, community factors, and individual motivation for change.

short of the initial step of taking action and do not address maintenance of change over time. There are exceptions. For example, TTM subscribes to stages of change and includes specific analysis of the maintenance stage. Still, this model has been criticized because it suggests that distinct behaviors are associated with that particular stage. TMM has been criticized because conceiving of behavior in stages may constrain our expectations and our notions of what interventions will work best.

With that said, theories to build an approach to behavioral change can be very useful. The purpose of theories is to shed light on why things occur, in what sequence, and under what conditions. They can either add simplicity or complexity. They are preferable to common sense or, in some cases, experience because they focus and organize thinking in systematic ways and provide not only content but structure to phenomena. Rather than producing a great deal of trivia, theories organize data in a meaningful way that allows for duplication and application in a number of situations. In this chapter, the major focus was on behavioral change from a psychosocial perspective. The chapter did not address physiological phenomena important in changing behaviors where indeed these phenomena are critical to behavior change, such as physical activity, dietary patterns, and smoking and drug use. In addition to understanding the psychosocial and environmental factors that influence such behaviors, elucidating the particular physiologic influences and how they interact with psychosocial and environmental factors is important but beyond the scope of the purpose of this chapter.

CHAPTER 23

Internet Use and Communications of Patients and Providers

Little is known about how the public accesses information about health on the Internet. How they process this information or even if they remember its source making it challenging to correct any misconceptions they have researched.
—Gwen van Servellen

CHAPTER OBJECTIVES

- Identify trends in the use of the Internet for healthcare information.
- Describe the various uses of Internet sites for information and support.
- Identify those individuals who are more likely to use the Internet for health-related information and how intensive their use might be.
- Describe the various kinds of health-related information and support Internet users are looking for.
- Differentiate the responses of providers to patients who bring Internet information to the patient–provider encounter, and describe how these response types influence patient–provider communications.
- Discuss why patient–provider online communications remain relatively uncommon.
- List three ethical concerns governing provider advice giving over the Internet.
- Discuss how patients turn to the Internet for information because they are inadequately informed in encounters with their provider.

Patients and their families have increasingly turned to other sources of information for their health and illness conditions. They may turn to Internet sites (e.g., search engines, including chat rooms). This chapter reviews and discusses these alternatives—including those that provide credible information and serve to expand patients' readiness to participate interactively in making healthcare decisions and those that provide inaccurate information or those that may be counter to the productive communication between patient and the healthcare provider. The opportunity to communicate with providers by e-mail in part increases patients' avenues to obtain and share important information. A critical issue is that communication that should occur with a health professional may not be heard in an appropriate venue. This chapter presents and analyzes several scenarios that may enhance or interfere with therapeutic communications and the opportunity to build the patient–provider alliance. It is clear that delivery channels affecting the way the provider communicates and the patient receives information will have a growing impact on communication between providers and patients.

The evolution of the use of the Internet to obtain health-related information over the last seven years reveals an increase in its use. Health providers must learn to accept that patients and families are ever more likely to use this source of communication about their healthcare needs. Early on, providers cautioned patients about the use of the Internet, and the American Medical Association warned patients not to obtain information from the Internet because it was believed that this information would change providers' relationships with patients and was likely to expose patients to inaccurate information about their condition. The assumption was that information from the Internet would misguide patients and cause them to rely less on the professional judgment of the provider. These assumptions have not held up, and instead of changing the patient–provider communications in deleterious ways, many providers now agree that the use of the Internet results in a more inquisitive and informed partner in managing care.

There are several avenues for health information through the use of the Internet: (1) e-mail communications; (2) community information (e.g., the use of bulletin boards, listservs, chat rooms, and electronic counseling and support groups); and (3) health information content found in articles and scientific, professional, and technical reports (McMullan, 2006). While there are several sources of information on the Internet, the healthcare provider must properly guide patients and families on the use of this information. Table 23–1 provides a list of do's and don'ts when discussing information from Internet sources.

USES OF THE INTERNET FOR HEALTH-RELATED INFORMATION AND SUPPORT

According to Fox and Rainie in 2000, the online healthcare information revolution was estimated to include as many as 10,000 medically related Web sites, indicating that the number of people who access the Internet for health-related information is rapidly growing. The growth in Internet use has been specified further by noting that there are groups for which use is not growing as rapidly. There is some question about whether the positive aspects of learning from websites is distributed equitably because not all patients and families have access to websites and not all will be comfortable and knowledgeable about searching for health information on the Web. The term used to infer that Internet further builds a wedge between who receives and who does not is the concept digital divide. Thus, a primary concern of the exploration of who is using the Internet to seek information about health is what impact it will have on disparities in health care. Will Internet use further widen the divide, or will it reduce the divide between those who do and those who don't receive access to healthcare information? Although there may have been some improvement, according to a report in the Journal of the American Medical Association (Berland et al., 2001), high reading levels are required to comprehend web-based health information and this may strengthen the divide, not reduce it. Gilmour (2006) aptly states that the challenge for healthcare providers is getting information to groups most disadvantaged, with an agenda of reducing inequalities in access to information. Table 23–2 displays standard approved sites for health information that can be trusted for accuracy and currency.

Table 23–1 Do's and Don'ts in Discussing Internet Information with Patients

Do's	*Don'ts*
Show interest in the content and source of the information.	Dismiss an invitation to discuss Internet information as invalid.
Interpret their use of Internet information as a positive attempt to engage in more informative conversations.	Interpret the gesture as a direct threat to your authority or medical judgment.
Direct patients to sources of good-quality consumer health information, including health-related Internet sites, but be aware of the educational level of the patient and whether he or she is likely to understand the information that will be provided.	Refer patients to medical sites that the provider has not personally reviewed both for content and ease of comprehension for the patient.
Be aware that in the course of searching the Internet, the patient may have become frustrated or fearful about what they read and may have abruptly discontinued but may still harbor some misconceptions.	If the patient does not raise the issue of discovery of information on the Internet or other health-related information, do not assume that he or she has not been exposed to this information.
Instruct the patient about how to do his or her own evaluation of the quality of the Internet information.	Assume that the quality of Internet data is at least acceptable; the quality of information on the Internet is quite variable.
Be aware that patients may be using aspects of online interactive sites to gain support and/or to obtain information for a friend or family member.	Assume that the patient is using the Internet solely to gain information and that this seeking is directly related to their own health or condition.

The report from the Pew Internet and American Life Project using a nationwide phone survey in the fall of 2006 (Available: http://www.pewinternet.org) provides some important data about Internet use and about its use among patients. According to this report, 128 million people accessed the Internet, or 63% of Americans; of these, 66% look for health-related information. This report also documented that people with disabilities and chronic illness are extensive users of the Internet. The Pew report states that persons with disabilities or chronic disease are less likely than others to go online, but when they do, they are avid Internet consumers of health information. The report estimates that about one-fifth of American adults say they have a disability, handicap, or chronic illness, and half (51%) go online—compared with 74% who report no chronic disease or disabilities. They report searching information about 17 different health topics, with the majority searching online for information about a specific disease or medical problem. The Pew report also indicates that since 2002 there has been increased interest in topics of diet, fitness, drugs, health insurance, experimental treatments, and particular information about doctors and hospitals. These patients, referred to as e-patients, are more likely to be 50 or older and do not use a computer on a regular basis. The population of persons with chronic illnesses are more likely to be older and less educated, raising the issue of how they use the Internet

Table 23–2 Recommended Internet Sites for Healthcare Information

Resource	*Focus*
Gateway site: Healthfinder (www.healthfinder.gov/)	Government site that provides health information from a wide range of resources, government agencies, voluntary groups, and professional healthcare organizations. The patient can gain access to Medline Plus through this site.
Medline Plus (PubMed) (www.nlm.nih.gov/medlineplus/)	Provides access to wide range of databases, including the abstracts of articles in Medline. Is supported by the National Library of Medicine.
National Institute of Health (www.nih.gov/health/consumer/)	Provides access to wide range of databases, including the abstracts of articles in Medline. Is supported by the National Library of Medicine.
American Medical Association through Medem.com	Wide array of medical information; offers the same news and information available from other sites (e.g., drkoop.com and America Online's Health Channel).
List of sites by disease or condition (National Cancer Institute, National Institute on Aging, National Institute of Arthritis and Musculosketetal and Skin Diseases, Centers for Disease Control and Prevention)	Provides access to update disease and illness and prevention and treatment specific information; Usually available in more than just English.

and how well they screen the information they receive (e.g., check the source and the date of the health information they find).

With an estimated 20,000 to 100,000 health-related websites available, Diaz and colleagues (2002) surveyed a randomly selected population of patients seen in an internal medicine private practice to determine who had used the Internet. With 53.5% of the patients returning surveys, those using the Internet for medical information were more educated and had higher incomes. Cotton and Gupta (2004), in an analysis of individuals responding to the 2000 General Social Survey cross-sectional study, revealed that key factors differentiating online users and offline information seekers were age, income, and education, in addition to the prior research factor. Younger individuals, with higher incomes and more education, were likely to use the Internet. Unlike previous studies, those individuals who were not as healthy would be desperate for information and would be online information seekers. This was not the case in this study. Cotton and Gupta referred to this phenomena as the "digital divide," meaning that larger societal issues influence who are online users and who are offline users of health information. They warn, however, that with greater numbers of older patients using the Internet, age as a factor may not remain a key discriminating factor. Age as a factor must also be understood from the standpoint that the elderly may be gaining from online information—but indirectly, as other family members are doing the searching and seeking of information.

In addition to the Pew report, which reported findings about chronic illness and disability in general, other studies report on Internet use by specific patient populations or through disease-specific surveys of Internet users. These surveys span a wide range of conditions including, studies by Schwartz and colleagues (2006) of family medicine patients; studies by Pereira and colleagues (2000), and Unruh and colleagues (2004) of Internet use by patients with cancer; studies by Wong and colleagues (2005) and Murero and colleagues (2001), of patients encountering cardiac surgery; and studies examining Internet use by patients with rheumatoid arthritis (Gordon, Capell, and Madhok, 2002), with infertility problems (Weissman et al., 2000), and with patients attending gastroenterology clinics (O'Connor and Johanson, 2000).

There is some indication that not only are there socioeconomic differences in Internet use, but there may be regional differences as well. For example, low-income populations in California were more likely than low-income populations in the United States as a whole to search for health information. It was reported that health insurance, alternative medical treatments, and experimental procedures were particularly popular among these Internet users, and this is the case whether they live in low- or high-income households. The contrary notion, that Internet services are not available and accessible to the low-income and less-educated populations, has been reported as well.

The prevalence of providers' use of the Internet to communicate with patients is not completely known; however, there are interesting national trends that seem to parallel patients' general use of Internet services to gather information on their own. Eysenbach (2000) refers to Internet exchanges between a patient and provider as type A and type B. Beckjord and colleagues (2007), using data from the Health Information National Trends Survey (HINTS) for 2003 and 2005, reported that in 2003 the prevalence was 7% of Internet users; this prevalence increased to 10% in 2005. Those who were Internet users with more years of education, who lived in metropolitan areas, who reported poorer health status, or who had a personal history of cancer were more likely to report use of patient–provider online communication. These investigators explain that while it is more accepted by the public and more Americans are online, patient–provider dialog remains uncommon due, in part, to provider concerns about confidentiality, reimbursement, and work time spent in online communication. Katz and colleagues (2004) suggest that online patient–provider communication is more acceptable to patients than it is to providers. Hesse and colleagues (2005), reporting on the HINTS survey data analysis, stated that health providers are the more trusted source of health information, but the Internet is the most sought-after source of health information.

HEALTHCARE INFORMATION SOUGHT BY INTERNET USERS

According to the Pew report, patients typically search for information about 17 different health topics, with the majority searching online for information about a specific disease or medical problem. The Pew report also indicates that since 2002, there has been increased interest in topics of diet, fitness, drugs, health insurance, experimental treatments, and particular information about doctors and hospitals. Further, the Pew survey results show changes over time in what patients are seeking; what remains important to them, however, is data on diet/nutrition/vitamins, exercise/fitness, prescription/over-the-counter drugs, health insurance, a particular doctor/hospital, and experimental treatments/medicines, in this order (Rice, 2005). In a study by Schwartz and colleagues (2006), findings were similar to that of the Pew project. The most commonly sought information was specific disease or conditions, medications, nutrition and exercise, illness prevention, and alternative therapies, in descending order. With the exception of illness prevention, these were also the most popular topics reported in the Pew project.

McMullan (2006) found that in general patients search the Internet before an encounter with the provider to handle their health care independently and/or to decide if they need help from their provider. After the encounter, they seek Internet information for reassurance or because they are dissatisfied with the information they received from their health professional during the clinical encounter. Studies early on of cancer patients indicated that patients search the Web for specific information and that this occurs after diagnosis and before beginning their treatment.

In a recent multivariate analysis of Pew surveys, Rice (2005) summarized the results from several major datasets and revealed that income and gender influence health seeking among Internet users, but more exposure to Internet use (usually between two to three years) and to other Internet activities also seem to be consistent predictors of health-seeking behaviors. Individual health concerns, poorer health conditions, more health-related reasons to go online, having a disability or chronic disease that prevents participation in activities, and information seeking on sensitive topics not easily discussed with providers can influence patients' Internet use.

There seems to be no single motivation that always drives Internet users to seek health information. There are many reasons behind the information seeking behaviors of Internet users. Fox and Fallows (2003) indicated that persons with disabilities and chronic conditions might gather information to challenge their providers' positions on health issues. In this case, they are looking for data to substantiate what they believe to be the case or what they hope to be the case. This kind of Internet information seeker may be more or less common, but it is difficult to judge. They may be arming themselves with information not so much to challenge the provider's assessment but to prepare themselves to communicate with the provider in ways that will more fully answer their questions. In a recent report by Stevenson and colleagues (2007), patients did not collect data to challenge their providers.

An increasing number of such requests are made to Web sites that provide "drive-up" "curb-side" medicine. Eysenbach (2000) states that these interactions for the most part constitute medical practice, and providers have the ethical responsibility not to respond to unsolicited e-mails. The flip side of the coin (providers should respond to such a request but do so carefully with ample hesitancy and referral to provider contact) is also important.

Diaz and colleagues (2002) reported that those 68% of their sample sought information about nutrition or diet. Another 58% reported using the Internet to investigate drug side-effects or complications from medical treatments. Still others sought information on complementary or alternative medicine or sought to obtain second opinions about medical conditions. In an interesting study by Hawkins and colleagues (2006), the motivation of Internet information seekers was described as both building knowledge and obtaining emotional support.

EFFECTS OF THE INTERNET ON PATIENT–PROVIDER RELATIONSHIPS

The use of the Internet in patient–provider relationships brings new challenges and exceedingly important opportunities. Patients' online activities entail several implications both for patients and healthcare providers but also for society in a larger perspective.

The motivations of Internet information seekers are frequently reflected in the manner they approach the Internet possibility. Eysenbach (2000) explains that there is the type A interchange, which is a form of consultation in the absence of preexisting relationship with the provider. Type B interactions are the traditional encounters, where there is a preestablished relationship; telemedicine is one form of this encounter. Eysenbach also noted that health information providers on the Internet and doctors with e-mail accounts have been confronted with receiving unsolicited e-mails from patients who are looking for advice but who do not have a preexisting relationship with the provider. This places the provider in a compromising position because to offer either a diagnosis or recommendation for treatment is an ethical violation. Patients have to be educated that it is unethical to diagnose and treat over the Internet in the absence of a preexisting patient–physician relationship. The recommended practice is not to ignore requests for help but to deal with them in an appropriate context. Health professionals need to protect the confidentiality of the individual and act within the limitations of the service provided. While e-mail is capable of dispensing general health information, diagnosis and treatment recommendations require the practice of medicine and, at the very least, advanced telemedical technology.

Of particular interest are the virtual communities that patients can form with others worldwide that share similar interests and concerns about disease and illness. Many of these activities include the use of interactive communications (e.g., chat rooms, discussion groups, support groups, and e-mail exchanges). Sharing of experience has been multiplied many times over, leading to exposure to many sources of information and advice. The sheer magnitude of potential information presents a challenge because providers are at a loss to really know what the patient has been exposed to and what the implications might be for the particular patient's health-seeking and disease management behaviors. These virtual communities serve the purpose of providing information, but support is also needed in the absence of clinical contacts that could address these needs.

The opportunity to communicate with others in the same situation is a critical contribution. When confronting an acute or chronic condition, individuals frequently feel the need to talk to other people, and this need goes beyond what the current healthcare arena can possibly provide them. Participation in the virtual community might be the only alternative to satisfying patients' needs that can appear at anytime, anywhere. Not only do these activities meet patients' needs for support they also direct patients as to how to find and evaluate what they have learned on the Internet about services, providers, and treatments. Patients without medical knowledge may learn more from others who themselves are not medical professionals. The possibility that patients can get various types of information has the potential of making patients more active partners in the assessment, diagnosis, and treatment process. If the user queries doctors through the Internet, it is possible that he or she might get information from several specialists worldwide versus just from his or her own geographical area. Consequently, the patient is obtaining a second opinion and has more information from which to draw when talking to his or her provider. With the possibility of interacting with large numbers of people, the patient can influence society and communities about health behaviors and disease management.

Just as Internet access to health-related information for knowledge and support presents major opportunities and has the potential of affecting communities not just individuals and families, there are major challenges facing the Internet age. Health professionals have been noted to respond in a variety of ways to the Internet-informed patient (McMullan, 2006). The first response would be the "authoritative" approach, where the provider is threatened by the information the patient brings to the clinical visit. Providers may steer patients away from the Internet information so as to accept their opinion, regardless of what the Internet suggests. The second response reflects a more patient-centered approach, where the patient and provider collaborate in issues about care. In this case, the provider may not have enough time to search the Internet and welcomes the eagerness of the patient to bring data to the encounter. The third option is where the provider actually recommends Web sites to the patient. In this case, the provider needs to be knowledgeable about how to navigate the Internet and must know how to judge the quality of the information provided. In this instance, the provider may also teach the patient how to judge the quality of the information on the Internet. This option maximizes the patient-centered professional-guided relationship (McMullan, 2006). In the Schwartz and colleagues (2006) study of family medicine patients who used the Internet, 90% attempted to verify the information they found, and the majority had discussed Web site information with their physician. This study concluded that physicians need critical appraisal skills to determine whether the information found by the patient is relevant to the patient's condition and is based on the best available evidence.

Patients forming virtual communities and their use of the Internet for medical information also involve a number of challenges. First, not all patients have access to the Internet, and an even smaller group have the knowledge and the resources necessary to find relevant and correct medical information on the Internet. This means that many patients cannot access or link to patients' virtual communities. Second, it is important that patients get access to the best evidence-based practice information. Patients need to know how to protect themselves from misinformation. Providers do not always have the skills or time it requires to counsel patients about Internet health information. The information on the Internet is constantly changing, and sites thought to be reliable may not be reliable on an ongoing basis. The use of government-sponsored Web sites is an alternative; however, not all patients know how to use these sites. Pharmaceutical sites may present information that is industry driven and, although easy to read, may not be helpful in personal application to the patient's condition. This raises the issue that not all of the information on the Internet is directed to lay use. Much of it is directed at professional healthcare providers. Thus, the data require certain academic credentials to interpret the science and statistics reported. Such would be the case in scientific publications. Additionally, much of the information is provided in English only, presenting further problems to patients whose primary language is not English. A significant problem rests in the patient's misinterpretation of information provided—for example, when the provider did not mean to diagnosis or treat a condition but the patient understands the information to apply directly to his or her condition and treatment needs. Patients need to be instructed about evaluating Web site information. There are various tools to assist them; some are listed in Table 23–3.

There is little doubt that the opportunities for using the Internet to gather health information offers added responsibility to the patient in the role of

Table 23–3 Tools to Use in the Evaluation of the Quality of Information on the Internet

Resource	*Service Provided*
The Health Information Quality Assessment Tool (hitiweb.mitretek.org/lg)	This service provides a tool for Internet users to use in evaluating Internet sites. The tool covers the credibility, content, disclosure, links, design, interactivity, and caveats addressing quality evaluations.
Health InSight: Taking Charge of Health Information (Harvard School of Public Health)	
Health on the Web: Finding Reliable Information (American Academy of Family Physicians)	Available in Spanish.
How to Evaluate Health Information on the Internet (NIH: National Cancer Institute)	
User's Guide to Finding and Evaluating Health Information on the Web (Medical Library Association)	
Ten Things to Know about Evaluating Medical Resources on the Web (NIH: National Center for Complementary and Alternative Medicine)	Available in Spanish.
Ten Tips for Evaluating Immunization Information on the Internet (Centers for Disease Control and Prevention)	
Understanding Risk: What Do Those Headlines Really Mean? (NIH: National Institutes of Health)	
Online Health Information: Can You Trust It? (NIH: National Institute of Aging)	

active participant in healthcare decision making. Patients are moving to be more than passive consumers of health provider advice and direction. Their access to Internet information influences the nature of their role with healthcare providers. Patients' new abilities to compare a variety of healthcare opinions also affects the nature of their relationship with primary providers. Providers and healthcare systems are required to be better prepared for this development. It is also the case that the expectations of patients about the nature of their collaboration will change what happens in the clinical encounter. More time may be required to address treatment options and discrepancies in recommended regimen requirements, and these issues will govern how the time is distributed in the clinical visit. It is also estimated that with the use of the Internet, patients will gain not only more responsibility but control and power for their care. Their access to information about care worldwide may further their scope of influence over care decisions because they will be informed of treatments available in foreign countries.

When the patient or patient's family member(s) brings data to the provider that they gathered in searching the Internet, another aspect of the relationship is interjected. How each deals with this "third party" will determine whether communication will be enhanced and successful or whether the outcome will be more disruptive of any trust and rapport. What is typically derived from the studies of Internet use in general is that patients are missing something from their relationship with their provider. They may be experiencing deficits in the information they received in provider encounters, or their emotional needs may not be sufficiently addressed in patient–provider encounters. Hawkins and colleagues (2006) revealed that perceived emotional insufficiency was positively associated with use of the Internet by women with cancer diagnoses. Increasing use of the Internet for information gathering but also for support in the form of chat rooms and so forth, provide at least two motivations driving Internet use. Another interpretation is that patients want to enrich their communications with their provider and seek online information to position themselves to be more active participants in conversations with their providers.

A Harris Interactive survey conducted in September 2006 elicited information from a cross section of adults' nationwide perceptions of providers who do and do not provide online services. The Health-Care Poll (available: www.harrisinteractive.com/healthcare) indicated that the availability of online services could play a part in patients' selections of a provider. For example, if given a choice, patients whose doctor provides an electronic medical record would be preferred in 54% of those surveyed. The availability of the provider via Internet was found to be more influential, with 62% of those surveyed reporting that it would greatly or to some extent influence their decision of who to see, compared with 29% who said it would not influence their decision of who they would see.

In the literature of patient–provider discussions about using Internet information, a number of different reactions have been described, some of which depict insecurity and feelings of being challenged. In a study by Bylund and colleagues (2007) of patient and provider responses, patients described as challenging were those who used Internet information for self-diagnosis or self-treatment or to test the provider's knowledge. Some physicians stated that they had limited Internet skills and attributed this to being too busy to improve on their computer skills. Even if the provider disagrees with the information the patient has found on the Internet, there is still the feeling that the provider is taking the information seriously—and this improves patients' satisfaction with the interaction. This study also revealed that the provider's responses are associated with the strategies that patients use in presenting the data they found. Otherwise, when the patient was more assertive and used a less face-threatening approach, the provider was more likely to engage in positive dialogue. Not worrying about a threat may facilitate more attention to the patient's needs rather than the authority of the provider.

Given the opportunity for Internet education, would the patient be more satisfied with Internet use than communications with their provider? The answer is probably no. In a national telephone study by Hesse and colleagues (2005), it was found that while the use of the Internet for healthcare information is increasing, patients are still likely to trust and desire information from their physician. However, the likelihood of using the Internet versus their physician as a primary source for cancer information was higher for those under 65 years of age. There may be contexts around which Internet exploration is preferred; however, the exact circumstances are not yet fully known or understood.

CONCLUSION

The scope and use of the Internet for healthcare information is increasing. While a growing number of patients bring Internet-based healthcare information to their encounters with health professionals, it is not fully known how this information is received and in what ways it changes the communications between providers and patients. Surveys thus far suggest that specific provider–patient online interactions are infrequent. However, the use of online patient–provider communication is likely to increase. The use of the Internet remains a barrier for those who have no access or for other reasons (age, health, literacy, linguistic, and socioeconomic status). And not only lack of access but lack of ability to search and screen for quality information remains a challenge.

Until recently, it appeared that the major benefit of Internet use was felt by patients and public consumers who wished to expand their knowledge of healthcare conditions, health promotion, and availability of specialists and hospitals offering specific treatments. There is the possibility that the healthcare industry could benefit from patients' Internet comments. One such new direction for the use of Internet communications is in reporting adverse events (Wasson, MacKenzie, and Hall, 2007). In this study, patients provided descriptive information about what went wrong in their care. This use of the Internet will provide new opportunities to investigate the cause and initiate remedies in cases of unsafe and poor care.

The document Healthy People 2010 (U.S. Department of Health and Human Services, 2000) (available: http://www.healthypeople.gov/document/HTML/Volume1/11HealthCom.htm) recognizes the importance of patient–provider communication and the value of the Internet to facilitate access to a wide array of health information and health-related support services and the extension of health communication. Objectives 11.1 of this document urges the increase in the proportion of households with access to the Internet at home, with a target of 80% and baseline of 26%.

Health communication contributes to all aspects of disease prevention and health promotion, and individuals' exposure to, search for, and use of this health information is germane not only to improving health but is relevant to the relationship and communications between providers and patients. The "paternalistic" era, when the provider had supreme knowledge and authority over healthcare decisions, is not likely to be revered nor seen in practice settings. While not the only force, the availability and accessibility of health-related information over the Internet contributes to this change, affecting not only specific patient–provider encounters but also society's view of appropriate and necessary patient–provider roles and communication. It is evident that implications for the training of health professionals include how to discuss information brought to the patient–provider encounter—not only how to encourage dialogue but how to appraise the information for accuracy and relevancy to the patient's condition—and how to understand the patient's need and use of the information while at the same time translating the information to the specific patient's health and well-being.

CHAPTER 24

Altering Systems of Care to Enhance Healthcare Communications

America's health care system is neither healthy, caring, nor a system.
—Walter Cronkite

Many of the problems with the U.S. healthcare system were exposed after Hurricanes Katrina and Rita when paper health records were lost and victims were unable to access their health information or provide complete medical histories to caregivers.
—Craig Barrett

Mr. Barrett is the Chairman of the Board with Intel Corporation, among other important committee work, he serves as the United Nations Global Alliance for Information and Communication Technologies and Development and is a presidential appointee to the American Health Information Community.

CHAPTER OBJECTIVES

- Define healthcare systems.
- Compare and contrast aspects of the U.S. healthcare system with healthcare systems in developed countries.
- Identify ways in which the U.S. healthcare system influences the nature of patient–provider communications.
- Identify needs for change in the healthcare system to enhance communications.
- Identify barriers in the system of healthcare delivery that affect the quality of healthcare communications.
- Discuss pilot projects that affect the nature of patient–provider and provider–provider communications, and discuss the implications for quality care.
- Identify strategies and programs that you believe would be feasible in changing the healthcare system to improve communications.
- Explain what steps you would take to improve the healthcare delivery system that would enhance communications and what specific outcomes you would expect.

If we are going to make a difference in the quality of care to patients, we must pay attention to the systems in which this care is carried out. Many providers and consumers alike, independently or collectively, are in a position

Acknowledgment: This chapter utilizes with permission excerpts from G. van Servellen, M. Fongwa, and E.M. D'Errico (2006). Continuity of care and quality care outcomes for people experiencing chronic conditions: A literature review. *Nursing and Health Sciences, 8*, 185–195.

to make at least minor changes in the organization of care delivery to enhance patient–provider communications. Systems of care can cause barriers to effective communications between patient and provider, but they can also set in motion processes that facilitate and improve communications. Problems in healthcare systems of care have been rigorously explored, with the recognition that communications between patient and provider do not occur in a vacuum. There are many factors that both enhance and impede communications, and these refer to how systems of care are organized. The most well-known issues include equitable access and utilization of healthcare systems for all.

This chapter discusses various system-level factors that promote therapeutic communication (e.g., the impact of continuity in building therapeutic alliances). A report of findings from selected research studies and a description of the program of change are examined. For example, programs such as transitional care, telephone based continuing care, and systematic care are discussed, and the methods of communication between provider and patients/families are detailed. The primary aim of these programs has been to improve continuity and coordination of care communications in hopes that quality of care will be advanced. There are several examples included in this chapter that illustrate what healthcare settings are doing to improve communications and reduce communication barriers. The objectives encourage you to critically appraise ways in which patients and families are treated and how well they are able to navigate the healthcare system with which you are most familiar.

OVERVIEW: SYSTEMS OF CARE

Systems of health care refer to institutions, organizations, and networks that have the exclusive function of healthcare delivery mandated by the values and goals of the society in question. Thus, systems of care include the organizations, processes, and methods by which health care is provided. The World Health Organization (WHO) refers to *health systems* as the combination of goods and services designed to promote health, including preventive, curative, and palliative interventions for individuals or populations (WHO, 2000). Not all health care could be said to be delivered by a single system. In most developed countries and in some developing countries, health care is provided to all regardless of their ability to pay. Not all systems are alike; for example, the United States, while it has many forms of private and public care, is the only developed country that does not have a universal healthcare system. Even within the United States, there is a great deal of diversity in the operations of healthcare organizations, which covers inpatient, outpatient, and partial care services at every phase of the prevention–treatment and palliative care cycle.

Healthcare system factors are generally known to affect outcomes of care. At the level of healthcare system, one of the most notable problems is the fact that care is often fragmented, consisting of multiple providers who may have little to no contact with one another. Without proper continuity and coordination of care, the patient is required to make several transitions over the course of a single illness and throughout his or her lifetime. The burden (and opportunity) is on the patient, and not all patients can adequately negotiate the healthcare system. However, the burden and opportunity is also levied at the provider as well, because of the inadequate flow of information across providers and within and outside settings. The skill levels of providers and patient advocates contribute to potential barriers, and financial disincentives contribute to the problem of lack of coordination and continuity. All of this results in poor quality of care. The following is a discussion of the basic principles of designing delivery systems to enhance communications between patients and providers and also to enhance providers' communications with one another.

SYSTEM CHARACTERISTICS TO ENHANCE PATIENT–PROVIDER AND PROVIDER–PROVIDER COMMUNICATIONS

The principles of care to be addressed are (1) coordination of care, (2) continuity of care, (3) comprehensiveness, and (4) accessibility. These guiding principles first codified by the Institute of Medicine outline the essentials of sound primary care practices but are also germane to the practice of health care in a variety of settings. Better patient care outcomes are associated with organizational properties and the way in which these properties affect processes of care. To further illustrate system impacts on communications we will examine several which are critically important to the quality of communications. System characteristics impact or are impacted by communication patterns and organizational attributes. Exhibit 24-1, for example, illustrates different organizational attributes and how they may affect internal relationships and communications.

COORDINATION OF CARE

To achieve *coordination of care*, all involved are required to practice as a coherent, harmonizing team with shared responsibility for patient care outcomes to achieve the most effective healthcare results. Coordinated care relies on the durability and effective interaction of many. With the recognition of the patient being a member of the healthcare team, coordination also relies on coordinated efforts with the patient and patient's family to achieve the best care possible. Effective provider–provider and patient–provider communication is essential to providing coordinated care.

Taking care of patients and then leaving the patient at the doorsteps of the hospital at discharge, or being nonchalant about any issues they may have transferring to a new provider, is problematic if not unethical. The goal of successfully handing off the patient in these circumstances is to provide good transitional care. Good transitional care whether from provider to provider, hospital to home, or between healthcare facilities requires coordination of care. It also requires adequate communications to ensure quality care. In a recent report of the 2005 Common Wealth international survey, a cross-national survey of individuals who had recently been hospitalized, had surgery, or had health problems were interviewed by telephone between March and June 2005. As stated in the report, while the United States performed better compared with other countries on the hospital transition measure, the United States had the highest rate of problems in coordination

Exhibit 24–1 Measuring Organizational Attributes

Communication

1. When there is a conflict in this practice, the people involved usually talk it out and resolve the problem successfully.
2. Our staff has constructive work relationships.
3. There is often tension between (among) people in this practice.
4. The staff and clinicians in this practice operate as a real team.

Decision Making

5. This practice encourages staff input for making changes and improvements.
6. This practice encourages nursing and clinical staff input for making changes and improvements.
7. All of the staff participate in important decisions about the clinical operation.
8. Practice leadership discourages nursing staff from taking initiative.
9. This is a very hierarchical organization: decisions are made at the top with little input from those doing the work.
10. The leadership in this practice is available for consultation on problems.
11. The practice defines success as teamwork and concern for people.
12. Staff are involved in developing plans for improving quality.

Stress / Chaos

13. It is hard to make any changes in this practice because we are so busy seeing patients.
14. The staff members of this practice very frequently feel overwhelmed by the work demands.
15. The clinicians in this practice very frequently feel overwhelmed by the work demands.
16. Practice experienced as "stressful."
17. This practice is almost always in chaos.
18. Things have been changing so fast in our practice that it is hard to keep up with what is going on.

History of Change

19. Our practice has changed in how it takes initiative to improve patient care.
20. Our practice has changed in how it does business.
21. Our practice has changed in how everyone relates.

Source: This survey is published in Ohman-Strickland and colleagues (2006). Measuring organizational attributes of primary care practices: Development of a new instrument. *Health Research and Educational Trust, 10*, 1257–1273.

Note: Higher scores indicate better communication. All items are formatted to use a 5-point Likert scale with 1 = strongly disagree and 5 = strongly agree. A practice score is calculated by averaging the scores for each individual staff member in the particular practice. The score for an individual was the average of the items belonging to the four factors listed. The scores range from 1 to 5 for each category.

during patient visits. These problems were reported to be test results or records not being available at the time of the visit or the physician performing duplicate tests. These findings suggested efficiency in this aspect of care delivery and a misuse of patient and physician time. In other developed countries, the rates of this type of coordination problem were much less, ranging from 20% to 25% compared to the U.S. rate of 33%.

Failure to coordinate care during transitional points due to or resulting in poor communication has significant consequences for quality of care. Coordination problems can negatively affect patient satisfaction, patient acceptance of and adherence to medical regimens, and eventually utilization of the very care that is offered. In the Common Wealth cross-national study (Schoen et al., 2005), at least one-fifth of those surveyed expressed gaps in communication between them and their providers, and one-sixth expressed the need to have greater involvement in decisions about their care. Also, conclusions addressing such problems will no doubt include policy innovations that go beyond current payment structures and the way healthcare delivery systems are configured today.

Coleman, Mahoney, and Parry (2005) explain that concerns about the quality and safety of patients during transitions of care remain and are growing. These investigators developed and tested a performance outcome measure based on the perceptions of patients obtained through the use of focus groups. The areas identified were information transfer, patient and caregiver preparation, self-management support, and empowerment to assert preferences (Coleman et al., 2002). Coleman and colleagues created a 15-item measure called the Care Transition Measure to clarify deficiencies in care during discharge from hospitals and to serve as a quality improvement measure. The National Quality Forum subsequently mounted a three-item version. Coleman, Parry, Chalmers, and Min (2006), in describing their randomized controlled trial of care transitions intervention, summarized the literature and suggested that quality and patient safety were compromised during periods of transition due to high risk for medication errors, incomplete or inaccurate transfer information, and lack of appropriate follow-up care. The program developed for transition of care at hospital discharge discusses more effective transitional care, including improvements in communication between inpatient and outpatient providers, reconciliation of prescribed medication regimens, adequate education of patients about prescribed medications, closer medical follow-up, engaging social support systems, and greater clarity in patient–provider communication.

CONTINUITY OF CARE

Continuity is coherent health care with an uninterrupted smooth transition over time. Continuity is possible when coordination is also present. For the patient and patient's family, the perception that someone(s) is in control of their care, is knowledgeable about them and their healthcare needs, and will follow them over time is the experience of continuity. Continuity of patient care, defined more broadly, signifies "coherent health care with a seamless transition over time between various providers in different settings" (Biem, Hadjustavropoulos, Morgan, Biem, and Pong, 2003, p. 1). Management of services to achieve seamless transitions has also been referred to as "continuance of care" (Preen et al., 2005), "continuum of care" (Wright, Litaker, Laraia, and DeAndrade, 2001), or "continuing care" (McKay et al., 2005). It has been described most often as either a structural dimension (Vrijhoef, Diederiks, Spreeuwenberg, and Wolffenbuttel, 2001; Kibbe, Phillips, and Green, 2004) or a process indicator (Beland, 1989; Saultz, 2003; van der Weide, Verbeek, and van Dijk, 1999). Guthrie and Wyke (2000) stated that there are at least two conflicting definitions of continuity. The first stresses the patient seeing the same healthcare provider at each visit (personal continuity). The second stresses consistency of care from the perspective of organizations, guidelines, and electronic medical records (care continuity), irrespective of whether the patient sees the same or a different provider.

Continuity can vary by type. And while one type might be present, another might not. Biem and colleagues (2003) explain that until recently continuity of care meant being cared for by the same provider. Continuity of patient care has been and continues to be associated with professional medical practice. Stokes and colleagues (2005) and Guthrie and Wyke (2000) assert that it is an official "core value" of primary care practice in the United Kingdom. According to Sparbel and Anderson (2000a, p. 17), it is "a fundamental tenet of professional nursing," but that with the advent of regionalizing and specializing health care as well as multidisciplinary issues with the delivery of care, continuity of care means much more. Saultz (2003) speaks of a hierarchy of dimensions including informational, longitudinal, and interpersonal continuity. Similar to Saultz, Haggerty, and colleagues (2003) examined continuity but with a multidisciplinary perspective. They identified informational, management, and relational (similar to interpersonal) continuity of care. Informational continuity refers to the "use of information on past events and personal circumstances to make current care appropriate for each individual" (Haggerty et al., 2003, p. 1220). Management continuity refers to "a consistent and coherent approach to the management of a health condition that is responsive to a patient's changing needs" (p. 1220). Finally, relational continuity of care refers to "an ongoing therapeutic relationship between a patient and one or more providers" (p. 1220). This dimension of relational continuity is said to be important because it provides the patient with a sense of predictability and coherence. Haggerty and colleagues also point out that management continuity is particularly important in chronic and complex diseases when care is provided by several providers who could potentially work at cross purposes. They also explain that processes designed to enhance continuity, such as care pathways and case management systems, do not mean that continuity is in place. Rather, it is the experience of care as "connected and coherent" that signals the presence of continuity of patient care.

Continuity of care is not absolute; patient care may be more or less continuous. Just how much continuity of care is desired and required is not known, but the value of continuity transcends all professions in health care.

COMPREHENSIVENESS

Comprehensive care has evolved over time to mean different things. Initially, it was used to describe a treatment perspective in which the patient would not be treated as a condition, disease, or surgical challenge, but as a "whole person." This meant that the physical, psychological, social, and spiritual needs of the patient would be appreciated. Subsequently, assessments of patient health-related quality of life and response to treatment incorporated all these domains in responding to the needs of a wide variety of patients. Like continuity and coordinated care, comprehensive care was also treated as a professional value in the assessment and design of patient care delivery systems.

Most recently, comprehensive patient care has been referred to as a number of resources "bundled together" to produce a "one-stop-shop" service; that is, case management, nutritional services, pharmacy, dental, women's health, and medical care would represent the range of services available at a single treatment facility. Another definition of comprehensive care delivery is that assessment, diagnosis, treatment, and case management and all indirect services for all complications could be contained under a single provider.

Integrated care has also been associated with comprehensive care. The idea that integrated care aims include continuity, coordination, and comprehensive care is clearly detailed in the recent Institute of Medicine report, *Crossing the Quality Chasm: A New Health System for the 21st Century* (2001). Integrated care systems entail complex communication linkages. The two options most often considered are that either the primary care provider or the patient shoulders the primary burden to achieve effective communication. There are two important avenues to consider: (1) the patient/family–provider unit and (2) the provider–provider communication channel. Gulmans and colleagues (2007) warn that gaps in communication should be monitored in both channels due to the complexity of integrated systems of care.

ACCESSIBILITY

Healthcare systems should embrace all aspects of goods and services, including preventive, curative, and palliative interventions (WHO, 2000). Operationally, this translates to equal access to all facets of health care *to all*. *Access* means equitable distribution of services of the highest caliber. Quality of care should not vary as a function of any personal characteristic.

The role of communication in accessing care is critical. There are several dimensions to consider. Accessibility means that important health communication is available but available to all. In the cross-national study previously discussed (Schoen et al., 2005) one-half of the adults in the United States surveyed said they did not see a doctor when sick, did not get recommended treatment, or did not fill a prescription because of cost. Respondents in both Canada and the United States reported that they were less likely to get a "same-day" appointment and more likely to wait six days or longer for an appointment.

An important prerequisite to access is that this communication be culturally appropriate. That is, communications must be designed to reach a wide range of populations including all ethnic, racial, literacy and educational levels, and those with a range of linguistic capabilities (U.S. Department of Health and Human Services [U.S. DHHS], 2000). Second, the information must not only be designed appropriately but must be made available to all.

Public health messages can be created and made available to target communities, but without access to prevention and treatment, appropriate follow-up is not possible. Accessibility inevitably includes available patient–provider interaction that itself is culturally competent and meets the criteria spelled out in *Healthy People 2010* criteria for attributes of effective health communication (U.S. DHHS, 2000). Effective counseling on the part of health providers requires these providers and patients to practice good communication skills—the provider exhibiting therapeutic communication skills and the patient being informed and motivated to ask questions and participate in healthcare decisions.

With the goal of increasing provider–patient communication skills in mind, some communications are more difficult to ensure. Health literacy levels of individuals and whole communities will hamper participatory interaction with health providers. Health literacy is critical in individuals' abilities to navigate the increasingly complex healthcare system and to manage their disease prevention and healthcare management activities. Low levels of healthcare literacy have been associated with increased risk of hospitalization, poorer adherence to treatment regimens, poorer health status, and incomplete knowledge of their health conditions and treatment plans. Health literacy shapes the communication between provider and patient and, in turn, increases with effective communication between them.

Advances in interactive health communication, such as the use of the Internet, health Web sites, and support groups, add to the possibility that accessibility challenges may be met more successfully than has previously been the case. This structure of networking capabilities provides an increasing number of opportunities to provide health information, self-management support, and services on demand. These channels increase the available options for patients and providers to communicate—and to communicate in new ways. The option to bring mass media campaigns to the level of individual application is enhanced in interactive health communication media.

The trends toward interactivity, customization, and multimedia have not been explored extensively, but there is evidence to suggest that these principles are important in individuals' access to health messages. Interactive health communications are being used to provide accessibility in a variety of ways: to exchange information, create informed decision making, promote healthy behaviors, encourage peer informational and social support, promote self-care management, address demands for healthcare services, and support clinical care.

STUDIES OF SYSTEM CHANGES AND THEIR POTENTIAL OUTCOMES

The provision of continuous, coordinated, comprehensive care that is also accessible to all is considered "a good thing" and something to be promoted in the design and delivery of healthcare services. The concept of continuity of patient care has been linked with quality care. Absence of these attributes has been linked to adverse events (e.g., medication errors and increased risk for rehospitalization). Literature addressing this linkage is found in studies of varied settings from inpatient units, extended care, and hospice services; in family practice; and in other outpatient settings. For example, continuity of care (defined as sustained contact with a primary provider), although disease specific, has been associated with early diagnosis of chronic disease (Koopman, Mainous, Baker, Gill, and Gilbert, 2003), decreased hospitalizations (Gill and Mainous, 1998), and improved quality of care (Parchman and Burge, 2002). Gill and Mainous found that after controlling for demographics, number of ambulatory visits, and case mix, higher provider continuity was associated with a lower likelihood of hospitalization for any condition. Parchman and Burge reported that patients with type 2 diabetes who had seen their usual providers within the past year were significantly more likely to have had an eye examination, a foot examination, two blood pressure measurements, and a lipid analysis. In a follow-up study, as the length of the relationship increased between patient and provider, scores on communication and accumulated knowledge of the patient by the physician and trust in the physician also increased (Parchman and Burge, 2003). Although equivocal, evidence of reductions in resource utilization and costs among health maintenance organization (HMO) patients receiving outpatient treatment for chronic illness has also been associated with continuity of care (Raddish, Horn, and Sharkey, 1999).

However, studies of the relationship of continuity of care and quality of care outcomes have revealed unexpected findings. Gill, Mainous, Diamond, and Lentard (2003) stated that while continuity might benefit some aspects of care for diabetic patients, provider continuity was not associated with completion of diabetic monitoring (receipt of a glycosylated hemoglobin test, a lipid profile, or an eye examination) in patients treated under a private national health plan. Pereira, Kleinman, and Pearson (2003) found that loss of continuity in care due to primary care system changes frequently addresses several of the phenomena discussed. The reason is that ensuring more than one element simultaneously is more likely to produce quality care outcomes and improved communications. In an extensive review of clinical studies altering systems to influence desired outcomes, several commonalities were noted. What these interventions have in common is the attempt to affect system elements that would improve communications: provider–provider and/or provider–patient/family.

The following is an overview of selected studies reporting on the impact of system changes. In general, the interventions piloted and described here were designed to improve patient care transitions, which would also improve communications, satisfaction, and coordination of care. Categories of outcome variables included in these studies were patient-level health and treatment behaviors, resource consumption, and provider influence. Virtually all focused on some aspect of affecting patients' health status and/or their satisfaction with care. Quality of life (either generic or disease specific) was a frequently cited outcome measure (Cowan, 2004; Fagerberg, Claesson, Gosman-Hedstrom, and Blomstrand, 2000; Fjaertoft, Indredavik, Johnsen, and Lydersen, 2004; Grunfeld et al., 1999; Harrison et al., 2002; Keitz, Box, Homan, Barlett, and Oddone, 2001; Moher, Yadkin, and Wright, 2001; Naylor et al., 2004; Neilsen, Palshof, Mainz, Jensen, and Olesen, 2003; Preen et al., 2005; Reynolds et al., 2004; Samet et al., 2003; Smeenk et al., 1998; Williams et al., 2001). Others addressed patient well-being and/or health status measures. For example, indicators included (1) patient satisfaction well-being, unmet needs, and health status (Byng et al., 2004); (2) symptom severity and symptom relapse (Atienza et al., 2004; Fjaertoft et al., 2004); (3) adverse events (Crotty, Rowett, Spurling, Giles, & Philips, 2004; Atienza et al., 2004); and (4) worsening condition or mobility (Crotty et al., 2004).

Of those addressing costs of care some focused on the nature and magnitude of resource use, such as overall or total direct costs of care (Atienza et al., 2004; Byng et al., 2004; Druss & Rhohrbaugh, 2001). Others addressed hospital, urgent care, or emergency visits and number and causes of readmissions (Atienza et al., 2004; Cowan, 2004; Harrison et al., 2002; Keitz et al., 2001; Reynolds et al., 2004; Smeenk et al., 1998); extent and speed of communications between hospital and practitioner (Preen et al., 2005); hospital length of stay (Preen et al., 2005); and efficiency or number of patients missed on rounds (van Eaton, Horvath, Lober, Rossini, & Pellegrini, 2005). Provider or caregiver factors (when associated with patient outcomes) were infrequently mentioned but included caregiver strain (Fjaertoft et al., 2004), communication and coordination of activities (van Eaton et al., 2005), processes of care (Byng et al., 2004), caregiver satisfaction (Byng et al., 2004), physician use of experimental intervention strategy or program (Williams et al., 2001), and physician knowledge of patient's disease and treatment (Neilsen et al., 2003). There was no single pattern of outcome measurement. Patient outcomes were examined most often, followed by some measure of resource consumption.

Analyses of selected studies are provided in Table 24–1. A focus on transition from hospital to home care was found in half these studies (Harrison et al., 2002; Naylor et al., 2004; Smeenk et al., 1998). A focus on shared care at the level of outpatient service was found in the remaining studies (Neilsen et al., 2003; Roy-Byrne, Katon, Cowley, & Russo, 2001; Simon, Ludman, Unutzer, & Bauer, 2002). The pivotal role of the nurse seemed to be integral in some of the studies. Quality of life or some measure of patient functioning was addressed in most studies.

In conclusion, while the principles of coordinated, continuous, and comprehensive care as well as accessible to all are valued, more research needs to be targeted to observe how these principles affect communications and, in turn, affect important quality care outcomes.

CONCLUSION

What differs most when comparing former systems of care to what is needed now is the new responsibilities for communication by both provider and patient. According to the IOM report *Fostering Rapid Advances in Health Care: Learning from System Demonstrations* (2002b), the patient has the right and the provider the responsibility to ensure that the patient receives safe, effective, patient-centered, timely, efficient, and equitable care. Profound changes in our concept of the role of the patient are needed, with the idea that patients will be collaborative partners in the enterprise. More research is needed to evaluate the effects of the organization and delivery of comprehensive, continuous, coordinated services on the health and utilization of services among a variety of populations. This includes the causes for disparities in healthcare use and in health among a variety of populations distinguished by

Table 24–1 Studies addressing coordination, continuity and comprehensive care provision

Author(s) names and location	*Study purpose and design*	*Intervention*	*Study population / setting*	*System elements*	*Major outcome variables examined*
Harrison et al. (2002) Kingston Ontario, Canada	Randomized trial to examine the effectiveness of hospital-to-home transitioning care program	Nurse-led intervention focusing on the transition from hospital-to-home and supportive care for self-management	Patients hospitalized for heart failure transitioning to home care	Nursing transfer letter to the home care nurse detailing patients' clinical status. Hospital to home transition program to increase coordination of care to improve the methods and processes of discharge care of heart failure patients. Continued relationship with nurse after discharge; phone outreach call by hospital nurse to patient within 24 hours of discharge home improved communication with patient/family.	Disease specific quality of life Generic quality of life Rates of hospital re-admission Emergency room use
Naylor et al., (2004) Philadelphia, Pennsylvania, USA	Randomized controlled trial to examine the effectiveness of a transitional care intervention delivered by advanced practice nurses to elders with heart failure	A follow-up post index hospital discharge to patients	Academic and community hospitals; elder patients hospitalized for heart failure transitioning to home care	Collaboration with physicians major focus of advanced practice nurses was to provide input to nursing staff regarding discharge needs of patients thus improving communication among staff. Face to face interactions with patient's physician during hospital and initial discharge visit. Program to follow up with specially trained advanced practice nurses within 24 hours of discharge. Continuity of visits conducted with the same nurses.	Time to first readmission or death Number of readmissions Total costs Short-term improvements in quality of life Patient satisfaction

continues

Table 24–1 Continued

Author(s) names and location	*Study purpose and design*	*Intervention*	*Study population/ setting*	*System elements*	*Major outcome variables examined*
Neilsen et al. (2003) Aarhus, Denmark	Randomized controlled trial to determine the effect of a shared care program on the attitudes of newly referred cancer patients towards the healthcare system	Shared care program included transfer of knowledge from oncologist to general practitioner, improved communications, and active patient involvement	Cancer patients referred to a university department of oncology practice	Transfer of knowledge of patient needs from oncologist to general practitioner. Discharge summary letters and information sent to the patient's general practitioner. Shared care program with three elements: knowledge transfer, communication channels, and active patient involvement. Intervention group had more contact with their general practitioners. Provided one more confidante.	Attitude towards the health care system Patients' perception of cooperation between primary and secondary healthcare sectors (GP's knowledge of their disease and treatment) Number of contacts with GP Health-related quality of life Performance status
Roy-Byrne et al. (2001) Seattle, Washington, USA	Randomized effectiveness trial of a collaborative care program for panic disorder patients in primary care	Collaborative care intervention included educational videotapes and pamphlets, pharmacotherapy, psychiatrist visits and telephone calls within the first eight weeks; and up to five telephone calls	Patients with panic disorder from primary care clinics	Coordinated, collaborative care intervention. Intervention program included multimodal approach with education, psychiatrist visits, telephone calls and psychopharmacologic intervention. Increased communication with continued contact with psychiatrist.	Adequate type, dose, and duration medication regimen Adherence to medication regimen Level of anxiety, depression, and disability over time

		between 3–12 months follow up versus usual care patients treated by their primary care physician			
Simon et al., (2002) Seattle, Washington, USA	Design of a randomized trial evaluating systematic program to improve quality and continuity of care for bipolar disorder	Multifaceted program including: collaborative treatment plan, monthly telephone monitoring by a dedicated nurse manager, feedback of monitoring results, and algorithm-based medication recommendations to treating mental health professionals, as needed outreach and care co-ordination, and a structured psychoeducational group program delivered by a nurse case manager	Population-based sample of patients with varying levels and subtypes of mood disorders	Coordinated, collaborative treatment plan to enhance communication and sharing of information about patients. Program with multifaceted intervention to enhance coordination of care and monthly telephone monitoring by dedicated nurse manager increased knowledge of and communication with patient.	Acceptance of regular telephone monitoring Contact with nurse case manager Completion of Life Goals Program Attendance at structured group sessions

continues

Table 24–1 Continued

Author(s) names and location	*Study purpose and design*	*Intervention*	*Study population / setting*	*System elements*	*Major outcome variables examined*
Smeenk et al. (1998) Eindhoven, The Netherlands	Quasi-experimental design to evaluate the impact of a trans-mural home care intervention program designed to optimize coordination and thereby improve continuity of care	Coordination of care or care not stopping at the walls of the hospital but adapting to the needs of the patient and occurs before, during, and after the hospital stay Program directed at optimizing communication, cooperation, and coordination, intra- and extra-mural health care	Terminal cancer patients receiving home care	Patients' wishes and care needs are assessed by the specialist nurse coordinator and communicated to the extramural care providers. Patient information available to 24-hour phone responders regarding patients via home care dossier. At the program level to provide trans-mural home care as a way of eliminating gaps in terminal patient's discharge from hospitalization and monitoring care at home by complementing, not duplicating, existing services through information sharing and phone support. Continuity of care by the specialist nurse before, during, and after hospitalization.	Re-hospitalization Quality of life Place of death for terminal patients

region, race, ethnicity, language, level of health literacy, and level of disability. It is important to understand, for example, what level of care coordination is needed to ensure the effective and efficient organization and utilization of resources that will, in turn, ensure access to comprehensive services.

Systems of health care refer to institutions, organizations, and networks that have the exclusive function of healthcare delivery mandated by the values and goals of the society in question. Systems of care include the organizations, processes, and methods by which health care is provided. Research is needed to create and evaluate models of care. Some models to improve the continuity and coordination of health care promise enhanced communication for both patient and provider. Still, these pilot projects have not been disseminated to a large degree, resulting in ill-managed care systems that result in some level of poor care delivery and dissatisfied patients and providers. Such experiments have occurred in academic settings or closed systems (e.g., the Veterans Affairs healthcare system), and the full value to those receiving community-based care is yet unknown. They have not been tested in the settings in which most people receive care. Without this kind of application and evaluation, there is no specific direction to guide policy at a more global level.

System reforms begin at the provider and patient level. And some patients might require different levels of care. It has been posited, for example, that continuity of the patient–provider relationship is most important for patients with co-morbid chronic conditions, who need or use more visits, and who cannot be easily engaged in their treatment plan. It could be argued that continuity of a single provider or provider team (relational continuity) is unnecessary for some and impractical to maintain over time. Guthrie and Wyke (2000) summarizing the literature on continuity of care and quality care outcomes, warned that current attempts to reorganize care delivery systems with an emphasis on technology to promote the development of general practice might, for example, reduce continuity of care.

Coordinated, continuous, and comprehensive care, together with accessibility of services, are purported to be necessary to ensure high-quality outcomes. Furthermore, organizing care to enhance these principles is believed to be critical and paramount in both the nursing (Sparbel and Anderson, 2000b) and medical professions (Guthrie and Wyke, 2000; Stokes et al., 2005). While few would argue with the need to enhance these aspects of care, providing and ensuring them might place considerable pressure on systems of care, especially those services extending over protracted periods of time as in the case of managing chronic disease and illness.

The literature review clearly indicated that systems of care were multimodal. It appeared that researchers did not think that one element operated in isolation of other important features of care. In the real world of designing and testing system interventions or programs, it is more likely that interventions are complex, using many elements. Effectiveness studies have to be feasible and flexible enough to be relevant to the "real-world" environment in which people are treated, yet defined and structured enough to be reliable and sufficient in detail to allow for replication.

An important area of future research is the question of whether these elements are needed for some but not equally for all patient populations. Along these same lines, for example, is continuity a clinical necessity or a patient region, race, ethnicity, language, level of health literacy, and level of disability. It is important to understand, for example, what level of care coordination is needed to ensure the effective and efficient organization and utilization of resources that will, in turn, ensure access to comprehensive services.

Systems of health care refer to institutions, organizations, and networks that have the exclusive function of healthcare delivery mandated by the values and goals of the society in question. Systems of care include the organizations, processes, and methods by which health care is provided. Research is needed to create and evaluate models of care. Some models to improve the continuity and coordination of health care promise enhanced communication for both patient and provider. Still, these pilot projects have not been disseminated to a large degree, resulting in ill-managed care systems that result in some level of poor care delivery and dissatisfied patients and providers. Such experiments have occurred in academic settings or closed systems (e.g., the Veterans Affairs healthcare system), and the full value to those receiving community-based care is yet unknown. They have not been tested in the settings in which most people receive care. Without this kind of application and evaluation, there is no specific direction to guide policy at a more global level.

System reforms begin at the provider and patient level. And some patients might require different levels of care. It has been posited, for example, that continuity of the patient–provider relationship is most important for patients with co-morbid chronic conditions, who need or use more visits, and who cannot be easily engaged in their treatment plan. It could be argued that continuity of a single provider or provider team (relational continuity) is unnecessary for some and impractical to maintain over time. Guthrie and Wyke (2000) summarizing the literature on continuity of care and quality care outcomes, warned that current attempts to reorganize care delivery systems with an emphasis on technology to promote the development of general practice might, for example, reduce continuity of care.

Coordinated, continuous, and comprehensive care, together with accessibility of services, are purported to be necessary to ensure high-quality outcomes. Furthermore, organizing care to enhance these principles is believed to be critical and paramount in both the nursing (Sparbel and Anderson, 2000b) and medical professions (Guthrie and Wyke, 2000; Stokes et al., 2005). While few would argue with the need to enhance these aspects of care, providing and ensuring them might place considerable pressure on systems of care, especially those services extending over protracted periods of time as in the case of managing chronic disease and illness.

The literature review clearly indicated that systems of care were multimodal. It appeared that researchers did not think that one element operated in isolation of other important features of care. In the real world of designing and testing system interventions or programs, it is more likely that interventions are complex, using many elements. Effectiveness studies have to be feasible and flexible enough to be relevant to the "real-world" environment in which people are treated, yet defined and structured enough to be reliable and sufficient in detail to allow for replication.

An important area of future research is the question of whether these elements are needed for some but not equally for all patient populations. Along these same lines, for example, is continuity a clinical necessity or a patient

Glossary

Accessibility (of care): Equitable care for all is a professional standard. Access problems in health care generally refer to the fact that health care is not provided equally to all citizens. The major deterrent is usually identified as a lack of adequate insurance coverage. It includes problems of certain persons being either uninsured or underinsured.

Accountability: Accountability in healthcare delivery refers to the process of knowing and controlling for outcomes. The issue refers to both efficiency and effectiveness of services.

Active listening: Active listening is the process of understanding fully what another is communicating. It enables providers to be fully attuned not only to what the patient is saying, but also to what the patient feels.

Active voice (versus passive voice): Active voice is an approach that is less wordy and clearer about what needs to happen. It positively stresses the individual's capacity to change. Rather than wording a directive passively (e.g., people who are over 40 need to watch their weight and exercise if they are to prevent premature cardiovascular problems), wording actively is easier to understand and usually less wordy (e.g., if you exercise three times a week and watch your weight, you can avoid premature cardiovascular disease).

Actualizing tendency: Carl Rogers's personality of change theory purports that change is a function of an underlying need for self-actualizing. Self-acceptance is key to growth and unconditional positive regard nurtures the individual's capacity to change.

Adverse drug event (ADE): Adverse drug events refer to injuries due to drug events and are found frequently in inpatient settings. Less is known about their occurrence in outpatient settings, but these are also considered to be problematic and frequently due to patients' lack of understanding of their condition and treatment regimen.

Advisement: The act of disclosing what you think another person should feel, think, or do. Less direct advice and providing rationale generally makes advice more palatable.

Affective sensitivity: This term is sometimes used synonymously with the term empathy. It refers to the ability to sense, at a feeling level, the experience of another.

Affordability: Affordability of healthcare services refers to the relative costs of rendering care as a portion of the gross national product (GNP). When accusations are made about healthcare costs being out of control, the context of the discussion includes not only percentage increases in expenditures but how this increase measures up in terms of increasing the proportion of the nation's GNP.

Aggression: This is a common negative stance that is displayed in blaming and/or attacking behaviors. Low self-esteem and feelings of inferiority may underlie behaviors of aggression.

Analogic communication: When we refer to objects as representations or likenesses and observe and respond nonverbally and contextually, we are using our analogic communication capacities.

Anonymity: Anonymity refers to the privacy rights of patients wherein their exact identity is not made known to others.

Arbitration: Arbitration is one solution to settling disputes. It involves an impartial third party who has been given the authority to present solutions.

Attribution theory: Attribution theory includes concepts and principles that explain the process of assigning meaning and character to events.

Autonomic nervous system: The nervous system that is responsible for regulating the functioning of internal organs is the autonomic nervous system.

Bargaining: Bargaining is the process of making trade-offs or coming to mutual compromise. It is one aspect of negotiation.

Biofeedback: By providing sensory feedback, it is believed that internal bodily responses (e.g., stress) can be controlled.

Care transition measure (CTM): This is a measure that can be used as a performance or quality improvement measure to evaluate the quality of care between transition points (e.g., between hospital and home). There are two versions of this measure: a 15-item version developed by Coleman and colleagues (2002) and a 3-item version mounted by the National Quality Forum.

Case management: Case management includes case assessment, treatment planning, referral, and follow-up to ensure comprehensive and continuous services and coordinated payment and reimbursement.

Chronic illness: Chronic illness refers to conditions that will not be cured by brief intervention. Chronic illnesses frequently have a downward course despite multiple remissions.

Classical conditioning: Classical conditioning refers to the Pavlovian principle of establishing a conditioned response by pairing a conditioned stimulus with an unconditioned stimulus.

Closed-ended questions: Questions that are phrased to evoke a narrow range of possible responses and that frequently elicit one-word or yes/no responses are closed-ended.

Coding: Coding is a term in neurophysiology that is used to describe the correspondence of some part of a stimulus and some aspect of action in the nervous system.

Coercion: Solutions reached through coercion have occurred because the alternatives have been severely restricted and fear or threats have underscored the process.

Commands: Like orders, commands are directives that must be followed. They are different from orders in that they demand immediate action.

Competition: Competition occurs when one disputant pursues his or her own interests, neglecting to consider the needs of the other.

Complainer: This is a common negative stance. Patients frequently exhibit unrealistic expectations, and fear and anxiety are often the inner feelings of dependent complaining patients.

Compliance/noncompliance/partial compliance: Compliance is the act of following medical orders as they are prescribed. Noncompliance refers to ignoring medical orders, at least the essential aspects. Partial compliance is inconsistency or incompleteness in following orders.

Comprehensive care: Comprehensive care is a critical element of quality patient care. It refers to the extent to which care includes attention to multiple factors that influence quality of life: psychological, physical, spiritual, and social domains.

Compromise: A compromise is a solution that produces relatively the same losses and gains for both parties.

Conciliation: Conciliation is a state or condition that is established to short-cut substantial discussion of issues wherein conflict could escalate.

Confidentiality: Confidentiality in healthcare communications implies that the patient may either assume or be explicitly assured that his private communications with the provider will not be transmitted to others except in specific instances. Providers have a moral, ethical, and legal responsibility to protect the confidentiality of these communications.

Confirmation: Confirmation is a way of communicating acknowledgment and acceptance of others. Confirming-communicative responses acknowledge and validate the other person.

Conflict: Conflict exists when two or more interdependent parties have opposing interests or positions on an issue. Conflicts can be latent, emerging, or manifest. They are characterized by disputes between two or more individuals. Whether latent or manifest, they are communicated.

Confrontation: Confrontation is the act of presenting differing observations. Patients may, for example, say one thing and do another. Telling patients that their behaviors are discrepant is an act of confrontation.

Continuity of care: Continuity of care is in place when coherent health care occurs with an uninterrupted smooth transition over time. Continuity is possible when coordination is also in place. Continuity of care is sometimes referred to as "continuance of care," "continuum of care," and "continuing care."

Consensus: Consensus refers to reaching an agreement on issues through the process of blending each party's views.

Coordinated care: To achieve coordinated care, all providers must practice as a coherent, harmonizing team with shared responsibility for patient care outcomes. Coordinated care refers to the durability and effective interaction of many, including patient and family.

Coping: Coping refers to that which an individual thinks and/or does in a particular stressful situation. It refers to efforts that help the individual to master, tolerate, or reduce the problem that is creating the stress and/or the emotional response to the problem.

Coping (maladaptive and adaptive): Coping, in crisis theory, refers to the sequential development of specific responses to stress and crisis. Crisis resolution is contingent on the development of effective adaptive responses. When these responses do not diminish the tension and anxiety or result in effective problem-solving behaviors, the responses are usually described as maladaptive.

Coping resources: Coping resources refer to both internal and external facilities that individuals in crisis have at their disposal. For example, they may possess a sense of hopefulness (an internal resource) or be recipients of social support (an external resource). Coping resources enhance individuals' abilities to deal with crisis situations. It is generally believed that individuals with low levels of resources will fare worse in crisis situations than persons with adequate resources.

Corpus callosum: The two hemispheres of the brain are connected by a large network of axons called the corpus callosum.

Crisis: The impact of stress can produce a state of crisis, placing an individual or entire family off balance. While emergencies are sudden, unforeseen, isolated incidences, crises may have been gathering momentum over time.

Cues to action: According to the Health Belief Model originating from the works of Rosenstock (1988), cues to action are important in eliciting behavior change and maintaining this change. Cues to action may be as simple as posting notes on a refrigerator to eat more vegetables and fruit.

Cultural blindness: While not as serious as cultural destructiveness and cultural incapacity, some individuals ignore cultural differences. These individuals are perceived as "unbiased" because they believe that "culture makes no difference"; they practice cultural blindness.

Cultural competence: Cultural competence refers to the capacity to function in an effective manner within the context of a multicultural society. Individuals who are culturally competent accept and respect differences, continually conduct self-assessments, pay attention to the dynamics of difference, and continually expand their knowledge of different groups.

Cultural destructiveness: Cultural destructiveness is one phase in the process of developing cultural competence. At the most negative end of the continuum, it refers to blatant attempts to destroy the culture of a given group. There is the assumption that one race or group is superior and that all others are inferior.

Cultural diversity: While there are many commonalities among, between, and within groups, there are also vast differences in individuals' communications and life views.

Cultural incapacity: Certain individuals do not intentionally seek to be culturally destructive but still lack the capacity to be responsive to differences. Ignorance and unrealistic fears are often the basis of the problem of cultural incapacity.

Cultural precompetence: Cultural precompetence implies movement toward cultural sensitivity. Characteristic of this phase is the active pursuit of knowledge about differences and attempts to integrate this information into the delivery of services.

Cultural proficiency: Cultural proficiency is represented at the most positive end of the continuum. Individuals at this end of the continuum hold cultures in very high esteem and are regarded as specialists in developing culturally sensitive practices.

Culture: The word *culture* refers to the integrated pattern of human behavior that includes the customs, values, beliefs, communications, and actions of a specific group. This group can be distinguished along racial, ethnic, religious, or social dimensions.

Customization (of care): Interactivity, customization, and multimedia trends must be explored for their impact on accessing health messages. By customizing health messages the likelihood that communities will access them and utilize them increases.

Deadlocks, stalemates, or impasses: These terms are used to refer to the state of inertia that is experienced by disputants. They are unable to move forward in resolving their issues and/or disagreements.

Decoding: The process of deciphering the meaning of a message is known as decoding. The receiver decodes messages.

Defensive communication: Defensive communication is that which addresses issues of personal interest in a rigid manner.

Denial: Denial is a coping response; it is also the first stage in the process of adaptation to illness. Denial helps patients minimize the threat (and, therefore, the painful, emotional reactions) associated with illness.

Digital communication: Humans utilize both digital communication and analogic communication; digital communication refers to perceiving and expressing oneself in concrete terms (e.g., referring to things by their names).

Digital divide: This is a term given to infer that the Internet further builds a wedge between who receives and who does not receive health care by virtue of the fact that not all individuals have access and can understand information on the web.

Directives: Directives are absolute statements made to patients about the preferred course of action. Providers expect directives to be followed. Directives are simply statements that tell patients what is expected of them. Directives are different from advice. Advice is offered without explicit expectations; directives describe what you want patients to do.

Disconfirmation: Disconfirmation denies the value of another's existence. Disconfirming-communicative responses are frequently irrelevant to the other person's communication. They cause the other person to feel devalued.

Disorganized families: Disorganized families are those in which appropriate role enactment is rarely attempted and never maintained. Dysfunction is more apparent in disorganized families than in marginally functioning families.

Double-barreled questions: This question format asks for one answer to multiple and separate questions. It is impossible to answer adequately with one response, although this is what is evoked.

"Drive-up" or "curb-side" medicine: Medical care practice conducted without full assessment of the patient is akin to obtaining fast-food at a drive-up window. Individuals get a rapid response to a request for information and direction. Information requested may include nutritional advice, how to locate a specialist, or may even ask for a second opinion about a healthcare problem. This kind of practice presents an ethical dilemma in that it might provide necessary information to those who do not have current access to health care but at the same time can delay treatment that needs further explanation and evaluation.

Dysfunctional communication: Dysfunctional communication may occur as a result of transient conditions or more permanent defects. Disturbances in perception, processing, or expression are manifested.

Dysfunctional families: In the broadest context, dysfunctional families are those that fail to be effective along various dimensions. Their communication and decision-making capacities are extremely limited.

Electronic counseling: Counseling that is delivered over the Internet in the form of e-mails, Web sites, or chat rooms is considered to be electronic counseling. This type of counseling is considered to be more immediate and absent of required assessment. Caution needs to be considered because delivering medical advice without firsthand assessment of the patient is unethical.

Electronic medical record: Medical records that can be transmitted to other healthcare providers or healthcare settings to inform providers about the patient's needs and health history are referred to as electronic medical records. These records may not be a full copy of the original record but a summary of essential current data.

Emotional knowing: Emotional knowing, often used to describe empathy, refers to the process of establishing objective awareness of another's thoughts and feelings through the process of entering the experiential world of the other.

Empathy/empathic understanding: Empathic understanding (or empathy) refers to the condition of knowing the other person through insight achieved in the process of identifying what it must be like to be that person.

Encoding: This is the process of forming a message that transmits a specific meaning. The sender encodes messages.

Experiential learning: Learning can occur through various approaches. Experiential learning refers to the learning that occurs when one experiences a phenomena in real life and is required to solve a particular problem or perceived need.

Feedback (feedback loop): Feedback generally refers to sensory information stemming from actions or activities; this information is fed back to affect sequential perceptions and actions (thus, the notion of a loop).

Functional communication: Functional communication is characterized by an absence of disturbance in perception, processing, and expression; it usually contains a great deal of clarification and qualification.

Functional health literacy: Rather than reflecting simply the reading level of the individual, health literacy refers to how the individual will be able to understand healthcare communications and will be able to successfully negotiate the healthcare system. When functional health literacy is low, further consideration of how to impart information is needed.

General Adaptation Syndrome (GAS): GAS refers to a specific description of the sequential responses to crisis events. Each of three stages, according to Selye (1978), have a corresponding level and type of behavioral disorganization. These stages, representing acute behavioral responses, include (1) alarm, (2) resistance, and (3) exhaustion.

Gestalt (e.g., in gestalt therapy): Gestalt therapy refers to an approach to therapy and counseling which recognizes personal growth as a function of "the here and now" experience of the individual. It is a holistic approach that recognizes the integration of mind, body, and culture.

Group content: In contrast to the process of the group, the content refers to the explicit tasks that the group addresses.

Group maintenance: Behavior in a group may be directed toward maintaining and encouraging the group. These behaviors include gate-keeping and harmonizing. Both behaviors encourage members to sustain their participation.

Group process: Group process refers to the dynamic unfolding of interaction within a group sequentially, over time. Stages of group development depict the process of the group at any one point in its history.

Healthcare delivery system: Healthcare delivery system describes the major way in which health care has been provided. One classical analysis is to consider the institutions in which the majority of services occur (e.g., inpatient or outpatient home-care programs).

Health Belief Model: The Health Belief Model originated from the works of Rosenstock (1988) and others and offers an expanded view of the change process, identifying the motivation for change and applied to health decisions, perception of severity of potential illness, perceived susceptibility to the illness, perceptions of the benefits of taking action, and the barriers of taking action interact to result in subsequent actions.

Health maintenance organizations (HMOs): HMOs are comprehensively designed structures for financing and delivering health care. These organizations provide services to enrollees within a geographical area through a panel of providers.

Health promotion: Health promotion versus disease prevention is an issue that is addressed in general healthcare policy. It is generally agreed that the ideal goal of the American healthcare system should be reflected in an increase in the years of healthy life of its citizens. This approach requires an investment not only in the treatment of disease but also in the prevention of illness.

Hemisphere: Hemisphere refers to either the right or left sphere of the brain; each sphere has decidedly different functions.

Humanistic psychology: Humanistic psychology is the school of psychology and psychotherapy that serves as the foundation of many current conceptual frameworks that address change in individuals' behavior. Theorists (e.g., Carl Rogers) believed in the individual's role in change and that man will solve his own problems once confronted with them. The provider is a facilitator in the process of change.

Hypochondriasis: This disorder is one form of a somatoform disorder. It includes excessive preoccupation with one's physical health. As with somatoform disorders in general, these somatic symptoms have no basis in a physical disorder.

Informational continuity of care: Informational continuity refers to the use of information about a patient on past events and personal circumstances to make the current patient care appropriate.

Informed choice: It is generally understood that patients who have the capacity to make decisions about their care must be permitted to do so. Patient choice is not absolute.

Informed consent: Informed consent is the permission from the patient to conduct a test, treatment, or procedure after the provider has fully informed the patient, in ways that the patient can understand, about the actions that will be taken. Informed consent can be obtained in writing or orally. Some conditions require written consent (e.g., in the case of research studies).

Informing: Informing refers to the process of offering data that are pertinent to the problem(s) that are confronting the patient.

Illiteracy: Illiteracy refers to the reading ability of the patient. Reading ability has been associated with low levels of health literacy. The problem of illiteracy in the United States continues to climb, suggesting that health care needs to consider literacy a critical problem in delivering equitable health care to all.

Interactivity (of care): Interactivity, customization, and multimedia trends must be explored for their impact on accessing health messages. Interactivity of health messages increases the exchange of patient-relevant information.

Integrated care: The aims of integrated care are continuity, coordination, and comprehensive care. In delivery of integrated care, both patient–provider and provider–provider channels of communication must be monitored.

Interest-based bargaining: With interest-based bargaining, as many needs or concerns as are presented are attempted to be addressed.

Interpersonal (relational) continuity of care: Interpersonal continuity of care refers to an ongoing therapeutic relationship between patient and one or more providers. It provides the patient with a sense of predictability and coherence.

Interpersonal group problems: Interpersonal group problems refer to discontent across groups. These problems also frequently include issues of power, status, and affiliation.

Interpersonal space: One way of conceiving of silence is to conceive of it as interpersonal space. This refers to a hypothetical, changing degree of psychosocial distance that occurs whenever two or more individuals communicate.

Interpretations: Convey an understanding of the individual that is not within his or her immediate awareness. In therapeutic encounters, interpretations are offered less frequently than reflections and when substantial data have been gathered.

Interresponse boundary: Interresponse boundary refers to the space after a speaker makes a statement and before another speaker replies or the same speaker talks again.

Interresponse time: The period of time that elapses after a speaker makes a statement and before another speaker replies or the same speaker talks again is the interresponse time. Interresponse times can vary; they include pauses as short as 1 to 2 seconds or therapeutic silences lasting up to 10 seconds.

Interruptive response: Interruptive responses are disruptions of another individual's speech that generally have the impact of cutting short the expression of the person's thoughts and feelings.

Intragroup problems: Healthcare delivery systems consist of many professional task groups that address larger organizational goals. Intergroup problems also reflect issues of power, status, and affiliation with groups.

Joint Commission on Accreditation of Healthcare Organizations (Joint Commission): The Joint Commission is a private, nonprofit organization whose purpose is the accreditation of hospitals and other provider facilities. The Joint Commission sets standards for the quality of health care by publishing national standards, evaluating facilities on request, and granting accreditation to those facilities that meet the standards.

Limbic system: The limbic system is responsible for emotional experience and expression; it consists of a set of subcortical structures in the forebrain that includes the hypothalamus, hippocorpus, amygdala, olfactory bulb, septum, part of the thalamus, and the cerebral cortex.

"Loaded" questions: Loaded questions are those that restrict or influence responses. The wording of these questions suggests which answers are appropriate or desirable.

Managed care: Managed care is an approach to providing a range of health services in such a way that both the services and the resulting costs are carefully scrutinized and controlled.

Management continuity of care: There are three types of continuity: interpersonal, informational, and management continuity. Management continuity refers to a consistent and coherent approach to the management of care that is responsive to the patient's changing needs and that can transcend healthcare settings.

Manipulator: Manipulative patients generally have self-centered attitudes. They attempt to control providers' actions, sometimes in passive-aggressive ways. Manipulators anticipate loss of control and are usually fearful.

Marginal families: Marginality refers to families who function below par due to illness, injury, or disability. Family needs exceed family resources. The family can function appropriately, but their level of functioning is tenuous.

Mediation: Mediation refers to the process by which an impartial third person with authority assists disputants to reach mutually acceptable solutions.

Meta-communication: Meta-communication is simply communication about the communication or message. It directs the receiver as to how to receive the content portion of the communication.

Meta-disclosure: Meta-disclosures are disclosures about a disclosure. An example would be, "I just told you that to see what you'd say."

Mistrust: Mistrust and trust can be viewed on a continuum. Mistrust can occur because providers are viewed as lacking competence. Mistrust can also occur if providers are deemed to have other than the patient's best interests in mind.

Motivational interviewing: Approaches to interviewing patients might facilitate change. Motivational interviewing is one such approach that recognizes that patients move from one stage to the next, from precontemplation to maintenance of change.

Multidimensional communication: The assumption that communication occurs on multiple levels (e.g., the verbal and nonverbal levels) exemplifies that interpersonal communication is indeed complex.

Multimedia messages: Interactivity, customization, and multimedia trends must be explored for their impact on accessing health messages. Multimedia messages will increase the accessibility of individuals to health and healthcare messages.

Multimodal strength: Modes refer to channels of communication; multimodal strength refers to exhibiting strength in more than one modality at a time (e.g., having strength in visual and auditory channels simultaneously).

Multiple-choice questions: These questions are phrased to evoke a response to simultaneously presented choices. One choice is made between two or more options (e.g., "Would you like to take your medication with or without juice?")

Mutual denial: When both the patient and the provider seem to enter into a conspiracy of denial about the prognosis of an illness, they exhibit mutual denial. One party's denial is dependent on the other party's need to avoid reality as well.

Newest vital sign (NVS): The NVS has been recently developed to measure health literacy in a primary care setting. It uses a nutrition label and asks six questions to assess patients' comprehension of the label.

Nondirective advice: Advice that is offered tentatively, as in the form of options or alternatives to be examined jointly by provider and patient and that refrains from projecting the provider's view onto the patient, is nondirective.

Nontherapeutic communication: Nontherapeutic communications are those that generally limit patients' expressions and cause patients to have negative reactions.

Nonverbal communication: Not all communication is expressed in the verbal exchange of messages and responses. A good deal is expressed through posture, facial gestures, spatial positioning, and the like; these components are aspects of nonverbal communication.

Normative beliefs: Normative beliefs are beliefs that individuals hold that represent the norms of their social group. In health care, if the norm is to exercise regularly, the individual's normative belief is that he or she should exercise regularly.

Online patient–provider communication: Rather than face-to-face communication, online patient–provider communication refers to medical care and advice discussed over the Internet, usually through e-mail exchanges.

Open-ended questions: Questions that are phrased to evoke a wide range of possible responses and that frequently begin with "what" phrases are open-ended.

Opinions: Opinions are expressions of thoughts or feelings about healthcare situations affecting patients and their families. Expressing opinions is not telling patients what to do, rather, it is offering them information and the benefit of the provider's professional views.

Orders: Orders are directives that the patient must follow. Giving orders is a critical aspect of providers' roles.

Outcome expectancies: Expectations about probable outcomes serve as motivators to change. Otherwise, when outcome expectancies are high and in a positive direction, the likelihood that the individual will pursue the change is increased.

Over-talk response: Over-talk occurs when both parties in a conversation speak simultaneously. It can occur at the beginning of a conversation, at the midpoint, or near the end of an expressed thought when these expressions trigger impulses in the other to respond. Over-talk usually indicates defensiveness in individuals, is rarely productive, and usually culminates in frustration for those trying to communicate.

Paraphrasing: Paraphrasing consists of selecting among several statements that the patient has made, summarizing these statements, and giving them meaning in another form.

Parasympathetic nervous system: This neuro-network to the internal organs tends to work to conserve energy and produce relaxation.

Patient-centered approach to care: Patient-centered approach to care is to be distinguished from care directed at a specific condition without consideration of the many individualized care needs of the individual and family.

Patient's bill of rights: There are several conceptual models of patients' rights that depict ethical and legal parameters for healthcare providers. Among the most well-known is the American Hospital Association's "Patient's Bill of Rights."

Plain language: Providers may use very complicated sentences to explain disease and treatment to patients. Using "plain language" increases the likelihood that the information will be understood. Plain language avoids jargon and expresses ideas simply.

Position-based bargaining: Position-based bargaining occurs when one or more disputants negotiate with a solution that satisfies that party's needs or interests.

Preferred provider organizations (PPOs): PPOs are managed care approaches that contract with independent providers (physicians, ancillary providers) for negotiated fees for services.

Prescription for danger: Many drugs are used inappropriately by patients. Prescriptions are also mis-prescribed. These dangers can be reduced by better communication between providers and across providers and patients. A good deal of the miscommunication factors relate to patients' failures to give information or to ask questions of providers.

Principle of utility: The principle of utility refers to the tendency of human needs to structure perception.

Privacy (and communication): The concept of privacy refers to the right of the patient to limit the knowledge of others about himself.

Privileged communication: Privileged communication refers to the legal right by statute that is provided to the patient from having confidences revealed publicly (e.g., from the witness stand without his expressed permission; Shah, 1969).

Process disclosure: Process disclosures describe reactions to the immediate interaction within the helping process. Process disclosures are helpful in clarifying patients' communications. "I notice that you interrupted me when I asked about how the treatment was working" is a process disclosure reflecting on the confusion that the provider has about the patient's reaction to treatment.

Projection: Projection applies to listeners' conscious or unconscious attempts to place on another their own thoughts and/or feelings. These thoughts and/or feelings, while they may be cogent, usually do not describe the patient's experience accurately. They have originated from the provider, not from the patient.

Quality care: The Institute of Medicine defines quality of care as the degree to which health services for individuals and populations increase the likelihood of desired health outcomes and are consistent with current professional knowledge. Sound patient–provider and provider–provider communications must be in place to ensure quality care.

Quality chasm: *Crossing the Quality Chasm* was an Institute of Medicine report about the needs for the 21st century. The chasm refers to the gap in care that exists when one measures where we are now and where we need to be to ensure better quality care to all.

REALM; REALM-R: The REALM refers to Rapid Estimate of Adult Literacy in Medicine and REALM-R is the revised measure of this instrument; it has eight items. The REALM assesses the level of health literacy by asking individuals about key medical terms and measuring both their recognition and ability to pronounce these terms. This ability has been associated with a ninth-grade reading level and when this is determined, it is assumed that the patient will need further explanation. The REALM is not a direct comprehensive measure of health literacy but a marker for determining deficits in health literacy.

Reception: Reception refers to the absorption of physical energy (e.g., light and sound).

Reflections: Responses that direct back to the patient the patient's ideas and feelings about the verbal content (as well as the verbal content itself).

Reframing: The strategy of reframing is used to substantially alter disputants' views on an issue. It is used to move parties out of a stalemate and toward new solutions.

Rephrasing: Rephrasing is an approach to encourage self-exploration of a phenomena. It is simply rewording with similar language what the patient has said and pausing for the patient to explain or expand on his or her communication.

Resolution (acceptance): Resolution is the last stage in the adaptation-to-illness process. In the case of death, it is a peaceful period wherein patients accept their impending demise. They no longer resist their diagnosis or prognosis and usually have given up hope that their illness will reverse its course.

Response burden: Response burden refers to the level of demand that is placed on the respondent to address a particular question format. Each question format requires of the respondent time, energy, and certain competencies. Questions that require a great deal from the respondent would be deemed high-response-burden questions, while those requiring little thought, time, or energy would be regarded as low-response-burden questions.

Response-matching: Response-matching refers to the tendency of the receiver to imitate the sender's level of disclosure.

Restatement: Stating again what the patient has said, or using a slightly different wording to reiterate what the patient has said, is making restatements. Restatements are limited to the expressed content. They do not require reference to the feelings that the patient is either expressing or may have expressed.

Role reversal: Role reversal is the reversal of the helper–helpee relationship wherein the provider is seeking assistance from the patient by disclosing some personal issue or problem. It is nontherapeutic and can lead to the patient's distrust of the provider.

SAHLSA-50: The SAHLSA-50, or Short Assessment of Health Literacy for Spanish-Speaking Adults, is based after the REALM and is intended to be used with Spanish-speaking adults only. It is used in the clinical setting to screen patients for low levels of literacy.

Salient attitudes: An individual holds many attitudes and beliefs that are shaped by experience. Those that pertain to a health issue they are facing are described as salient in the context of health behaviors.

Self-disclosure: Self-disclosure refers to instances of openly sharing personal information, including personal preferences, experiences, attitudes, and feelings. It should be used judiciously by the provider and be purposeful.

Self-efficacy: Self-efficacy is the individual's level of confidence that he or she can master a particular challenge. Self-efficacy about a health behavior (e.g., adherence to treatment) is the individual's belief that he or she can be adherent to treatment or will successfully master the actions required to be adherent to their treatment regimen.

Self-management: Self-management refers to the extent to which the patient can successfully manage the treatment and assessment of his or her current medical condition. If self-management behaviors are adequate, the patient may experience improved health-related quality of life and control potential morbidity and early mortality.

Self-reference statements: Self-reference statements are usually spontaneous and reveal a limited amount of personal data. Self-disclosure is not the aim.

Settlement: Settlements are those agreements that come with resolution. Settlements can be either binding or nonbinding decisions.

Significant other (SO): Significant other refers to individuals who may or may not be related by blood or marriage but who act as family members.

Social Ecological Model (Behavioral Ecological Model): This model emphasizes change from the perspective of a multitude of factors, including sociocultural and physical environmental factors. These factors are placed on an equal basis as individual characteristics that create change.

Social learning theory: Social learning theory suggests that change occurs as a function of an individual's experience of his or her social environment in which case situations are experienced and result in a sense of self-efficacy that subsequently shapes whether change will be approached. Bandura (1977) and others suggest that a personal sense of control or self-efficacy enhances behavioral change.

Social network: Social network refers to the structure of social relationships of an individual.

Social penetration: Social penetration is a process in which the depth and breadth of personal disclosures increases over time.

Social support: Social support is a generic term that specifies emotional and/or instrumental support provided by others.

Split-brain: This term is used to refer to conditions wherein a portion of the corpus callosum has been damaged or destroyed.

Stage of action: Stage of action is one phase of the process of behavioral change in the Transtheoretical Model of Change. Action refers to individuals taking steps to change a behavior.

Stage of contemplation: Contemplation of change, according to the Transtheoretical Model of Change, is the stage that indicates that individuals are thinking about changing their behavior but have not started to take action.

Stage of maintainance: According to the Transtheoretical Model of Change, this stage refers to the actions taken to sustain the behavior change.

Stage of pre-contemplation: The stage of pre-contemplation is the stage before contemplating a need or desire for change. The patient is usually not aware of the need for change.

Stage of preparation (for action): Preparation for change follows contemplation of change in the Transtheoretical Model of Change. In this stage, individuals are gathering information and skills to increase their success with the change of behavior.

Stress: Almost any event can pose a threat to the needs or goals of an individual. Every stressful event or situation does not lead to a crisis; a great deal depends on the meaning of the stress to the patient and the extent to which the stressful situation taxes the individual's current capabilities to cope.

Stressors: Stressors are specific stimuli that cause stress. In crisis situations, they are often referred to as stressful events or precipitating events. Newer ideas about stressors suggest that daily hassles and major strains may be as lethal to individuals as the occurrence of major stressful life events.

Supportive self-management: Supportive self-management refers to the actions a provider will take to support the self-management activities a patient will practice. This may include surveys, patient diaries, or measures to assist the patient in coming to a better understanding of his or her condition over time.

Sympathetic nervous system: The sympathetic nervous system includes the neuro-network to the internal organs; this system prepares the body for vigorous activity (e.g., running, lifting, exercising).

Sympathy: This is a term used to refer to the act of feeling the feelings or needs of another. It is usually accompanied by responses of sadness or pity.

Systems of care: Systems of care refer to institutions, organizations, and networks that have the exclusive function of healthcare delivery. Systems of care can facilitate or deter from effective patient–health provider communications.

Teach-back: Teach-back refers to the process of teaching a patient a procedure or explaining a phenomena, and then asking the patient to do a return demonstration or explain in his or her own words what the provider has said. This procedure better ensures that the patient has heard and understands the teaching provided.

Temporal continuum: Self-disclosures can be categorized by their temporal characteristics. Self-disclosures about an individual's current experience include such statements as "I feel cold" or about immediate or distant past experiences such as, "I remember feeling very nervous when I found out my diagnosis."

Theory of reasoned action (TRA): The Theory of Reasoned Action explains why people behave as they do. Fishbein and Ajzen defined and revised this model. The theory expands on how attitudes influence behavior and how some attitudes, norms, and intentions are directly related to behaviors.

Therapeutic communication: Therapeutic communication can occur between any two persons; healthcare providers employ it intentionally to give support, present reality, elicit full descriptions from patients, and so on.

TOPLA and S-TOPLA: The TOPLA is a marker of literacy; and S-TOPLA a shorter version of this measure. Along with the REALM, it is considered a "gold standard" in assessing level of literacy in patients, which would suggest their needs for further explanation of medical conditions and procedures. It is a measure of reading fluency and evaluates both reading prose and numeracy. It has a section to assess labels on prescription vials.

Transduction: Transduction refers to our capacities to change the energy from the physical stimulus to an electrochemical pattern in the brain's neurons.

Transitional care: Transitional care refers to the care that must occur as patients transition from one facility to another (e.g., hospital to home, hospital to nursing home, or outpatient to inpatient care). Transitional care is important in ensuring quality and safe patient care.

Transtheoretical Model of Change: The Transtheoretical Model of Change (Prochaska and others) describes behavior change in stages. The theory supports five phases of change that occur sequentially are considerably more dynamic. Patient–provider communications should be stage specific.

Treatment adherence: Adherence to treatment refers to the degree to which the patient follows the treatment as prescribed by the health provider. More often than not, the term is used to express adherence to medication regimen where the patient follows the prescribed directions and dosage indicated in the physician's recommendation. Adherence also refers to keeping clinic appointments and following recommendations for exercise, diet, self-management of disease, and appropriate preventive measures.

Trust: Trust is the reliance on the veracity and integrity of another individual. In patient–provider relationships, it includes both confidence in providers' competence and perceptions that providers have patients' best interests in mind.

Underlying meaning: Underlying meaning refers to the context in which behaviors occur; they include not-so-obvious thoughts, feelings, and attitudes that explain behavioral responses.

Victim patient: Patients who present as victims are generally self-pitying. They appear somewhat immobilized by a perceived real or anticipated threat. They exhibit low levels of self-esteem and fear rejection. Patients who take on the role of victim without a clear and present threat should be distinguished from those who have been victimized.

Virtual communities (in patient care): Patients who are dealing with an acute or chronic healthcare condition may have the need to frequently talk about their condition with other people who may not be their healthcare providers. Participation in a virtual community might be the only other alternative they have in satisfying their needs that can appear at anytime, anywhere. These services, including chat rooms, provide necessary support as well as information about treatment and how to navigate the healthcare system.

Wellness versus illness: The goal of health promotion stresses the number of years of healthy life that individuals experience. It does not rely heavily on estimates of mortality, or even morbidity, to judge the adequacy of care, because these measures minimize quality-of-life indicators.

White-coat adherence: This type of adherence is used to describe the behaviors immediately proceeding a visit to the provider. Otherwise, it is presumed that the patient will exhibit better adherence immediately before a visit with the provider and that this level of adherence is not a true picture of adherence over time.

References

Abramson, L. Y., Metalsky, F. I., & Alloy, L. B. (1989). Hopelessness depression: A theory based subtype of depression. *Psychological Review, 96*(2), 358–372.

Acosta, F., Jamamoto, J., & Evans, L. A. (1991). *Effective psychotherapy for low-income and minority patients.* New York: Plenum Press. (Epigraph from p. vii)

Agency of Healthcare Quality and Research (AHRQ) (2004). National Health Disparities Report. Accessed August 27, 2007, from http://www.ahrq.gov/qual/nhdr03/nhdrsum03.htm

Agosta, L. Quoted in J. Lichtenberg, M. Bornstein, and D. Silver, eds. 1984. *Empathy*. London: The Analytic Press. (Epigraph from p. 49)

Ajzen, I., & Fishbein, M. (1977). Attitude-behavior relations: A theoretical analysis and review of empirical research. *Psychological Bulletin, 84,* 888–918.

Ajzen, I., & Fishbein, M. (1980). *Understanding attitudes and predicting social behavior*. Englewood Cliffs, NJ: Prentice-Hall.

American Medical Association (AMA). (1999). Ad Hoc Committee on Health Literacy for the Council of Scientific Affairs.

American Medical Association (AMA). (2007). Patient confidentiality. Division of Health Law. Accessed June 19, 2008, from http://www.ama-assn.org/ama/pub/category/4610.html

American Pain Association. (2004). Racial and ethnic identifiers in pain management: The importance to research, clinical practice, and public policy. APS Pain Care Coalition. Accessed May 21, 2008, from http://www.ampainsoc.org/advocacy/ethnoracial.htm

American Psychiatric Association. (2000). *Diagnostic and statistical manual of mental disorders (DSM-IV- TR*). Washington, D.C.: American Psychiatric Association.

Arnold, E., & Boggs, K. (1995). *Interpersonal relationships: Professional communication skills for nurses.* 2nd ed. Philadelphia: W. B. Saunders Co.

Atienza, F., Anguita, M., Martinex-Alzamora, N., Osca, J., Ojeda, S., Almenar, L., et al. (2004). Multicenter randomized trial of a comprehensive hospital discharge and outpatient heart failure management program. *European Journal of Heart Failure*, *6*(5), 643–652.

Auvil, C. A., & Silver, B. W. (1984). Therapist self-disclosure: When is it appropriate? *Perspectives in Psychiatric Care, 22*(2), 57–61.

Averill, J. (1973). Personal control over aversion stimuli and its relationship to stress. *Psychological Bulletin 88*:29. Cited in J. D. Miller, *Coping with chronic illness—overcoming powerlessness*. Philadelphia: F. A. Davis, 1983, p. 23.

Axelrod, D. A., & Goold, S. D. (2000). Maintaining trust in the surgeon-patient relationship: Challenges for the new millennium. *Archives of Surgery, 135*(1), 55–61.

Azoulay, E. (2005). Editorial: The end-of-life family conference: Communication empowers. *American Journal of Respiratory Critical Care Medicine, 171*, 803–805.

Bagozzi, R. P., & Edwards, E. A. (1998). Goal setting and goal pursuit in the regulation of body weight. *Psychology and Health, 13*, 593–621.

Bakan, F. (1971). The eyes have it. *Psychology today, 4*(11), 64–67.
Baker, D. W., Gazmararian, J. A., Williams, M. V., Scott, T., Parker, R. M., Green, D., et al. (2004). J. Health literacy and use of outpatient physician services by Medicare managed care enrollees. *Journal of General Internal Medicine, 19*, 215–220.
Baker, D. W., Parker, R. M., Williams, M. V., Pitkin, K., Parikh, N. S., Coates, W., et al. (1996). The health care experience of patients with low health literacy. *Archives of Family Medicine, 5*(6), 329–334.
Baker, D. W., Parker, R. W., Williams, M. V., Clark, W. S., & Nurss, J. (1997). The relationship of patient reading ability to self-reported health and use of health services. *American Journal of Public Health, 87*, 1027–1030.
Baker, D. W., Parker, R. M., Williams, M. V., & Clark, W. S. (1998). Health literacy and the risk of hospital admission. *Journal of General Internal Medicine, 13*, 791–798.
Baker, D. W., Williams, M. V., Parker, R. M., Gazmararian, J. A., & Nurss, J. R. (1999). Development of a brief test to measure functional health literacy. *Patient Education and Counseling, 38*, 33–42.
Bandler, R., & Grinder, J. (1982). *Reframing: Neurolinguistic programming and the transformation of meaning.* Moab, Utah: Real People Press.
Bandura, A. (1997). *Self-efficacy: The exercise of control.* New York: W.H. Freeman.
Bandura, A. (1986). *Social foundations of thought and action: A social cognitive theory.*Englewood Cliffs, NJ: Prentice-Hall.
Bandura, A. (2000). Exercise of human agency through collective efficacy. *Current Directions in Psychological Science, 9*, 75–78.
Barbara, D. A. (1958). *The art of listening.* Springfield, Ill.: Bannerstone House.
Barbe, W. B., & Milone, M. N. (1980). Modality. *Instructor,* 44–47.
Bass, P. F., Wilson, J. F., Griffith, C. H., & Barnett, D. R. (2002). Residents' ability to identify patients with poor literacy skills. *Academy of Medicine, 77*(10), 1039–1041.
Bass, P. F., Wilson, J. F., & Griffith, C. H. (2003). A shortened instrument for literacy screening. *Journal of General Internal Medicine, 18*(12), 1036–1038.
Bateson, G. (1972). *Steps to an ecology of mind.* New York: Ballantine Books.
Beck, C. K., Rawlins, R. P., & Williams, S. R. (1988). *Mental health–psychiatric nursing: A holistic life-cycle approach.* 2nd ed. St. Louis, MO: C.V. Mosby Co.
Beckjord, E. B., Rutten, L. J. F., Squiers, L., Arora, N. K., Volchmann, L., Moser, R. P., et al. (2007). Use of the internet to communicate with health care providers in the United States: Estimates from the 2003 and 2005 Health Information National Trends Survey (HINTS). *Journal of Medical Internet Research, 9* (3). Accessed November 19, 2007, from http://www.jmir.org/2007/3/e20
Beland, F. (1989). A descriptive study of continuity of care as an element in the process of ambulatory medical care utilization. *Canadian Journal of Public Health, 80*(4), 249–254.
Belle, D. (1982). *Lives in stress.* Beverly Hills, CA: Sage Publications, Inc.
Benjamin, M., & Curtis, J. (1992). *Ethics in nursing.* New York, NY: Oxford University Press.

Berland, G. K., Elliott, M. N., Morales, L. S., Algazy, J. I., Kravitz, R. L., Broder, M. S., et al. (2001). Health information on the internet: Accessbility, quality, and readability in English and Spanish, *JAMA, 285*, 2612–2621.

Bernstein, L. S., & Bernstein, R. S. (1985). *Interviewing: A guide for health professionals*. New York: Appleton Century-Crofts.

Berren, M. R., Santiago, J. M., Zent, M. R., & Carbone, C. P. (1999). Health care utilization by persons with severe and persistent mental illness. *Psychiatric Services, 50*, 559–561.

Berry, L. L., Parish, J. T., Janakiraman, R., Ogburn-Russell, L., Couchman, G. R., Rayburn, W. L., et al. (2008). Patients' commitment to their primary physicians and why it matters. *Annals of Family Medicine,* 6, 6–13.

Bertakis, K. D., Roter, D., & Putnam, S. M. (1991). The relationship of physician medical interview style to patient satisfaction. *Journal of Family Practice, 32*(2), 175–181.

Biem, H. J., Hadjustavropoulos, H. D., Morgan, D., Biem, D., & Pong, R.W. (2003). Breaks in continuity of care and the rural senior transferred for medical care under regionalization. *International Journal of Integrated Care, 3*, 1–16.

Bilu, Y., & Witztum, E. (1994). Culturally sensitive therapy with ultra-orthodox patients: The strategic employment of religious idioms of distress. *Israel Journal of Psychiatry and Related Sciences, 31*(3), 170–182.

Blackburn, J. A. (1992). Achieving a multicultural service orientation: Adaptive models in service delivery, and race and culture training. *Caring, 11*(4), 22–26.

Bluhm, J. (1991a). *How to work with difficult people.* Phoenix, AZ: Judy Bluhm Seminars.

Bluhm, J. (1991b). *The healing triangle in working with difficult people.* Santa Clara, CA: California. (Epigraph from p. 6)

Bok, S. (1978). *Lying—Moral choice in public and private life.* New York, NY: Pantheon Books.

Bokinskie, J. C. (1992). Family conferences: A method to diminish transfer anxiety. *Journal of Neuroscience Nursing, 24*(3), 129–133.

Bolton, R. (1979). *People skills: How to assert yourself, listen to others, and resolve conflicts.* New York: Simon & Schuster.

Bradford, L. P., Stock, D., & Horowitz, M. (1978). How to diagnose group problems in communication and group process. In *Group development*, edited by L. Bradford. Washington, D.C.: National Training Laboratories, National Education Association.

Bradley, J. C., & Edinberg, M. A. (1990). *Communication in the nursing context.* Norwalk, CT: Mosby Year Book.

Brafford, L. P., & Beck, K. P. (1991). Factor analysis of the Condom Use Self-Efficacy Scale among multicultural college students. *Health Education Research, 15*(4), 485–489.

Brock, C. D., & Salinsky, J. V. (1993). Empathy: An essential skill for understanding the physician-patient relationship in clinical practice. *Family Medicine, 25*(4), 245–248.

Brodal, A. (1981). *Neurological anatomy*. 3rd ed. New York: Oxford University Press.

Brown, M., Frost, R., Ko, Y., & Woosley, R. (2007). Diagramming patients' views of root causes of adverse drug events in ambulatory care: An online tool for planning education and research. *Patient Education and Counseling, 62*(3), 302–315.

Brown, S. J. (1995). An interviewing style for nursing assessment. *Journal of Advanced Nursing, 21*, 340–343.

Brown, S. L., Teufel, J. A., & Birch, D. A. (2007). Early adolescents perceptions of health and health literacy. *The Journal of School Health, 77*(1), 7–15.

Buber, M. (1957). Distance and relation. *Psychiatry, 20*, 97–104.

Buchholz, W. (1990). A piece of my mind: Hope. *JAMA, 263*(17), 2357–2358.

Buhl, H. S. (posted 2001). Autonomic nervous system and energetic medicine. The Science of Wilhelm Reich. Accessed from http://www.orgon.articles/article1.htm

Burgess, D., van Ryn, M., Dovidio, J., & Saha, S. (2007). Reducing racial bias among health care providers: Lessons from social-cognitive psychology. *Journal of General Internal Medicine, 22*(6).

Bylund, C. L., Gueguen, J. A., Sabee, C. M., Imes, R. S., Li, Y., & Sanford, A. A. (2007). Provider-patient dialogue about internet health information: An exploration of strategies to improve the provider-patient relationship. *Patient Education and Counseling,* 66(3), 346–352.

Byng, R., Jones, R., Leese, M., Hamilton, B., McCrone, P., & Craig, T. (2004). Exploratory cluster randomized controlled trial of shared care development for long-term mental illness. *British Journal of General Practice, 54*(501), 259–266.

Cable, D. G. (1991). Caring for the terminally ill: Communicating with patients and family. *Henry Ford Hospital Medical Journal, 39*(2), 85–88.

Cade, J. (1993). An evaluation of early patient contact for medical students. *Medical Education, 27*(3), 205–210.

Carkhuff, R. T. (1969). *Helping and human relations: A primer for lay and professional helpers.* Vol. 1, Selection and training. New York: Holt, Rinehart, & Wilson.

Carkhuff, R., & Rordan, J. W. (1987). *The art of helping.* Philadelphia: W. B. Saunders Co.

Centers for Disease Control and Prevention. (1999). National Center for Health Statistics: Preliminary Data for 1999. Accessed September 19, 2007, from http://www.cdc.gov/nccdphp/overview.htm

Cherry, D. K., Woodell, D. A., & Rechtsteiner, E. A. (2007). National ambulatory medical care survey: 2005 summary. *CDC Advance Data, Vital and Health Statistics, 287*, 1–40.

Chilingaryan, L. I. (2001). Pavlov's theory of higher nervous activity: Landmarks and developmental trends. *Neuroscience and Behavioral Physiology, 31*(1), 39–47.

Chisolm, D. J., & Buchanan, L. (2007). Measuring adolescent functional health literacy: A pilot validation of the Test of Functional Health Literacy in Adults. *Journal of Adolescent Health, 41*(3), 312–314.

Christiansen, M., Vik, P., & Jarchow, A. (2002). College student heavy drinking in social contexts versus alone. *Addictive Behaviors, 27*(3), 393–404.

Clark, K. B. (1980). Empathy: A neglected topic in psychological research. *American Psychologist, 35*(2), 187–190.

Cohen, S., & Wills, T. A. (1985). Stress, social support, and the buffering hypothesis. *Psychological Bulletin, 98*(2), 310–357.
Cole-Kelly, K. (1992). Illness stories and patient care in the family practice context. *Family Medicine, 24*(1), 45–48.
Coleman, E. A., Smith, J. D., Frank, J. C., Ellertsen, T. B., Thiare, J. N., & Kramer, A. M. (2002). Development and testing of a measure designed to assess the quality of care transitions. *International Journal of Integrated Care,* April–June, 2, e02.
Coleman, E. A., Mahoney, E., & Parry, C. (2005). Assessing the quality of preparation for posthospital care from the patient's perspective: The care transitions measure. *Medical Care, 43*(3), 246–255.
Coleman, M. T., & Newton, K. S. (2005). Supporting self-management in patients with chronic illness. *American Family Physician, 72*(80), 1503–1510.
Coleman, E. A., Parry, C., Chalmers, S., & Min, S. J. (2006). The care transition intervention: Results of a randomized controlled trial. *Archives of Internal Medicine, 166*(17), 1822–1828.
Coleman, T., Cheater, F., & Murphy, E. (2004). Qualitative study investigating the process of giving anti-smoking advice in general practice. *Patient Education and Counseling, 52,* 159–163.
Collins, M. (1977). *Communication in health care: Understanding and implementing effective human relationships*. St. Louis, Mo: C.V. Mosby Co.
Conlin, K. K., & Schumann, L. (2002). Research. Literacy in the health care system: a study on open heart surgery patients. *Journal of the American Academy of Nurse Practitioners, 14*(1), 38–42.
Cotton, S. R, & Gupta, S. S. (2004). Characteristics of online and offline health information seekers and factors that discriminate between them. *Social Science and Medicine, 59*, 1795–806 [Medline].
Cournoyer, B. (1991). *The social work skills workbook*. Belmont, CA: Wadsworth Publishing Co.
Cowan, M. J. (2004). Hallmarks of quality: Generating and using knowledge. *Communicating Nursing Research,* 37(1), 3–12.
Crate, M. A. (1965). Nursing functions in adaptation to chronic illness. *The American Journal of Nursing, 65*(10), 72–76.
Cross, T. L., Bazron, B. J., Dennis, K. W., & Isaacs, M. R. (1989). Towards a culturally competent system of care. Washington, D.C.: CASSP Technical Assistance Center, Georgetown University Child Development Center.
Crotty, M., Rowett, D., Spurling, L., Giles, L. C., & Philips, P. A. (2004). Does the addition of a pharmacist transition coordinator improve evidence-based medication management and health outcomes in older adults moving from the hospital to a long-term care facility? Results of a randomized, controlled trial. *American Journal of Geriatric Pharmacotherapy, 2*(4), 257–264.
Crowther, D. J. (1991). Metacommunications: A missed opportunity? *Journal of Psychosocial Nursing and Mental Health Services, 29*(4),13–16.
Curtis, J. R., Engelberg, R. A., Nielsen, E. L., Au, D. H., & Patrick, D. L. (2004). Patient-physician communication about end-of-life care for patients with COPD. *European Respiratory Journal, 24*, 200–205.
Davidhizar, R., & Giger, J. R. (1994). When your patient is silent. *Journal of Advanced Nursing, 20*(4), 703–706.

Davis, C. M. (1990). What is empathy, and can empathy be taught? *Physical Therapy, 70*(11), 707–711.

Davis, T. C., Michielutte, R., Askov, E. N., Williams, M. V., & Weiss, B. D. (1998). Practical assessment of adult literacy in health care. *Health Education and Behavior, 25*(5), 613–624.

Davis-Martin, S. (1994). Perceived needs of families of long-term critical care patients: A brief report. *Heart and Lung, 23*(6), 515–518.

Day, M. E. (1964). An eye movement phenomenon relating to attention, thought, and anxiety. *Perceptual and Motor Skills, 19*, 443–446.

Debate, R. D., & Pyle, G. F. (2003). Early entry into WIC: Ethnic perceptions and cues to action. Abstract Academy of Health Meet. 20, abstract no. 721. (Available National Library of Medicine).

Del Mar, C. B. (1994). Communicating well in general practice. *The Medical Journal of Australia, 160*(21), 367–370.

Denny, M. R., & Ratner, S. C. (1970). *Comparative psychology: Research in animal behavior*. Rev. ed. Homewood, IL: Dorsey Press.

Diaz, J. A., Griffith, R. A., Ng, J. J., Friedmann, P. D., & Moulton, A. W. (2002). Patients' use of the internet for medical information. *Journal of General Internal Medicine, 17*(3), 180–185.

Diette, G. B., & Rand, C. (2007). The contributing role of health-care communication to health disparities for minority patients with Asthma. *Chest, 132*, 802S–809.

Dilorio, C., Dudley, W. N., Soet, J., Watkins, J., & Maibach, E. (2000). A social cognitive-based model for condom use among college students. *Nursing Research, 49*(4), 208–214.

Dilts, R. (1983). *Applications of neuro-linguistic programming*. Cupertino, CA: Meta Publications.

Dilts, R. B., Grinder, J., Bandler, R., Delozier, J., & Cameron-Bandler, L. (1979). Neurolinguistic programming.(Vol 1). Cupertino, CA: Meta Publications.

Di Noia, J. D., Schinke, S. P., Prochaska, J. O., & Contento, I. R. (2006). Application of the Transtheoretical Model to fruit and vegetable consumption among economically disadvantaged African-American adolescents: Preliminary findings. *American Journal of Health Promotion, 20*(5), 342–348.

Doescher, M. P., Saver, B. G., Franks, P., & Fiscella, K. (2000). Racial and ethnic disparities in perceptions of physician style and trust. *Archives of Family Medicine, 9*(10), 1156–1163.

Donovan, H. S., Hartenbach, E. M., & Method, M. W. (2005). Patient-provider communication and perceived control for women experiencing multiple symptoms associated with ovarian cancer. *Gynecological Oncology. 99*(2), 404–411.

Downey, L. A., & Zun, L. (2007). Testing of a verbal assessment tool of English proficiency for use in the healthcare setting. *The Journal of the National Medical Association, 99*(7), 795–798.

Drossman, D. A., Leserman, J., Li, Z., Keefe, F., Hu, Y. J. B., & Moomey, T. C. (2000). Effects of coping on health outcome among women with gastrointestinal disorders. *Psychosomatic Medicine, 62*, 309–317.

Druss, B. G., & Rhohrbaugh, R. M. (2001). Integrated medical care for patients with serious psychiatric illness: A randomized trial. *Archives of General Psychiatry, 58*(9), 861–868.

Dunham-Taylor, J. (2000). Nurse executive transformational leadership found in participative organizations. *Journal of Nursing Administration, 30*(5), 241–250.

Dutta-Bergman, M. J. (2005). The relation between health-orientation, provider-patient communication, and satisfaction: An individual-difference approach. *Health Communications, 18*(3), 291–303.

Duvall, E. M. (1977). *Marriage and family development*. 5th ed. Philadelphia: J.B. Lippincott, Inc.

Egger, G., & Swinburn, B. (1997). An "ecological" approach to the obesity pandemic. *British Medical Journal, 317*, 477–480.

Ehmann, V. (1971). Empathy. Its origin, characteristics and process, *Perspectives in Psychiatric Care 9*(77). Cited in S. J. Sundeen, G. W. Stuart, E. A. D. Rankin, and S. A. Cohen, Nurse-client interaction—Implementing the nursing process. St. Louis, MO: Mosby Yearbook, Inc., 1994, p. 176.

Elder, J. P., Ayala, G. X., & Harris, S. (1999). Theories and intervention approaches to health-behavior change. Available online. Adapted from: Theories and intervention approaches to health behavior in primary care. *American Journal of Preventive Medicine, 17*(4), 275–284.

Engel, G. L. (1960). A unified concept of health and disease. *Perspectives in Biology and Medicine, 3*, 459–485.

Erikson, E. H. (1963). *Childhood and society.* New York: Norton, Inc.

Ervin, M. G. (2004). Unequal access to hospice and palliative care. *Journal of Palliative Medicine, 7*(2), 301–302.

Evans, B. J., Stanley, R. O., & Burrows, G. D. (1993). Measuring medical students' empathy skills, part 2. *British Journal of Medical Psychology, 66*,121–133.

Evans, D. R., Hern, M. T., Uhlemann, M. R., & Ivey, A. E. (1989). *Essential interviewing: A programmed approach to effective communication.* Pacific Grove, CA: Brooks/Cole.

Eysenbach, G. (2000). Towards ethical guidelines for dealing with unsolicited patient emails and giving teleadvice in the absence of a pre-existing patient-physician relationship–Systematic review and expert survey. *Journal of Medical Internet Research, 2*(1). Accessed from http://www.jmir.org/2000/1/el/

Fagerberg, B., Claesson, L., Gosman-Hedstrom, G. B., & Blomstrand, C. (2000). Effect of acute stroke unit care integrated with care continuum versus conventional treatment: A randomized 1-year study of elderly patients: The Goteborg 70+ Stroke Study. *Stroke, 11*, 2578–2584.

Fishbein, M., & Ajzen, I. (1975). *Belief, attitude, intention, and behavior: An introduction to theory and research*. Reading, MA: Addison-Wesley.

Fishbein, M. (1967). Readings in attitude theory and measurement. New York: Wiley.

Fjaertoft, H., Indredavik, B., Johnsen, R., & Lydersen S. (2004). Acute stroke unit care combined with early supported discharge. Long-term effects on quality of life. A randomized controlled trial. *Cliinical Rehabilitation, 18*(5), 580–586.

Fleishman, P. R. (1989). *The healing zone*: *Religious issues in psychotherapy*. New York: Paragon House.

Fordham, C. C., III. (1994). Issues of trust in medicine. *Southern Medical Journal, 87*(7), 770. (Epigraph from p. 770)

Foster, W. A. Accessed December 11, 2007, from WorldofQuotes.com, http://www.worldofquotes.com/topic/Quality/1/index.html

Fox, S., & Rainie, L. (2000). The online health care revolution: How the web helps Americans take better care of themselves. Washington DC: Pew Internet & American Life Project (cited 2007 November from: http://www.pewinternet.org/ppf/r/26/report_display.asp)

Fox, S., & Fallows, D. (July 16, 2003). Internet health resources. Health searches and email have become more commonplace, but there is room for improvement in searches and overall Internet access. Washington, D.C.:Pew Internet & American Life Project. Accessed from http://www.pewinternet.org/

Frankel, R. M. (1995). Emotion and the physician-patient relationship. *Motivation and Emotion, 19*(3). Accessed from http://www.springerlink.com/content/y35hg48130mh4912/

Freud, S. (Brill, A.A., Translator). (1995). *The basic writings of Sigmund Freud*. New York: Random House.

Fuchs, R. (1996). Causal models of physical exercise participation: Testing the predictive power of the construct "pressure to change". *Journal of Applied Social Psychology, 26*, 1931–1960.

Gadacz, T. R. (2003). A changing culture in interpersonal and communication skills. *American Surgery, 69*(6), 453–458.

Gardner, E. R., & Hall, R. C. W. (1981). The professional stress syndrome. *Psychosomatics, 22*, 672–680.

Gazda, G. M., Childers, W. C., & Walters, R. P. (1982). *Interpersonal communication: A handbook for health professionals.* Gaithersburg, MD: Aspen Publishers, Inc. (Epigraph from pp. 141–142)

Geisser, M. E., Robinson, M. E., Keefe, F. J., & Weiner, M. L. (1994). Catastrophizing, depression, and the sensory, affective and evaluative aspects of chronic pain. *Pain, 59*, 79–83.

Geschwind, N., & Levitsky, W. (1968). Human brain: Left-right asymmetries in temporal speech region. *Science, 161*, 168–187.

Giger, J. N., & Davidhizar, R. (2002). The Giger and Davidhizar Transcultural Assessment Model. *Journal of Transcultural Nursing, 13*(3), 185–188.

Gill, J. M., & Mainous, A. G. (1998). The role of provider continuity in preventing hospitalizations. *Archives of Family Medicine, 7*(4), 352–357.

Gill, J. M., Mainous, A. G., Diamond, J. J., & Lentard, M. J. (2003). Impact of provider continuity on quality of care for persons with diabetes mellitus. *Annals of Family Medicine, 1*, 162–170.

Gilmour, J. A. (2007). Reducing disparities in the access and use of internet health information. A discussion paper. *Journal of Nursing Studies, 44*(7), 1270–1278.

Gladstein, G. A. (1987). *Counselor empathy and client outcomes, in Empathy and counseling: Explorations in theory and research,* edited by G. A. Gladstein. New York: Springer-Verlag. Cited in S. J. Sundeen, G. W. Stuart, E. A. D. Rankin, and S. A. Cohen, *Nurse-client interaction—Implementing the nursing process.* St. Louis, MO: Mosby Yearbook, Inc., 1994, p. 178.

Glassby, P. F. (2002). Health illiteracy-the hidden handicap. *Journal of IR Dental Association, 48*(2), 67–68.

Gold, M. (2004). Ethics in medicine: Is honesty always the best policy? Ethical aspects of truth telling. *Internal Medicine Journal, 34*, 578–580.

Goldman, J. (1967). *A comparison of sensory modality preference of children and adults.* Ph.D. diss., Yeshiva University, New York.
Goodman, G., & Esterly, G. (1988). *The talk book: The intimate science of communicating in close relationships.* Emmaus, PA: Rodela.
Gordon, D. (1978). *Therapeutic metaphors: Helping others through the looking glass*. Cupertino, CA: Meta Publications.
Gordon, M. M., Capell, H. A., & Madhok, R. (2002). The use of the internet as a resource for health information among patients attending a rheumatology clinic. *Rheumatology, 41*, 1402–1405.
Grunfeld, E., Gray, A., Mant, D., Yudkin, P., Adewuyi-Dalton, R., Coyle, D., et al. (1999). Follow up of breast cancer in primary care vs specialist care: Results of an economic evaluation. *British Journal of Cancer, 79,* 1227–1233.
Gulmans, J., Vollenbroek-Hutten, J. E., van Gemert-Pijnen, W. C., & van Harten, W. H. (2007). Evaluating quality of patient care communication in integrated care settings: A mixed method approach. *International Journal for Quality in Health Care,* July, 1–8.
Gur, R. E. (1975). Conjugate lateral eye movements as an index of hemispheric activation. *Journal of Personality and Social Psychology, 31*, 751–757.
Guthrie, B., & Wyke, S. (2000). Does continuity in general practice really matter? *British Medical Journal, 321*, 734–736.
Haas, J. S., Weissman, J. S., Cleary, P. D., Goldberg, J., Gatsonis, C., Seage, G. R., et al. (1993). Discussion of preferences for life-sustaining care by persons with AIDS: Predictors of failure in patient-physician communication. *Archives of Internal Medicine, 153*(10), 1241–1248.
Haggerty, J. L., Reid, R. J., Freeman, G. K., Starfield, B. H., Adair, C. E., & McKendry, R. (2003). Continuity of care: A multidisciplinary review. *British Medical Journal, 327*, 1219–1221.
Hahn, S. R. (2001). Physical symptoms and physician-experienced difficulty in the patient-physician relationship. *Annuals of Internal Medicine, 134*,897–904.
Halbert, C. H., Armstrong, K., Gandy, O. H., & Shaker, L. (2006). Racial differences in trust in health care providers. *Archives of Internal Medicine, 166*(8), 896–901.
Haley, J., & Haley, M. R. (2000). Directive Family Therapy. *The Family Journal, 9*, 227. (DVs of Haley's work available online)
Hall, M. A., Zheung, B., Dugan, E., Camacho, F., Kidd, K. E., Mishra, A., et al. (2002). Measuring patients' trust in their patient care providers. *Medical Care Research and Review, 59*(3), 293–318.
Halpern, J. (2003). What is clinical empathy? *Journal of General Internal Medicine, 18*, 670–674.
Hames, C. C., & Joseph, D. H. (1986). Basic concepts of helping. In *Communications in nursing*, edited by S. B. Smith. St. Louis, MO: Mosby Year Book, 1992.
Hammer, E. F., ed. (1968). *Use of interpretation in treatment.* New York: Grune & Stratton, pp. 1–41. (Epigraph from p. 6)
Han, B., & Haley, W. E. (1999). Family caregiving for patients with stroke: Review and analysis. *Stroke, 30*, 1478–1485.
Hanes, C. C., & Joseph, D. H. (1986). *Basic concepts of helping: A holistic approach*. Norwalk, CT: Appleton-Century-Crofts.
Harrison, M. B., Browne, G. B., Roberts, J., Tugwell, P., Gafni, A., & Graham, I. D. (2002). Quality of life of individuals with heart failure: A randomized

trial of the effectiveness of two models of hospital-to-home transition. *Medical Care, 40*(4), 271–282.

Hawkins, R. P., Lee, S., & Hwang, H. (2006). Why do patients use the internet? The effects of insufficiency on patients' health-related internet use. Accessed November 19, 2007, from http://www.allacademic.com/meta/p92971_index.html

Haynes, D. F., & Watt, P. (2008). The lived experience of health behaviors in people with debilitating illness. *Holistic Nursing Practice, 22*(1), 44–53.

Hazavehei, S. M., Taghdisi, M. H., & Saidi, M. (2007). Application of the Health Belief Model for osteoporosis prevention among middle school girl students, Garmsar, Iran. Education for Health. Accessed from http://www.education-forhealth.net/

Hein, E. C. (1980). *Communication in nursing practice*. 2d ed. Boston, MA: Little, Brown & Co.

Herth, K. (1989). The relationship between level of hope and level of coping response with other variables in patients with cancer. *Oncology Nursing Forum, 16*, 67–72.

Hesse, B. W., Nelson, D. E., Kreps, G. L., Croyle, R. T., Arora, N. K., et al. (2005). Trust and sources of health information: The impact of the internet and its implications for health care providers: Findings from the first Health Information National Trends Survey. *Archives of Internal Medicine, 165*, 2618–2624.

Hill, C. E., & Gormally, F. (1977). Effects of reflection, restatement, probe, and nonverbal behaviors on client affect. *Journal of Counseling Psychology, 24*(2), 92–97.

Hojat, M., Gonnella, J. S., Nasca, T. J., Mangione, S., Vergare, M., & Magee, M. (2002). Physician empathy: Definition, components, measurement, and relationship to gender and specialty. *American Journal of Psychiatry, 159*(9), 1563–1569.

Holmes, T. H., & Masuda, M. (1974). Life changes and illness susceptibility. In *Stressed life events: The nature and effects,* edited by B. S. Dohrenwend and B. H. Dohrenwend. New York: John Wiley & Co.

Holmes, T. H., & Rahe, R. H. (1967). The Social Readjustment Rating Scale. Journal of Psychosomatic Research, 11(2), 213–218.

Howell, J. B., & Schroeder, D. P. (1984). *Physician stress: A handbook for coping.* Baltimore, MD: University Park Press.

Hull, S. K., & Broquet, K. (2007). How to manage difficult patient encounters. *Family Practice Management, 14*(6).

Institute of Medicine. (2000). *To Err Is Human: Building a Safer Health System.* Kohn, K. T., Corrigan, J. M., Donaldson, M. S. (Eds).Washington, DC: National Academy Press.

Institute of Medicine. (2001). *Crossing the Quality Chasm: A New Health System for the 21st Century.* Washington, DC: National Academy Press.

Institute of Medicine. (2002a). *Unequal treatment: Confronting racial and ethnic disparities in health care.* Washington DC: National Academies Press.

Institute of Medicine. (2002b). Committee on Rapid Advance Demonstration Projects: Health Care Finance and Delivery Systems, Janet M. Corrigan, Ann Greiner, Shari M. Erickson (Eds.). Fostering rapid advances in health care: Learning from system demonstrations. Accessed from www.nap.edu

Institute of Medicine. (2004a). *Keeping Patients Safe: Transforming the Work Environment of Nurses.* Accessed from www.iom.edu/cms/3809/4671/16173.aspx

Institute of Medicine. (2004b). *1st Annual Crossing the Quality Chasm Summit: A Focus on Communities.* Accessed from www.iom.edu.CMS/3809/9868/22344/aspx

Institute of Medicine. (2004c). *Health Literacy: A Prescription to End Confusion.* Washington, DC: National Academic Press.

Institute of Medicine. (2004d). *Improving Medical Education: Enhancing the Behavioral and Social Science Content of Medical School Curriculum.* Accessed from http://www.iom.edu/CMS/3775/3891/19413.aspx

Institute of Medicine/National Academy of Service (IOM/NAS). (2004). *Crossing the Quality Chasm Report.* Washington, DC: IOM.

Institute of Medicine. (2006a). *The Chasm in Quality: Select Indicators from Recent Reports.* Accessed September 6, 2007, from http://www.iom.edu/CMS/8089/14980.aspx

Institute of Medicine. (2006b). *Identifying and Preventing Medication Errors.* Accessed from http://www.iom.edu/CMS/3809/22526.aspx

Jackson, J. L., & Kroenke, K. (1999). Difficult patient encounters in the ambulatory clinic: Clinical predictors and outcomes. *Archives of Internal Medicine, 159*, 1069–1075.

Jackson, S. W. (1992). The listening healer in the history of psychological healing. *The American Journal of Psychiatry, 149*(12), 1623–1632.

Janosik, E. H. (1984). *Crisis counseling: A contemporary approach.* Monterey, CA: Wadsworth Health Sciences Division. (Epigraph from p. 5)

Johnson, S. S., Driskell, M. M., Johnson, J. L., Dyment, S. J., Prochaska, J. M., & Bourne, L. (2006). Transtheoretical model intervention for adherence to lipid-lowering drugs. *Disease Management, 9*, 102–114.

The Joint Commission. (2007). *"What did the doctor say?:" Improving health literacy to protect patient safety.* Oakbrook Terrace, IL. The Joint Commission., Accessed May 21, 2008, from http://www.jointcommission.org/NR/rdonlyres/D5248B2E-E7E6-4121-8874-99C7B4888301/0/improving_health_literacy.pdf

Jourard, S. M. (1971). *The transparent self.* New York: Van Nostrand Reinhold.

Kaiser Family Foundation. (2006). Accessed October 4, 2007, from http://www.imshealth.com

Kaiser Family Foundation. (2007). Prescription drug trends. Accessed October 4, 2007, from http://www.imshealth.com

Kalichmann, S. C., & Rompa, D. (2000). Emotional reactions to health status changes and emotional well-being among HIV-positive persons with limited reading literacy. *Journal of Clinical Psychology in Medical Settings, 7*(4), 203–211.

Kao, A. C., Green, D. C., Davis, N. A., Koplan, J. P., & Cleary, P. D. (1998). Patient' trust in their physicians effects of choice, continuity, and payment method. *Journal of General Internal Medicine, 13*(10), 681–686.

Katz, R. L. (1963). *Empathy: Its nature and uses.* New York: Free Press.

Katz, S. J., Nissan, N., & Moyer, C. A. (2004). Crossing the digital divide: evaluating online communication between patients and their providers. *The American Journal of Managed Care, 10*(9), 593–598.

Kavan, M. G., Guck, T. P., & Barone, E. J. (2006). *American Family Physician, 74*, 1159–1166.

Keitz, S. A., Box, T. L., Homan, R. K., Barlett, J. A., & Oddone, E. Z. (2001). Primary care for patients infected with Human Immunodeficiency Virus. *Journal of General Internal Medicine, 16*, 573–582.

Kercher, E. E. (1991). Crisis intervention in the emergency department. *Emergency Medicine Clinics of North America, 9*(1), 219–232.

Khanna, N., & Phillips, M. D. (2001). Adherence to care plan in women with abnormal papanicoloa smears: A review of barriers and interventions. *Journal of the American Board of Family Practice, 14*, 123–130.

Kibbe, D. C., Phillips, R. L., & Green, L. A. (2004). The continuity of care record. *American Family Physician, 70*, 1220–1223.

Kimura, D. (1961). Cerebral dominance and the perception of verbal stimuli. *Canadian Journal of Psychology 15*,166–171.

Kinsler, J. J., Wong, M. D., Sayles, J. N., Davis, C., & Cunningham, W. E. (2007). The effect of perceived stigma from a health care provider on access to care among a low-income HIV-positive population. *AIDS Patient Care and STDs, 21*(8), 584–592.

Kirlin, D. (2007). Truth telling, autonomy and the role of metaphor. *Journal of Medical Ethics, 33*, 11–14.

Kirsch, I. S., Jungeblut, A., Jenkins, L., & Kolstad, A. (1993). *Adult literacy in America: A first look at the findings of the National Adult Literacy Survey.* 2nd ed. Washington DC: Department of Education (U.S.), Office of Educational Research and Improvement.

Knafl, K., Breitmayer, B., Gallo, A., & Zoeller, L. (1992). Parents' views of health care providers: An exploration of the components of a positive working relationship. *Childrens Health Care 21*(2), 90–95.

Knauft, M. E., Nielsen, E. L., Engelberg, R. A., Patrick, D. L., & Curtis, J. R. (2005). Barriers and facilitators to end-of-life care communication for patients with COPD. *Chest, 127*, 2188–2196.

Koopman, R. J., Mainous, A. G., Baker, R., Gill, J. M., & Gilbert, G. E. (2003). Continuity of care and recognition of diabetes, hypertension, and hypercholestrolemia. *Archives of Internal Medicine, 163*(11), 1357–1361.

Krashen, S. D. (1977). The left hemisphere. In *The human brain*, edited by M. C. Wittrock. Englewood Cliffs, NJ: Prentice-Hall, Inc.

Kübler-Ross, E. (1969). *On death and dying*. New York: Macmillan.

Lane, R. C., Koetting, M. G., & Bishop, J. (2002). Silence as communication in psychodynamic psychotherapy. *Clinical Psychology Review, 22*(7), 1091–1104.

Lang, F., & McCord, R. S. (1999). Agenda setting in the patient-physician relationship. *The Journal of the American Association of Medicine, 282*(10), 942–943.

Lavizzo-Mourey, R., & Jung, M. (2005). Fighting unequal treatment: The Robert Wood Johnson Foundation and a quality-improvement approach to disparities. *Circulation, 111*, 1208–1209.

Lax, D., & Sebenius, J. (1986). *The manager and negotiator*. New York: Free Press.

Lazarus, R., & Folkman, S. (1984). *Stress, appraisal and coping.* New York: Springer Publishing.

Lee, S. Y., Bender, D. E., Ruiz, R. E., & Cho, Y. I. (2006). Development of an easy-to-use Spanish health literacy test. *Health Services Research, 41*(4, Part 1), 1392–1412.

Lee, Y., & Lin, J. (2008). Linking patients' trust in physicians to health outcomes. *British Journal of Hospital Medicine, 69*(1), 42–46.

Levine, S. M. (2001). Positive results from clinician-patient communication programs at Kaiser Permante: A physician's view. *The Permanente Journal, 5*(2).

Levinson, W. (1994). Physician-patient communication: A key to malpractice prevention. *JAMA, 272*, 1619–1620.

Levinson, W., Gorawara-Bhat, R., Dueck, R., Egener, B., Kao, A., Kerr, C., et al. (1999). Resolving disagreements in the patient-physician relationship: Tools for improving communication in managed care. *The Journal of the American Medical Association, 282*(15), 1477–1483.

Liegner, E. (1971). The silent patient. *Psychoanalytic Review, 61*, 229–245.

Lin, P., Simoni, J. M., & Zemon, V. (2005). The health belief model, sexual behaviors, and HIV risk among Taiwanese immigrants. *AIDS Education and Prevention, 17*(5), 469–483.

Lipps, T. (1935). *Empathy, I . . . , Imitation and Sense. Feelings*. In *A modern book of esthetics: An anthology*, edited by M. M. Rader. New York: Henry Holt.

Lloyd, K. B., & Berger, B. A. (2002). Communicating with the allergic rhinitis patients. *U.S. Pharmacist, 27*(10),. Accessed May 20, 2008, from http://www.uspharmacist.com/index.asp?show=article&page=8_962.htm

Lussier, M. T., & Richard, C. (2007). Feeling understood: Expression of empathy during medical consultations. *Canadian Family Physician, 53*(4), 640–641.

MacLean, P. D. (1962). New findings relevant to the evolution of psychosexual functions of the brain. *Journal of Nervous and Mental Disease, 135*, 289–301.

MacLean, P. D. (1970). The limbic brain in relation to the psychoses. In *Physiological correlates of emotion*, edited by P. Black. New York: Academic, pp. 129–146.

MacLean, P. D. (1973). *A triune concept of the brain and behavior*. Toronto: University of Toronto Press.

Maguire, P., & Pitceathy, C. (2002). Key communication skills and how to acquire them. *British Medical Journal, 325*, 697–700.

Martyres, G. (1995). On silence: A language for emotional experience. *Australian and New Zealand Journal of Psychiatry, 29*(1), 118–123.

Marwick, C. (1997). Patients' lack of literacy may contribute to billions of dollars in higher hospital costs. *Journal of the American Medical Association 278*, 971–972.

Massachusetts Coalition for the Prevention of Medical Errors. MEDLIST. Massachusetts Medical Society. Accessed October 4, 2007, from http://www.macoalition.org/

Masson, V. (2005). Here to be seen: Ten practical lessons in cultural consciousness in primary health care. *Journal of Cultural Diversity, 12*(3), 94–98.

Matthews, D. A., Suchman, A. L., & Branch, W. T. (1993). Making "connexions": Enhancing the therapeutic potential of patient-clinician relationships. *Annals of Internal Medicine, 118*(12), 973–977.

Mayeaux, E. J., Murphy, P. W., Arnold, C., Davis, T. C., Jackson, R., & Maslach, C. (1982). *Burnout: The cost of caring*. Englewood Cliffs, NJ: Prentice-Hall.

McCleary, R. A. (1966). Response-modulating functions of the limbic system: Initiation and suppression. In *Progress on physiological psychology*, edited by E. Steller and J. M. Sprague. New York: Academic.

Mc Daniel, S. H., Beckman, H. B., Morse, D. S., Silberman, J., Seaburn, D. B., & Epstein, R. M. (2007). Physician self-disclosure in primary care visits: Enough about you, what about me? *Archives of Internal Medicine, 167*(12), 1321–1326.

McKay, J. R., Lynch, K. G., Shepard, D. S., Morgenstern, J., Forman, R. F., & Pettinatic, H. M. (2005). Do patient characteristics and initial progress in treatment moderate the effectiveness of telephone-based continuing care for substance use disorders? *Addictions,* 100, 216–226.

McKinley, R. K., Stevenson, K., Adams, S., & Manku-Scott, T. K. (2002). Meeting patient expectations of care: The major determinant of satisfaction with out-of-hours primary medical care? *Family Practice, 19*(4), 333–338.

McLeroy, K. R., Bibeau, D., Steckler, A., & Glanz, K. (1988). An ecological perspective on health promotion programs. *Health Education Quarterly, 15*(4), 351–377.

McMillan, S. C., & Mahon, M. (1994). Measuring quality of life in hospice patients using a newly developed Hospice Quality of Life Index. *Quality of Life Research, 3*(6), 437–448.

McMullan, M. (2006). Patients using the internet to obtain health information: How this affects the patient–health professional relationship. *Patient Education and Counseling 63*, 24–28.

Meredith, L. S., Orlando, M., Humphrey, N., Camp, P., & Shelbourne, C. D. (2001). Are better ratings of the patient-provider relationship associated with higher quality of care for depression. *Medical Care, 39*(4), 349–360.

Miller, D., Brownlee, C. D., McCoy, T. P., & Pignone, M. P. (2007). The effect of health literacy on knowledge and receipt of colorectal cancer screening: A survey study. *BioMed Central Family Practice 8,* 16. Published online 2007 March 30. doi: 10.1186/1471-2296-8-16.

Miller, G. A. (1956). The magical number seven, plus or minus two: Some limits on our capacity for processing information. *Psychological Review, 6*, 81–97.

Miller, J. F. (1983). *Coping with chronic illness: Overcoming powerlessness.* Philadelphia: F. A. Davis Company. (Epigraph from p. 15)

Miller, L. G., Liu, H., Hays, R. D., Golin, C. E., Ye, Z., et al. (2003). Knowledge of regimen dosing and medication adherence: A longitudinal study of antiretroviral medication use. *Clinical Infectious Diseases, 36*, 514–518.

Miller, M., & Degenholtz, H. (2003). The relationship between general functional literacy and use of preventive health care services among the elderly. *Gerontologist, 43*, 74–75.

Miller, W. L. (1992). Routine, ceremony or drama: An exploratory field study of the primary care clinical encounter. *Journal of Family Practice, 34*(3), 289–296.

Miller, W. R., & Rollnick, S. (1991). *Motivational interviewing: Preparing people to change addictive behavior*. New York: Guilford Press.

Miller, W. R., & Rollnick, S. (2002). *Motivational interviewing.* New York: Guilford Press.

Minuchin, S. (1974). *Families and family therapy*. Cambridge, MA: Harvard University Press.

Mirotznik, J., Ginzler, E., Zagon, G., & Baptiste, A. (1998). Using the Health Belief Model to explain clinic appointment-keeping for the management of a chronic disease condition. *Journal of Community Health, 23*(3),195–210.

Modlin, C. S. (2003). Culture, race, and disparities in health care. *Cleveland Clinic Journal of Medicine, 70*(4), 283–288.

Moher, M., Yadkin, P., & Wright, L. (2001). Cluster randomized controlled trial to compare three methods of promoting secondary prevention of coronary heart disease in primary care. *British Medical Journal, 322*, 1–7.

Molassiotis, A. (1997). A conceptual model of adaptation to illness and quality of life for cancer patients treated with bone marrow transplants. *Journal of Advanced Nursing, 26*(3), 572–579.

Mooney, K. H., Beck, S. L., Friedman, R. H., & Farzanfar, R. (2002). Telephone-linked care for cancer symptom monitoring. *Cancer Practice, 10*(3), 147–154.

Moore, C. W. (1986). *The mediation process.* Boulder, CO: Communication/Decisions/Results (CDR) Associates, pp. 1–87.

Morales, L. S., Cunningham, W. E., Liu, H., Brown, J. A., & Hays, R. D. (1999). Are Latinos less satisfied with communication by health providers? *Journal of General Internal Medicine, 14*(7), 409–417.

Mullally, L. (1977). Educational cognitive style: Implications for instruction. *Theory Into Practice, 16*, 238–242.

Murero, M., D'Ancona, G., & Karamanoukian, H. (2001). Use of the internet by patients before and after cardiac surgery: Telephone survey. *Journal of Medical Internet Research, 3*, pe27.

National Cancer Institute. Accessed October 4, 2007, from hpp://www.cancer.gov/cancertopics/pdq/supportivecare/depression/HealthProfessional/

National Cancer Institute. (2004). Addressing areas of public health emphasis: Improving the quality of cancer care. Accessed May 21, 2008, from http://plan2004.cancer.gov/public/quality.htm

National Institutes of Health (NIH). (2002). Accessed October 4, 2007, from http://www.nih.gov/news/pr/jul2002/od-17.htm

Naylor, M. D., Brooten, D. A., Cambell, R. L., Maislin, G., McCaulety, K. M., & Schwartz, J. S. (2004). Transitional care of older adults hospitalized with heart failure: a randomized, controlled trial. *Journal of the American Geriatric Society, 52*(5), 675–684. Erratum in: *Journal of the American Geriatric Society* 2004, *52*(7), 1228.

Nebes, R. D. (1977). Man's so-called minor hemisphere. In *The human brain*, edited by M. C. Wittrock. Englewood Cliffs, NJ: Prentice-Hall, Inc.

Neilsen, J. D., Palshof, T., Mainz, J., Jensen, A. B., & Olesen, F. (2003). Randomised controlled trial of a shared care programme for newly referred cancer patients: Bridging the gap between general medical practice and hospital. *Quality and Safe Health Care, 12*(4), 263–272.

Northouse, L. L., & Northouse, P. G. (1985). *Health communication: A handbook for health professionals*. Englewood Cliffs, NJ: Prentice-Hall, Inc.

Northouse, L. L., & Northouse, P. G. (1992). *Health communication—Strategies for health professionals*. 2nd ed. East Norwalk, CT: Appleton and Lange.

Norton, B. A., & Miller, A. M. (1986). *Skills for professional nursing practice*. East Norwalk, CT: Appleton-Century-Crofts.

Nunnolly, E., & Moy, C. (1989). *Communication basics for human service professionals.* Newbury Park, CA: Sage Publications.

O'Connor, J.B. & Johanson, F.J. (2000) Use of the web for medical information by a gastroenterology clinic populations. *Journal of the American Medical Association, 284,* 1962-1964.

O'Malley, A. S., Sheppard, V. B., Schwartz, M., & Mandelblatt, J. (2004). The role of trust in use of preventive services among low-income African-American women. *Preventive Medicine, 38*, 777–785.

Olnick, S. L. (1984). A critique of empathy and sympathy (chapter 6). In J. Lichtenberg, M. Bernstein, and D. Silver, eds. *Empathy* Vol. 1. London: The Analytic Press, pp. 137–166.

Olson, R. M., Blank, D., Cardinal, E., Hopf, G., & Chalmers, R. K. (1996). Understanding medication-related needs of low-literacy patients. *Journal of American Pharmacists Association, NS36*(7), 424–429.

Onibokun, A. (2002). Applying the theory of reasoned action to acquired immune deficiency syndrome risk behaviour: Condom use among sex workers. *International Conference AIDS*. Jul 7–12; 14: abstract no. WePeD6401.

Osterberg, L., & Blaschke, T. (2005). Adherence to medication. *The New England Journal of Medicine, 353*(5), 487–497.

Paasche-Orlow, M. K., Schillinger, D., Greene, S. M., & Wagner, E. H. (2006). How health care systems can begin to address the challenge of limited literacy. *Journal of General Internal Medicine, 21*, 884–887.

Page, J. B. (2005). The concept of culture: A core issue in health disparities. *Journal of Urban Health, 82*(2), iii35–iii43.

Paice, J. A., Ferrell, B. R., Coyle, N., Coyne, P., & Callaway, M. (2008). Global efforts to improve palliative care: The international end-of-life nursing education consortium training programme. *Journal of Advanced Nursing, 61*(2), 173–180.

Paquette, V., Levesque, J., Mensour, B., Leroux, J. M., Beaudoin, G., et al. (2003). Change the mind and you change the brain": Effects of cognitive-behavioral therapy on the neural correlates of spider phobia. *Neuroimaging, 2*, 401–409.

Parchman, M. L., & Burge, S. K. (2002). Residency Research Network of South Texas Investigators. Continuity and quality of care in type 2 diabetes: A Residency Research Network of South Texas study. *Journal of Family Practice, 51*(7), 619–624.

Parchman, M. L., & Burge, S. K. (2003). The patient-physician relationship, primary care attributes, and preventive services. *Family Medicine, 36*(1), 22–27.

Parikl, N. S., Parker, R. M., Nurss, J. R., Baker, D. W., & Williams, M. V. (1996). Shame and health literacy: The unspoken connection. *Patient Education and Counseling, 27*(1), 33–39.

Parkerton, P. H., Smith, D. G., & Straley, H. L. (2004). Primary care practice coordination versus physician continuity. *Family Medicine, 36*(1), 15–21.

Patrick, K., Intille, S. S., & Zabinski, M. F. (2005). An ecological framework for cancer communication: Implications for research. *Journal of Medical Internet Research, 7*(3), e23. Accessed http://www.jmir.org/2005/3/e23

Pawar, M. (2005). Five tips for generating patient satisfaction and compliance. *Family Practice Management. 12*(6).

Pearce, W. B. (1974). Trust in interpersonal communication. *Speech Monographs 41*, 236–244.

Pearlin, L., & Schooler, C. (1978). The structure of coping. *Journal of Health and Social Behavior, 19*, 2–21.

Pearson, S. D., & Raeke, L. H. (2000). Patients' trust in physicians: Many theories, few measures, little data. *Journal of General Internal Medicine, 15*, 509–513.

Pereira, A. G., Kleinman, K. P., & Pearson, S. D. (2003). Leaving the practice: Effects of primary care physician departure on patient care. *Archives of Internal Medicine, 163*, 2733–2766.

Pereira, J. L., Koski, S., Hanson, J., Bruera, E. D., & Mackey, J. R. (2000). Internet usage among women with breast cancer: An exploratory study. *Clinical Breast Cancer, 1*, 148–153.

Pettigrew, J. (1990). Intensive nursing care: The ministry of presence. *Nursing Clinics of North America, 2*(3), 503–508.

Pew Report & American Life (cited 2007 November). Accessed http://www.pewinternet.org

Pinderhughes, E. (1989). *Understanding race, ethnicity and power: The key to efficiency in clinical practice.* Southfield, MI: National Center for Special Needs Adoption.

Preen, D. B., Bailey, B. E., Wright, A., Kendall, P., Phillips, M., et al. (2005). Effects of a multidisciplinary, post-discharge continuance of care intervention on quality of life, discharge satisfaction, and hospital length of stay: A randomized controlled trial. *International Journal for Quality in Health Care, 17*(1), 43–51.

President's Commission for the Study of Ethical Problems in Medicine and Biomedical and Behavioral Research. (1983). *Securing access to care.* Vol. 1. Washington, DC: U.S. Government Printing Office.

Prochaska, J. O., & DiClemente, C. C. (1983). Stages and processes of self-change of smoking: Toward an integrative model of change. *Journal of Consulting and Clinical Psychology, 51*, 390–395.

Prochaska, J. O., DiClemente, C. C., Velicer, W. F., Ginpil, S., & Norcross, J. C. (1985). Predicting change in status for self-changers. *Addictive Behaviors, l0*, 395–406.

Prochaska, J. O., DiClemente, C. C., & Norcross, J. C. (1992). In search of how people change: Applications to addictive behavior. *American Psychologist, 47*, 1102–1114.

Prochaska, J. O., DiClemente, C. C., Velicer, W. F., & Rossi, J. S. (1993). Standardized, individualized, interactive and personalized self-help programs for smoking cessation. *Health Psychology, 12*, 399–405.

Prochaska, J. O., & Velicer, W. F. (1997). The Transtheoretical Model of health behavior change. *American Journal of Health Promotion, 12*, 38–48.

Psychopathology Committee of the Group for the Advancement of Psychiatry. (2001). This month's highlights: Evidence-based practices. *Psychiatric Services, 52*, 1425.

Quo, G., Johnson, C. A., Unger, J. B., Lee, L., Xie, B., Chou, C., et al. (2007). Utility of the theory of reasoned action and theory of planned behavior for predicting Chinese adolescent smoking. *Addiction, 32*(5), 1066–1081.

Raatikainen, R. (1991). Dissatisfaction and insecurity of patients in domiciliary care. *Journal of Advanced Nursing, 16*(2), 154–164.

Raddish, M., Horn, S., & Sharkey, P. D. (1999). Continuity of care: is it cost effective? *American Journal of Managed Care, 5*, 727–734.

Rees, A. M. (1993). Communication in the physician-patient relationship. *Bulletin of the Medical Library Association, 81*(1), 1–10.

Reik, T. (1951). *Listening with the third ear: The inner experiences of a psychoanalyst.* Garden City, NJ: Garden City Books. (Epigraph from p. 144)

Reynolds, W., Lauder, W., Sharkey, S., Maciver, S., Veitch, T., & Cameron, D. (2004). The effects of a transitional discharge model for psychiatric patients. *Journal of Psychiatric Mental Health Nursing, 11*, 82–88.

Riccardi, B. M., & Kurtz, S. M. (1983). *Communication and counseling in health care*. Springfield, IL: Charles C. Thomas Publisher.

Ridsdale, L., Morgan, M., & Morris, R. (1992). Doctors' interviewing technique and its response to different booking time. *Family Practice, 9*(1), 57–60.

Roberts, G. W. (1994). Nurse/patient communication within a bilingual health care setting. *British Journal of Nursing, 3*(2), 60–64, 66–67.

Rogers, C. (1951). *Client-centered therapy*. Boston: Houghton-Mifflin Co.

Rogers, C. (1957). The necessary and sufficient conditions of therapeutic personality change. *Journal of Consulting Psychology, 21*, 95–100.

Rogers, C. (1980). *A way of being*. Boston: Houghton-Mifflin Co.

Rogers, C. R. (1959). A theory of therapy, personality and interpersonal relationships, as developed in the client-centered framework. In S. Koch (ed.), *Psychology: A study of science (pp. 184–256)*. New York: McGraw Hill.

Rogers, C. R. (1961). *On becoming a person*. Boston: Houghton Mifflin.

Rogers, C. R. (1977). *Carl Rogers on personal power*. New York: Delacorte Press.

Rogers, C. R., & Freiberg, H. J. (1994). Freedom to learn 3rd ed. Columbus, OH: Merrill/Macmillan.

Rooda, L. A. (1992). The development of a conceptual model for multicultural nursing. *Journal of Holistic Nursing, 10*(4), 337–347.

Rosenstock, I. M., Strecher, V. J., & Becker, M. H. (1988). Social learning theory and the health belief model. *Health Education Quarterly, 15*, 175–183.

Roter, D. L. (2000). The outpatient medical encounter and elderly patients. *Clinics in Geriatric Medicine,* 16(1), 95–107.

Roter, D. L., & Ewart, C. K. (1992). Emotional inhibition in essential hypertension: Obstacle to communication during medical visits? *Health Psychology, 11*(3), 163–169.

Roter, D. L., & Hall, J. A. (1992). *Doctors talking with patients/patients talking with doctors—improving communication in medical visits*. Westport, CT: Auburn House.

Rothman, R., Malone, R., Bryant, B., Horlen, C., DeWalt, D. A., & Pignone, M. (2004). The relationship between literacy and glycemic control in a diabetes disease-management program. *Diabetes Education, 30*(2), 263–273.

Rovniak, L. S., Anderson, E. S., Winett, R. A., & Stephens, R. S. (2002). Social cognitive determinants of physical activity in young adults: A prospective structural equation analysis. *Annals of Behavioral Medicine, 24*(2), 149–156.

Rowland-Morin, P. A., & Carroll, J. G. (1990). Verbal communication skills and patient satisfaction: A study of doctor-patient interviews. *Evaluation and the Health Professions, 13*(2), 168–185.

Roy-Byrne, P., Katon, W., Cowley, D., & Russo, J. (2001). A randomized effectiveness trial of collaborative care for patients with panic disorder in primary care. *Archives of General Psychiatry, 58*(9), 869–876.

Ruesch, J. (1961). *Therapeutic communication*. New York: W. W. Norton. (Epigraph from p. xiv)

Sable, M. R., Schwartz, L. R., Kelly, P. J., Lison, E., & Hall, M. A. (2006). Using the theory of reasoned action to explain physician intention to prescribe emergency contraception. *Perspectives on Sexual and Reproductive Health, 38*(1), 20–27.

Safeer, R., & Keenan, J. (2005). Health literacy: The gap between physicians and patients. *American Family Physician, 72*(3), 463–468.

Safran, D. G. (2003). Defining the future of primary care: What can we learn from patients? *Annals of Internal Medicine, 138*, 248–255.

Saltman, D. C., O'Dea, N. A., & Kidd, M. R. (2006). Conflict management: A primer for doctors in training. *Postgraduate Medical Journal, 82*, 9–12.

Samet, J. H., Larson, M. J., Horton, N. J., Doyle, K., Winter, M., & Saitz, R. (2003). Linking alcohol-and-drug dependent adults to primary medical care: A randomized controlled trial of a multi-disciplinary health intervention in a detoxification unit. *Addiction, 98*, 509–551.

Sarkar, U., Fisher, L., & Schillinger, D. (2006). Is self-efficacy associated with diabetes self-management across race/ethnicity and health literacy? *Diabetes Care, 29*(4), 823–829.

Satir, V. (1967). *Conjoint family therapy.* Palo Alto, CA: Science and Behavior Books.

Satterfield, J. M., & Hughes, E. (2007). Emotion skills training for medical students: A systematic review. *Medical Education, 41*, 935–941.

Saultz, J. W. (2003). Defining and measuring interpersonal continuity of care. *Annals of Family Medicine, 1*, 134–143.

Saultz, J. W., & Albedaiwi, W. (2004). Interpersonal continuity of care and patient satisfaction. *Annals of Family Medicine,* 2, 445–451.

Schacter, D. L. (1990). Project on the Decade of the Brain; Panel: The Science of Memory and Emotion–Executive Summary. Memory: The fragile power. Library of Congress. Accessed from http://www.loc.gov/loc/brain/emotion/Schacter.html

Schatz, I. J. (1995). Empathy and medical education. *Hawaii Medical Journal, 54*(4), 495–497.

Schifter, D. E., & Ajzen, I. (1985). Intention, perceived control, and weight loss: An application of the theory of planned behavior. *Journal of Personality and Social Psychology, 49*, 843–851.

Schillinger, D., Barton, L. R., Karter, A. J., Wang, F., & Adler, N. (2006). Does literacy mediate the relationship between education and health outcomes: A study of a low-income population with diabetes. *Public Health Reports, 121*, 245–254.

Schillinger, D., Grumback, K., Piette, J., Wang, F., Osmond, D., Daher, C., et al. (2002). Association of health literacy with diabetes outcomes. *JAMA, 288*, 475–482.

Schillinger, D., Piette, J., Grumbach, K., Wang, F., Wilson, C., Daher, C., et al. (2003). Closing the loop: Physician communication with diabetic patients who have low health literacy. *Archives of Internal Medicine, 163*(1), 83–90.

Schoen, M. S., Osborn, R., Huynh, P. T., Doty, M., Zapert, K., Peugh, J., et al. (2005). Taking the pulse of health care systems: Experiences of patient with health problems in six countries. *Health Affairs Web Exclusive* November 3, 2005 W5-509–W5-525.

Schumacher, K. L., Dodd, M. L., & Paul, S. M. (1993). The stress process in family caregivers of persons receiving chemotherapy. *Research in Nursing & Health, 16*, 395–404.

Schwartz, K. L., Roe, T., Northrup, J., Mezsa, J., Seifeldin, R., & Neale, V. N. (2006). Family medicine patients' use of the internet for health information: A metronet study. *The Journal of the American Board of Family Medicine, 19*, 39–45.

Schwarzer, R., & Jerusalem, M. (1995). Generalized Self-Efficacy scale. In J. Weinman, S. Wright, & M. Johnston. Measures in health psychology: A user's portfolio. Causal and control beliefs (pp. 35–37). Windsor, UK: NFER-NELSON.

Selye, H. (1976). *The stress of life*. New York: McGraw-Hill.

Sentell, T. L., & Halpin, H. A. (2006). The importance of adult literacy in understanding health disparities. *Journal of General Internal Medicine, 21*, 862–866.

Shah, S. A. (1970a). Privileged communication, confidentiality and privacy: *Confidentiality. Professional Psychology, 1*, 159–164.

Shah, S. A. (1970b). Privileged communication, confidentiality and privacy: Privacy. *Professional Psychology, 1*, 243–252.

Sharpe, N. F. (1994). Informed consent and Huntington's disease: A model for communication. *American Journal of Medical Genetics, 50*(3), 239–246.

Sharpe, L., Sensky, T., Timberlake, N., Allard, S., & Brewin, C. R. (2001). The role of cognitive e behavioural therapy in facilitating adaptation to illness in rheumatoid arthritis: Case series. *Behavioural and Cognitive Psychotherapy, 29*, 303–309.

Shenolikar, R. A., Balkrishman, R., & Hall, M. A. (2004). How patient-physician encounters in critical medical situations affect trust: Results of a national survey. *BMC Health Services Research, 4*, 4–24.

Sherbourne, C. D., Meredith, L. S., Rogers, W., &. Ware, J. E. (1992). Social support and stressful life events: Age differences in their effects on health-related quality of life among the chronically ill. *Quality of Life Research, 1*, 235–246.

Sherman, J. J., & Cramer, A. (2005). Measurement of changes in empathy during dental school. *Journal of Dental Education, 69*(3), 338–345.

Sieburg, E. (1969). *Dysfunctional communication and interpersonal responsiveness in small groups*. Ph.D. diss., University of Denver. Abstract in Dissertation Abstracts International, 1969, *30*(2622A).

Silbersweig, D. A., & Stern, E. (1998). Towards a functional neuroanatomy of conscious perception and its modulation by volition: Implications of human auditory neuroimaging studies. *Philosophical Transactions of the Royal Society, 353*, 1883–1888.

Simmons, L. E., & Blount, R. L. (2007). Identifying barriers to medication adherence in adolescent transplant recipients. *Journal of Pediatric Psychology*. Accessed October 4, 2007, from http://jpepsy.oxfordjournals.org/cgi/content/abstract/jsm030v3

Simon, G. E., Ludman, E., Unutzer, J., & Bauer, M. S. (2002). Design and implementation of a randomized trial evaluating systematic care for bipolar disorders. *Bipolar Disorders, 4*(4), 226–-236.

Singer, L. L. (1976). *Daydreaming and fantasy*. London: George Allen & Unwin, Ltd.

Skelton, J. R. (2002). A concordance-based study of metaphoric expressions used by general practitioners and patients in consultation. *The British Journal of General Practice, 52*(475), 114–118.

Smeenk, F. W., de Witte, L. P., van Haastregt, J. C. M., Schipper, R. M., Biezemans H. P. H., & Crebolder, H. F. (1998). Transmural care: A new approach in the care for terminal cancer patients: Its effects on rehospitalization and quality of life. *Educational Counseling, 35*, 189–199.

Smith, A. A., & Friedemann, M. L. (1999). Perceived family dynamics of persons with chronic pain. *Journal of Advanced Nursing, 30*(3), 543–551.

Smith, M. C. (1984). The client who is anxious. In *The American Handbook of Psychiatric Nursing*, S. Lego, (Ed.). Philadelphia: J.B. Lippincott Company, p. 389.

Smith, M. E., & Hart, G. (1994). Nurses' responses to patient anger: From disconnecting to connecting. *Journal of Advanced Nursing, 20*(4), 643–651.

Smith, R. C., & Hoppe, R. B. (1991). The patient's story: Integrating the patient- and physician-centered approaches to interviewing. *Annals of Internal Medicine, 115*(6), 470–477.

Smith, S. (1992). *Communications in nursing*. 2nd ed. St. Louis, MO: Mosby Yearbook.

Sparbel, K. J. H., & Anderson, M. A. (2000a). Integrated literature review of continuity of care: Part 1, conceptual issues. *Journal of Nursing Scholarship, 32*(1), 7–24.

Sparbel, K. J. H., & Anderson, M. A. (2000b). A continuity of care integrated literature review, Part 2: Methodological issues. *Journal of Nursing Scholarship, 32*(2), 131–135.

Spiro, H. (1992). What is empathy and can it be taught? *Annals of Internal Medicine, 116*(10), 843–846.

Steinglass, P., & Horan, M. E. (1987). Families and chronic medical illness. In *Chronic disorders and the family*, edited by F. Walsh and C. M. Anderson. New York: Haworth Press, pp. 127–142.

Stern, S. B. (1990). Privileged communication: An ethical and legal right of psychiatric clients. *Perspectives in Psychiatric Care, 26*(4), 22–25.

Stevenson, F. A., Kerr, C., Murray, E., & Nazareth, I. (2007). Information from the internet and the doctor-patient relationship: The patient perspective–a qualitative study. *BMC Family Practice, 8*. Accessed from http:///www.biomedcentral.com/1471-2296/8/47/prepub

Stevenson, S. (1991). Heading off violence with verbal de-escalation. *Journal of Psychosocial Nursing and Mental Health Services, 29*(9), 6–10.

Stokes, T., Tarrant, C., Mainous, A. G., Schers, H., Greeman, G., & Baker, R. (2005). Continuity of care: Is the personal doctor still important? A survey of general practitioners and family physicians in England and Wales, the United States, and the Netherlands. *Annals of Family Medicine, 3*, 353–359.

Stumpf, S. H., & Bass, K. (1992). Cross-cultural communication to help physician assistants provide unbiased health care. *Public Health Reports, 107*(1), 113–115.

Suchman, A. L., Roter, D., Green, M., & Lipkin, M. (1993). Physician satisfaction with primary care office visits: Collaborative study group of the American Academy on Physician and Patient. *Medical Care, 31*(12), 1083–1092.

Sudore, R. L., Yaffe, K., Satterfield, S., Harris, T. B., Mehta, K. M., Simonsick, E. M., et al. (2006). Limited literacy and mortality in the elderly: The health, aging, and body comparison study. *Journal of General Internal, 21*, 806–812.

Sullivan, H. S. (1953). *The interpersonal theory of psychiatry.* New York: W.W. Norton & Co.

Sundeen, S. J., Stuart, G. W., Rankin, E. A. D., & Cohen, S. A. (1994). *Nurse-client interaction—Implementing the nursing process* (5th ed.). St. Louis, MO: Mosby Co.

Sussman, M. B. (1982). Family-organizational linkages. In *The psychiatric hospital and the family*, edited by H. T. Harbin. Jamaica, NY: Spectrum Publications, Inc., pp. 277–96.

Tarn, D. M., Meredith, L. S., Kagawa-Singer, M., Matsumura, S., Bito, S., Liu, H., et al. (2005). Trust in one's physician: The role of ethnic match, autonomy, acculturation, and religiosity among Japanese and Japanese Americans. *Annals of Family Medicine, 3*, 339–347.

Taylor, L., &. Adelman, H. S. (1989). Reframing the confidentiality dilemma to work in children's best interest. *Professional Psychology: Research and Practice, 26*(2), 79–83.

Teutsch, C. (2003). Patient-doctor communication. *Medical Clinics of North America, 87*(5), 1115–1145.

Thom, D. H. (2001). Physician behaviors that predict patient trust. *Journal of Family Practice, 50*, 32–328.

Thom, D. H., Hall, M. A., & Pawlson, L. G. (2004). Measuring patients' trust in physicians when assessing quality of care. *Health Affairs, 23*(4), 124–132.

Thompson, J. E., & Thompson, H. O. (1985). *Bioethical decision-making for nurses.* Norwalk, CT: Appleton-Century-Crofts.

Thyer, G. L. (2003). Dare to be different: Transformational leadership may hold the key to the nursing shortage. *Journal of Nursing Management, 11*, 73–79.

Todres, I. D., Earle, M., & Jellinck, M. S. (1994). Enhancing communication: The physician and family in the pediatric intensive care unit. *Pediatric Clinics of North America, 41*(6), 1395–1404.

Tong, K. L., & Spicer, B. J. (1994). The Chinese palliative patient and family in North America: A cultural perspective. *Journal of Palliative Care, 10*(1), 26–28.

Tongue, J. R., Epps, H. R., & Forese, L. L. (2005). Communication skills for patient-centered care. *The Journal of Bone and Joint Surgery, 87*, 652–658.

Travaline, J. M., Ruchinskas, R., & D'Alonzo, G. E. (2005). Patient-physician communication: Why and how. *The Journal of American Osteopathic Association, 105*(1), 13–18.

Truax, C. B., & Carkhuff, R. (1967). *Toward effective counseling and psychotherapy*. Chicago, IL: Aldine.

Tulsky, J. A. (2005). Beyond advance directives: Importance of communication skills at the end of life. *JAMA,* 294, 359–365.

Unruh, H. K., Bowen, D. J., Meischket, H., Bus, N., & Woldridge, J. A. (2004). Wineb's approaches to the use of new technology for cancer risk information. *Women Health, 40*, 59–78.

Ury, W. L., Brett, J. M., & Goldberg, S. B. (1988). *Getting dispute resolved: Designing systems to cut the costs of conflict.* San Francisco, CA: Jossey-Bass.

U.S. Department of Health and Human Services. (2000). Healthy People 2010. Accessed October 4, 2007, from www.healthypeople.gov/Document/HTML/Volume 1/11HealthCom.htm

Usherwood, T. (1993). Subjective and behavioral evaluation of the teaching of patient interview skills. *Medical Education, 27*(1), 41–47.

Vaillot, M. C. (1970). Hope: The restoration of being. *American Journal of Nursing, 70*(2), 268–273.

van der Weide, W. E., Verbeek, J. H., & van Dijk, F. J. (1999). Relation between indicators for quality of occupational rehabilitation of employees with low back pain. *Occupational and Environmental Medicine, 56*(7), 488–493.

van Eaton, E. G., Horvath, K. D., Lober, W. B., Rossini, A. J., & Pellegrini, C. A. (2005). A randomized, controlled trial evaluating the impact of a computerized rounding and sign-out system on continuity of care and resident work hours. *Journal of the American College of Surgeons, 200*(4), 538–545.

van Servellen, G., Carpio, F., Lopez, M., Garcia-Teague, L., Herrera, G., Monterrosa, F., et al. (2003). Program to enhance health literacy and treatment adherence in low-income HIV-infected Latino men and women. *AIDS Patient Care and STDs, 17*(11), 581–594.

van Servellen, G., Fongwa, M., & D'Errico, E. M. (2006). Continuity of care and quality care outcomes for people experiencing chronic conditions: A literature review. *Nursing and Health Sciences, 8*, 185–195.

Vrijhoef, H. J., Diederiks, J. P., Spreeuwenberg, C., & Wolffenbuttel, B. H. (2001). Substitution model with central role for nurse specialist is justified in the care for stable type 2 diabetic outpatients. *Journal of Advanced Nursing, 36*(4), 546–555.

Wada, J. A. (1977). Fundamental asymmetry of the infant brain. In S. J. Dimond and D. A. Blizard, eds., *Annals of the New York Academy of Sciences, 299*, 370–379.

Wade, C., & Tauris, C. (1990). *Psychology*. 2nd ed. St. Louis, MO: Harper and Row.

Wasson, J. H., MacKenzie, T. A., & Hall, M. (2007). Patients use of internet technology to report when things go wrong. *Quality and Safety in Health Care, 16*, 213–215.

Watzlawick, P. J., Beavin, J., & Jackson, D. D. (1967). *Pragmatics of human communication*. New York: W.W. Norton & Company, Inc. (Epigraph from p. 13)

Watzlawick, P., Weakland, J. H.,& Fisch, R. (1974). *Changing a system*. Change, NY: W.W. Norton and Company, Inc.

Weiner, J. S., & Cole, S. A. (2004). Three principles to improve clinician communication for advance care planning: Overcoming emotional, cognitive, and skill barriers. *Journal of Palliative Medicine, 7*(6), 817–829.

Weisman, A. D. (1972). *On dying and denying: A psychiatric study of terminality*. New York: Behavioral Publications.

Weisman, A. D., & Worden, J. W. (1976). *Coping and vulnerability in cancer patients*. Boston: Project Omega, Harvard Medical School.

Weisman, C. S. (1986). Women and their health care providers: A matter of communication. *Public Health Reports Supplement,* July–August, 147–151.

Weiss, B. D., Mays, M. Z., Martz, W., Castro, K. M., DeWalt, D. A., Pignone, M. P., et al. (2005). Quick assessment of literacy in primary care: The newest vital sign. *Annals of Family Medicine, 3*(6), 514–522.

Weissman, A., Gotlieb, L., Ward, S., Grennblatt, E., & Casper, R. F. (2000). Use of the internet by infertile couples. *Fertility and Sterility, 73*, 1179–1182.

Whitaker, C. (1996). Let it flow: Carl Whitaker's philosophy of becoming. *Journal of Marital and Family Therapy, 22*(3), 317–319.

Williams, J. G., Cheung, W. Y., Chetwynd, N., Cohen, D. R., El-Sharkawi, S., Finlay, I., et al. (2001). Pragmatic randomized trial to evaluate the use of patient held records for the continuing care of patients with cancer. *Quality Health Care, 10*(3), 159–165.

Williams, M. V., Baker, D. W., Honig, E. G., Lee, T. M., & Nowlan, A. (1998). Inadequate literacy is a barrier to asthma knowledge and self-care. *Chest, 114*, 1008–1015.

Williams, M. V., Baker, D. W., Parker, R. M., & Nurss, J. R. (1998). Relationship of functional health literacy to patients' knowledge of their chronic disease. A study of patients with hypertension and diabetes. *Archives of Internal Medicine, 158*, 166–172.

Wilson, L. (1982). *The skills of ethnic competence*. Seattle: University of Washington. Resource paper.

Winslow B. (1997). Effects of formal supports on stress outcomes in family caregivers of Alzheimers patients. *Research in Nursing & Health, 20*, 27–37.

Witelson, S. F., & Pallie, W. (1973). Left hemisphere specialization for language in newborn: Neuroanatomical evidence of asymmetry. *Brain, 96*, 641–646.

Wong, B. M., Yung, B. M., Wong, A., Chow, C. M., & Abramson, B. L. (2005). Increasing internet use among cardiovascular patients: New opportunities for heart health promotion. *Canadian Journal of Cardiology, 21*, 349–354.

World Health Organization (WHO). (2000). *The World health report 2000: Health systems: Improving performance*. Accessed from www.who.int/healthsystems

Wright, L. K., Litaker, M., Laraia, M. T., & DeAndrade, S. (2001). Continuum of care for Alzheimer's disease: A nurse education and counseling program. *Issues in Mental Health Nursing, 22*(3), 231–252.

Youmans, S. L., & Schillinger, D. (2003). Functional health literacy and medication use: The pharmacist's role. *Annals of Pharmacotherapy, 37*(11), 1726–1729.

Young, C. M. (2004). *Health literacy a national epidemic* [Internet]. Louisville, KY: University of Louisville; [modified 2004 Feb 13; cited 2004 Apr 30]. Accessed from http://www.louisville.edu/~cmyoun02/firstpage.htm

Young, R. M., Connor, J. P., Ricciardelli, L. A., & Saunders, J. B. (2006). The role of alcohol expectancy and drinking refusal self-efficacy beliefs in university student drinking. *Alcohol and Alcoholism, 41*(1), 70–75.

Zimmerman, G. L., Olsen, C. G., & Bosworth, M. F. (2000). A 'Stages of Change' approach to helping patients change behavior. *American Family Physician, 61*(5), 1409–1416.

Index

I

N

O

Q